CANCER IS A PARASITE

CANCER IS A PARASITE

Kill It with the Safe, Over-the-Counter Antiparasitic Fenbendazole

William F. Supple Jr., PhD

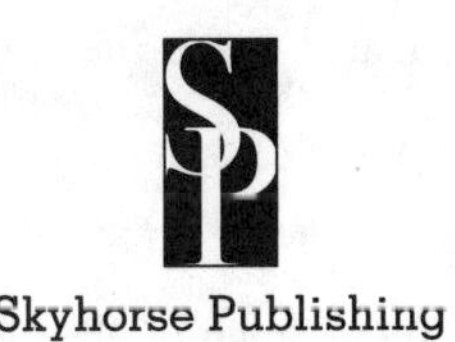

Skyhorse Publishing

A portion of the proceeds goes to MAHA Action 501(c)4.

MAHA Books books may be purchased in bulk at special discounts for sales promotion, corporate gifts, fund-raising, or educational purposes. Special editions can also be created to specifications. For details, contact the Special Sales Department, Skyhorse Publishing, 307 West 36th Street, 11th Floor, New York, NY 10018 or info@skyhorsepublishing.com.

MAHA Books is an imprint of Skyhorse Publishing, Inc.®, a Delaware corporation.

Visit our website at www.skyhorsepublishing.com.

Please follow our publisher Tony Lyons on Instagram @tonylyonsisuncertain.

10 9 8 7 6 5 4 3 2

Library of Congress Cataloging-in-Publication Data is available on file.

Cover design by David Ter-Avanesyan

Print ISBN: 978-1-5107-8513-7
Ebook ISBN: 978-1-5107-8514-4

Printed in the United States of America

The purpose in life is to contribute in some way to making things better. —Robert F. Kennedy

To Roberta, whose determination to avoid traditional chemotherapy started the journey to where we are today.

Contents

Contents

Disclaimer

All facts presented in this book are based on publicly available published research papers, documents, and studies, the majority of which have been linked in the references. Nevertheless, in some places the author has also expressed personal opinions, where it seems to him that the facts can be assembled to form a larger, albeit partly speculative picture. The author has made every effort to clearly separate facts and such interpretations in terms of language.

The publisher and author have checked the information in this work to the best of their knowledge and belief for correctness, accuracy, and completeness sufficient for reasonable interpretation. However, neither the publisher nor the author explicitly takes any responsibility for the content of the work or for any errors.

This also applies to quantities of micronutrients, drugs, vitamins, and other supplements, as there may be differences in dosage and administration that can result from lifestyle, gender, age, body size, and possible preexisting conditions. Therefore, any use of any of the substances mentioned in this book should only be carried out after consultation with a trusted physician or other medical professional, and in any case on one's own responsibility—the publisher and author accept no liability.

The author does not endorse the contents of any of the cited websites except for the Substack publication *Fenbendazole Can Cure Cancer*, which he publishes. Reference is made to their status at the time of initial publication. All citations have been carefully checked for accuracy at the time of this writing in summer of 2025. It is not uncommon for the content of an online source to change or even disappear completely. Unfortunately, the integrity of scientific material that is on the internet can no longer be blindly trusted.

Preface

Our journey into the world of fenbendazole and cancer began with a single, anonymous comment online. On a website article discussing the role of bacteria in stomach cancer, a reader wrote: "Look into fenbendazole, it cured my prostate cancer."

That was it. But it was enough.

Just one day earlier, my eighty-three-year-old mother-in-law had been diagnosed with metastatic breast cancer. The tumors had spread everywhere—liver, lungs, and so many bones the radiological report simply stated they were "too numerous to list." Having lived a long, full life, she refused to endure the brutal side effects of chemotherapy and radiation. She was ready to let go.

Her family was not.

That one comment regarding fenbendazole sparked an urgent search for a different path. What we discovered was nothing short of astonishing. I am a neuroscientist by training, not an oncologist, but the preclinical science I found was solid enough for a last-ditch effort. My mother-in-law had nothing to lose. After my wife and I tested the animal dewormer on ourselves to ensure its safety, her mother began taking it mixed into her morning yogurt.

Within two weeks, she started to feel better. Her appetite returned, and her energy levels soared. Within a month, she was strong enough to be released from hospice care. And within six months of starting a simple protocol with fenbendazole—and no other treatment—her cancer was gone. Completely eradicated. Four years later, she has just celebrated her eighty-seventh birthday, vibrant and cancer-free. No side effects, no suffering. Just results. I would not have believed it if I had not witnessed it with my own eyes.

Good news of this magnitude travels fast. As word of my mother-in-law's recovery spread, my phone began ringing constantly. Family, then friends, then friends of friends, were all asking the same questions. To share her story and answer the flood of inquiries, I launched a Substack publication in October 2022 called *Fenbendazole Can Cure Cancer*. I wrote under the pseudonym Ben Fen, because the messenger wasn't important—the information was.

The response was explosive. The Substack grew into a community of hundreds of thousands of subscribers. Readers began submitting their own powerful stories of using fenbendazole to treat breast, prostate, lung, colon, skin, and brain cancers, often after being failed by the conventional medical system. These case reports, many of which you will read in this book, provide not only inspiration but also practical, how-to guidance for those who may choose to self-treat their own cancers. This grassroots movement has now broken into the mainstream, with figures like Joe Rogan, Mel Gibson, and Roger Stone speaking about fenbendazole curing people they know of terminal cancers. Importantly, the oncology community is beginning to take notice, with three of our early case reports recently being published in the peer-reviewed cancer journal, *Case Reports in Oncology*.

This book is the culmination of that journey. It is the story of a powerful, effective, safe, and inexpensive cancer treatment that has been hiding in plain sight for decades.

What is fenbendazole? It's a veterinary antiparasitic drug for animals, often dismissed as "dog medicine." This dismissal is a mistake that has cost countless lives. We have discovered that the medical establishment has been accidentally stumbling upon the anticancer power of fenbendazole and its chemical cousins for years, only to dismiss, ignore, or suppress the findings.

In 2002, scientists at the MD Anderson Cancer Center discovered that mebendazole, a nearly identical drug to fenbendazole that is approved for use in humans, destroyed human lung, breast, ovary, colon, and bone cancer cells. It was a stunning breakthrough that went nowhere.

In 2008, researchers at Johns Hopkins University were baffled when their lab mice would not grow the lymphoma tumors they had implanted. The cause? The mice were being dewormed as part of routine veterinary care with fenbendazole. The scientists issued an alert, not to announce a potential cure, but to warn other researchers that the drug might "confound research results." They saw an inconvenience, not a miracle.

In 2009, in another once-in-a-lifetime "accident" at Johns Hopkins, a different team of scientists couldn't get experimental brain cancer tumors to grow in their mice. They connected the dots and found the same culprit: veterinary administration of fenbendazole.

This time, the discovery finally stuck, leading to more research into how fenbendazole prevented their cancer cells from growing. But the world shouldn't have had to wait for lightning to strike three times. We've also discovered that fenbendazole's power as a cancer cure was known as far back as the 1970s. And we can prove it. Furthermore, we will show you that many of today's blockbuster chemotherapy drugs are based on the anticancer mechanisms of the safe and inexpensive antiparasitic drug fenbendazole.

How can a dewormer be so effective against cancer? The answer is both simple and revolutionary. Cancer cells and parasites share a fatal flaw: they both rely on tiny internal structures called microtubules to survive, grow, and replicate. Fenbendazole is designed to attack and dismantle the specific type of microtubules found in parasites but not healthy mammalian cells. In what can only be described as a gift from God, cancer cells are built with the very same vulnerability in their microtubule design.

While traditional chemotherapy is a blunt instrument that poisons the whole body, fenbendazole is a precision-guided missile. It targets and dismantles cancer cells while leaving healthy cells untouched, which is why it is free of toxic side effects. Fenbendazole has all of the characteristics of an ideal cancer treatment: specificity, lethality, and no toxic side effects. It is the Holy Grail of cancer treatment.

But its power doesn't stop there. Fenbendazole launches a multifront war on cancer. It not only dismantles the cancer cell's structure but also starves it of glucose, cuts off its blood supply, blocks its ability to replicate, and reawakens the patient's own immune system to identify and attack the invaders, among other mechanisms. Cancer can't adapt to this overwhelming, all-out assault, which is why fenbendazole is also so effective against the deadly cancer stem cells that survive chemotherapy and cause recurrence and ultimately kill us.

This book is your guide to understanding this groundbreaking treatment using fenbendazole on cancer. In it, you will discover:

1. The Science Justifying Fenbendazole as a Cancer Treatment, Simplified: We present the evidence for how fenbendazole works to kill cancer in language anyone can understand.
2. The Real-World Proof that Fenbendazole Can Cure Cancer: You will read the powerful case report accounts of people who took control of their health and successfully self-treated their cancers with fenbendazole.
3. The Global Evidence That Fenbendazole-like Drugs May Also Prevent Cancer: We reveal how countries with mass public health deworming programs using antiparasitic drugs have dramatically lower cancer rates, suggesting these programs are also preventing cancer on a massive scale.

4. The Fifty-Year Cover-Up of Fenbendazole as a Cure for Cancer: We uncover the story of international intrigue, greed, and suppression that has kept this safe and effective cancer cure from the public for half a century.
5. A Revolutionary New Theory to Help Understand Why Fenbendazole Kills Cancer: We make the case that cancer behaves just like a parasite. This new framework provides a road map for developing even more effective cancer treatments based on this observation.

When I began writing this book, I thought I knew most of the story on fenbendazole and cancer. But as I pulled the thread connecting parasites and cancer, a breathtaking picture emerged. My contribution has been to simply combine the science of parasitology with the science of oncology to answer the "how" and "why" of fenbendazole's success in killing cancer.

This book will educate you and give you hope. But most of all, I think that it will lessen the deep-seated fear of cancer that we all carry. The journey of fenbendazole from a humble dewormer to a potent cancer cure transforms our view of this dreaded disease—from a terrifying, larger-than-life opponent to that of a mere bug that we already know how to squash.

—William F. Supple Jr., PhD, a.k.a. Ben Fen
Author of the Substack *Fenbendazole Can Cure Cancer*

CHAPTER 1

An Accidental Discovery: Fenbendazole, Mebendazole, and Their Shared History as Parasite Killers

The story of fenbendazole and mebendazole—two drugs now at the center of the intense world of cancer research—does not begin in a sterile cancer lab. Their story begins on farms and in villages, in the long and difficult war against parasitic worms, a battle that has shaped human and animal life for thousands of years.[1, 2] This history is about the relentless search for safe and powerful drugs, called anthelmintics, to defeat the devastating worm infections that have caused immense suffering and economic loss throughout history.[3, 4]

Parasites, especially worms like nematodes (roundworms), cestodes (tapeworms), and trematodes (flukes), are a powerful force of nature. For humans, these infections are a crippling public health crisis, whether they are diagnosed or not.[5] They are a major cause of malnutrition, anemia, stunted growth, and learning difficulties.[6, 7] History books are filled with descriptions of diseases caused by parasites, which shortened lifespans and held back entire societies.[8] Even today, the World Health Organization reports that over a billion people, mostly in the world's poorest regions, suffer from these infections.[9]

The damage to livestock and farm animals is just as severe. Worms in cattle, sheep, and other farm animals lead to staggering economic losses worldwide.[10] Infected animals produce less meat, milk, and eggs, and are more likely to die or get other diseases.[11] The cost to agriculture runs into the hundreds of billions of dollars every year.[12] For pets like dogs and cats, parasites like heartworms and intestinal worms are a serious threat, making regular deworming a basic part of responsible pet ownership.[13,14] The widespread and harmful impact of these organisms created a desperate need for a solution.

Early attempts to fight worms used crude and often toxic substances from plants and minerals, like tin, turpentine, or chenopodium oil.[15] These remedies were unreliable and often poisoned the patient as much as the parasite. The mid-twentieth century was a turning point. Pharmaceutical companies began using modern chemistry to screen thousands of compounds, looking for molecules that could kill parasites without harming the host.[16]

This intense search led to a major breakthrough: the discovery of a chemical structure called the benzimidazole.[17] This simple structure became the foundation for a new generation of powerful parasite-killing drugs. The first success was thiabendazole, introduced in 1961 by researchers at Merck.[18] It revolutionized parasite control in livestock, but it wasn't perfect. This pushed scientists to refine the benzimidazole structure to create even better drugs with fewer side effects.

Through a systematic process of creating and testing thousands of chemical variations, researchers developed a series of highly effective drugs.

Fenbendazole and Mebendazole: The Two Pillars of a Medical Revolution

The most successful and long-lasting drugs to emerge from this research were fenbendazole and mebendazole. They were developed separately but share the same core structure and the same fundamental method of attack.

Fenbendazole for Animals: Developed in the early 1970s, fenbendazole quickly proved its worth.[19] It was exceptionally effective against a wide range of parasites in farm animals and pets, including roundworms, lungworms, and tapeworms.[20, 21, 22, 23] Because it was so safe and easy to administer (often mixed in feed), fenbendazole became a cornerstone of veterinary medicine, sold under brand names like Panacur and Safe-Guard.[24] Decades of global use provided an enormous amount of real-world data on its effectiveness and remarkable safety, even when used for many days in a row.

Mebendazole for Humans: At the same time, scientists at Janssen Pharmaceuticals, led by the legendary Dr. Paul Janssen, created mebendazole specifically for people. Introduced around 1971, mebendazole was a powerful weapon against common human parasites like pinworms, whipworms, and hookworms.[25, 26] This was a monumental achievement for public health. Marketed as Vermox, mebendazole offered a safe, effective, and simple oral treatment for infections that affected hundreds of millions of people, especially children. The drug is poorly absorbed by the body, which is actually a benefit: it stays in the intestines to kill the worms there, which makes it incredibly safe for humans.[27] Mebendazole became so vital that it was used in mass deworming programs around the globe, providing decades of clinical data on its reliability and safety.[28, 29]

The parallel success of fenbendazole in animals and mebendazole in humans made the benzimidazole family the most important group of antiparasitic drugs of the twentieth century. They dramatically improved animal health, reduced human suffering, and generated a massive library of safety data. This legacy of safety is exactly what, decades later, made them prime candidates for fighting a completely different enemy: cancer.[30] Their journey from parasite killers to potential cancer drugs is a perfect example of drug repurposing—using established, safe medicines in new ways to provide faster, cheaper, and safer treatments.[31]

The Benzimidazole Family: Different Versions of the Same Weapon

While we focus on fenbendazole and mebendazole in this book, they are part of a larger family. Each member has small structural differences from the others that affect how it works in the body. It is important to realize that while there may be slight chemical variations between the antiparasitic drugs that end in "azole" that they function very similarly as antiparasitic and anticancer agents. Key members include:

- Albendazole: Developed shortly after fenbendazole and mebendazole, albendazole has a very broad range of action against worms and flukes in both humans and animals.[32] Unlike mebendazole, it is well-absorbed into the bloodstream, making it effective against parasites living in tissues throughout the body, such as in the brain or liver.[33] Like mebendazole, it is on the WHO's List of Essential Medicines.
- Flubendazole: Structurally very similar to mebendazole, flubendazole is used mainly in pigs and poultry, but also in humans in some parts of the world.[34, 35, 36]
- Thiabendazole: The original benzimidazole developed in the early 1960s. Its use has declined because newer drugs like fenbendazole and albendazole work better and have fewer side effects.[37]
- Oxfendazole: The active form that fenbendazole turns into in the body. It is also used directly as a dewormer in animals.[38]

- Ricobendazole: The active form of albendazole, sometimes used directly in veterinary medicine.

Despite these minor variations in chemical structure, the core mechanism is the same for all major benzimidazoles. They work by attacking the internal structure of the parasite's cells. In simple terms, they destroy the parasite's cellular skeleton, causing the cell to collapse from within.[39, 40]

For our purpose of exploring their anticancer potential, we will treat fenbendazole, mebendazole, albendazole, and flubendazole as functionally the same yet we will call attention to their differences in function when relevant. They share the same core structure and the same primary weapon: attacking a protein called tubulin that makes up microtubules in parasite and cancer cells.[41, 42] While there are differences in how they are absorbed—fenbendazole and albendazole enter the bloodstream more easily than mebendazole, and fenbendazole is better at crossing into the brain—their effects on cancer cells are remarkably similar.[43, 44] Ironically, most lab research on cancer uses the "human" drug mebendazole, while most personal success stories where people self-treat their cancers involve the "animal" drug fenbendazole.[45, 46] This overlap reinforces that they are functionally interchangeable in this new fight against cancer.

As we will see, fenbendazole stands out as the best of the group for human use against cancer. Its ability to be absorbed orally and penetrate the brain and its proven safety profile make it the superior choice. It is the drug most often chosen by people who decide to self-treat their cancers, and future clinical trials for cancer should focus on fenbendazole directly.

Fenbendazole: The Biochemical Weapon That Starves and Paralyzes Parasites

The incredible success of these drugs as antiparasitics comes from their ability to attack a critical part of the parasite's cells: microtubules. Think of microtubules as the cell's internal scaffolding and highway system. They give the cell its shape and are used to transport vital supplies like nutrients and waste.

Microtubules are built from protein building blocks called tubulin. These tubulin blocks link together, like stacking Lego bricks, to form long, hollow tubes. This building process is constant and dynamic, with microtubules always growing and shrinking as needed. This process is absolutely essential for the cells to function, multiply, and survive.[47]

The key roles of microtubules include:

- Maintaining Cell Shape: They act as an internal skeleton.
- Transporting Cargo: They are the tracks for moving nutrients, waste, and other materials around the cell.
- Cell Division: They form the machinery that pulls duplicated chromosomes apart when a cell divides.
- Movement: In some cells, they form the structures used for swimming-like movements.

Fenbendazole and mebendazole kill parasites by attacking their microtubules. Their specific target is the beta-tubulin building block of microtubules.[48] They bind tightly to a specific spot on the parasite's beta-tubulin, which is different from the beta-tubulin in mammalian or human cells.[49] This spot is known as the "colchicine-binding site, which is where the drug colchicine attaches." Knowing exactly where fenbendazole binds shows us why it is so effective against parasite cells but safe for healthy human cells—it simply doesn't attach to human beta-tubulin.[50]

Here is how these antiparasitic drugs destroy the parasite:

- They Stop the Building Process: By binding to the tubulin Lego "brick," the drug prevents it from linking with other bricks. It acts like a cap, stopping microtubules from growing and causing existing ones to fall apart. Early microscope studies visually showed this happening in real time, as the internal structure of parasite cells simply vanished after being treated with the drug.[51]
- They Cause a Catastrophic Collapse: Without functional microtubules, the parasite's entire internal system breaks down, killing the parasite.

The key to the success of these drugs is selective toxicity. These drugs bind to the parasite's tubulin hundreds of times more strongly than they do to human or animal tubulin.[52] This biochemical difference is what makes them so safe for use in animals and humans. By safe, we mean no adverse side effects. The dose needed to kill the parasite is far too low to have any effect on the host.[53] It is targeted killing of the parasite, leaving healthy cells untouched.

Physiological Havoc: How a Broken Cell Structure Kills the Parasite

This attack on the parasite's cellular skeleton leads to a total system failure, ultimately causing paralysis, starvation, and death.

- **Starvation:** The intestinal cells of worms rely on microtubules to absorb nutrients, especially glucose (sugar), from their host. By destroying these microtubules, the drugs cut off the parasite's food supply. The parasite literally starves to death.
- **Halted Growth and Reproduction:** Since microtubules are needed for cells to divide, the parasite can no longer grow, develop, or reproduce. Its life cycle is broken.[54]
- **Toxic Waste Buildup:** The cell's highway system is gone, so the parasite can no longer transport waste out of its cells or secrete enzymes. It becomes poisoned from the inside.
- **Paralysis:** Without microtubules, the parasite's cells lose their shape and strength. Its muscles and nerves stop working, leading to paralysis. Unable to hold on, the weakened parasite is simply flushed out of the host's body.[55]
- **Programmed Cell Death:** All this cellular stress—starvation, poisoning, and structural collapse—triggers the parasite's cells to self-destruct in a process called apoptosis.[56]

This combination of failures makes survival impossible. The elegant genius of these drugs is that they target a system so vital to the parasite, yet just different enough from our own to ensure our safety when using these drugs.

A Legacy of Safety: The Foundation for a New Purpose

A major reason for the excitement around repurposing fenbendazole and mebendazole for cancer is their incredible safety record, proven over fifty years of use in billions of animals and people. This gives these antiparasitic medicines a huge advantage over brand-new drugs that have no safety history.

- **Selective Toxicity:** As we've seen, the foundation of their safety is that they target parasite cells, not host cells.
- **Proven Safety in Animals:** Fenbendazole has been used widely in veterinary medicine, often at high doses for many days, with very few reports of any side effects.[57, 58] It is considered exceptionally safe for a wide range of animals.

- **Proven Safety in Humans (Mebendazole):** Mebendazole's safety is extremely well-documented from its use in global deworming programs. Side effects are rare and, if they occur are usually mild, such as an upset stomach, which is often caused by the death and elimination of the worms themselves. Both mebendazole and albendazole are on the WHO's List of Essential Medicines for a reason: they are safe and effective.
- **Predictable Behavior in the Body:** We have a very good understanding of how these medicines are absorbed, distributed, and removed by the body.
- **Absorption:** Fenbendazole is absorbed into the bloodstream better than mebendazole, especially when taken with a fatty meal.[59, 60]
- **Distribution:** Fenbendazole is known to cross the blood-brain barrier much more effectively than mebendazole, which makes it the logical choice for treating cancers in the brain.[61]
- **Metabolism and Excretion:** Both drugs are processed by the liver and mostly removed through feces.
- **Tolerated at High Doses:** In some human studies for rare parasitic diseases or early cancer trials, patients have taken very high doses of mebendazole or albendazole for long periods.[62, 63, 64] While these high doses require medical monitoring, the studies show that the drugs are often well-tolerated, further supporting the push to repurpose them for cancer.[65, 66]

This massive amount of safety data provides a strong foundation of confidence. It dramatically lowers the risk of exploring these drugs as cancer treatments compared to starting from scratch with a new, unknown molecule· The journey from fighting worms in pastures to targeting cancer cells in patients is a powerful story of scientific discovery. The story begins with parasites, but the tools developed to fight them have abilities that reach far beyond, into the modern battle against cancer.

CHAPTER 2

How Fenbendazole and Mebendazole Fight Cancer: A Multifaceted Attack

Disrupting Tubulin: The Core Weapon Against Cancer Cells

The proven power of fenbendazole and mebendazole to kill parasites comes from one profound ability: they interfere with a process called tubulin polymerization. This is the same core mechanism that is now recognized as the key to their incredible anticancer potential.

To understand this, think of microtubules as the internal scaffolding and highway system of a cell. These structures are built from smaller protein units called α- and β-tubulin. In all complex cells, including cancer cells, microtubules are essential. They provide the cell's shape, act as tracks for transporting vital materials, and form the critical machinery needed for cell division. This makes them a perfect target for anticancer therapy.

Cancer cells are defined by their out-of-control growth, which is fueled by chaotic and unstable microtubules.[1] While healthy cells carefully manage their microtubule scaffolding, cancer cells have dysregulated and hyperactive systems that support their rapid division and spread.[2] Fenbendazole and mebendazole exploit this dependency. They bind directly to a specific spot on β-tubulin, effectively putting a cap on the microtubule and stopping it from growing.[3] This action slams the brakes on microtubule activity.

This disruption puts immense, cell-killing pressure on rapidly dividing cancer cells, which are desperately dependent on a functional microtubule network. This gives these drugs a powerful therapeutic advantage, as they have a much smaller effect on healthy, less active, or resting cells. The simple act of binding to tubulin sets off a chain reaction of powerful anticancer effects that attack multiple aspects of the cancer cell, ultimately leading to its death.

Sabotaging Cell Division by Disrupting Microtubules

For a cell to divide, it must first accurately copy its chromosomes and then pull them apart into two new daughter cells. This process is managed by the mitotic spindle, a complex machine built almost entirely of microtubules.[4] Cancer cells, which are notoriously unstable, rely on this spindle to continue multiplying.

By binding to tubulin and halting microtubule construction, fenbendazole and mebendazole prevent the cancer cell from building a working mitotic spindle.[5] This interference stops the chromosomes from lining up correctly, throwing the entire process of cell division into chaos. The cell's internal safety systems detect this failure and trigger the spindle assembly checkpoint, which freezes the cell in the G2/M phase of the cell cycle, a critical stage of division.[6] If the cell cannot fix this problem and restart division, it is forced to self-destruct through a process called apoptosis. This is the exact same mechanism used by many of the most successful chemotherapy drugs on the market today.

Stopping Metastasis in Its Tracks by Disrupting Tubulin

Metastasis—the spread of cancer from its original site to other parts of the body—is responsible for the vast majority of cancer-related deaths. For cancer to metastasize, a cell must be able to move and invade surrounding tissue. These actions require a dynamic and constantly changing internal skeleton, where microtubules are central to providing direction and forming invasive "feet" that burrow into new territory.

Microtubules also serve as the transport highways that deliver the proteins and materials needed for a cell to move and invade. By destabilizing these microtubule highways, fenbendazole and mebendazole directly cripple a cancer cell's ability to move and break through tissue barriers. This powerful anti-metastatic action is a profound and critically important therapeutic benefit of these drugs.

Triggering Cell Suicide (Apoptosis) by Disrupting Tubulin

The combination of assaults from fenbendazole and mebendazole—the disrupted cell division and the shattered internal skeleton—sends powerful stress signals throughout the cancer cell. These signals activate the cell's own internal self-destruct program, known as apoptosis.

Cancer cells are masters of survival and are famous for developing ways to shut down this self-destruct program. This is a key reason why they can grow uncontrollably and resist treatment. Fortunately, fenbendazole and mebendazole have a demonstrated ability to override these survival mechanisms and force the cancer cell to undergo apoptosis. Their primary attack on microtubules is the trigger that unleashes a cascade of events, firmly establishing them as potent, multipronged anticancer agents. Their unique ability to simultaneously halt cell division and stop metastasis makes them highly compelling candidates for comprehensive cancer treatment.

Beyond Microtubules: The Expanded Anticancer Arsenal of Benzimidazole Drugs

While microtubule disruption is the foundational mechanism, a growing body of evidence proves that fenbendazole and mebendazole launch additional, powerful attacks by targeting completely different cellular pathways. These non-tubulin actions dramatically broaden their effectiveness and confirm their ability to fight cancers using a variety of different complementary mechanisms.

Metabolic Sabotage: Starving Cancer Cells

A defining feature of aggressive cancers is a unique metabolic state known as the Warburg effect. This is a cancer cell's preference for burning sugar (glucose) for quick energy, even when plenty of oxygen is available.[7] This process not only provides fast fuel but also the raw building blocks needed for endless growth characteristic of cancer.

Fenbendazole strikes directly at this metabolic Achilles' heel. Definitive studies confirm that fenbendazole dramatically blocks cancer cells from taking up glucose, effectively cutting off their primary fuel source.[8] It also interferes with key enzymes inside the cell, further crippling its ability to generate energy.[9] This metabolic crisis creates profound stress, which is a major contributor to the fenbendazole's overall cancer-killing effect.[10]

Crippling the Warburg Engine: A Strategy Against Resistance

Fenbendazole's attack on glucose metabolism is a strategic strike against a core cancer dependency. By blocking glucose uptake, it drains the cell of its energy currency (ATP). This also leads to a sharp drop in the production of lactate, a toxic waste product. High levels of lactate in a tumor are not simply harmless by-products; lactate creates an acidic environment that shields the tumor from the immune system, fuels the growth of new blood vessels, promotes metastasis, and makes the cancer resistant to other therapies.[11] Increased lactate levels associated with cancer are a major factor not only related to growth of the cancer but also to defending it from outside threats like chemotherapy drugs.

By blocking glucose and slashing lactate production, fenbendazole dismantles a key engine of tumor growth and drug resistance. This potent metabolic attack offers a powerful way to kill cancer cells that have become resistant to traditional chemotherapy drugs.

Targeting Key Enzymes and Signaling Pathways

Hexokinase 2 (HK2) is a critical enzyme that jumpstarts the sugar-burning process in cancer cells. It is a key link between the cell's metabolism and its ability to resist self-destruction. Both mebendazole and fenbendazole directly target and inhibit this pivotal enzyme.[12, 13]

Furthermore, fenbendazole activates the master tumor suppressor protein, p53. As the "guardian of the genome," p53 responds to cellular stress by halting the cell cycle, repairing DNA, and triggering apoptosis. Fenbendazole-induced p53 activation is a central event that contributes to the shutdown of the cell's defective metabolism.[14] At the same time, fenbendazole disrupts other cancer-promoting signals, like the Hedgehog pathway. By hitting key enzymes like HK2 and controlling major signaling networks like p53 and Hedgehog, fenbendazole wages a multifront war on cancer's metabolism.

Inducing Lethal Oxidative Stress

Fenbendazole potently induces massive oxidative stress inside cancer cells. It does this by flooding the cell with damaging molecules called reactive oxygen species (ROS), which are like cellular rust. Under normal conditions, cells can manage ROS, but the flood caused by fenbendazole overwhelms the cancer cell's defenses, causing devastating damage to its DNA, proteins, and membranes, which ultimately leads to cell death.[15]

In response to this oxidative assault, the cell activates stress pathways that can lead to the cell's demise. Fenbendazole triggers a strong and sustained activation of the p38 MAPK pathway. While brief activation of this pathway can be a survival signal, the intense and prolonged signal caused by fenbendazole is overwhelmingly a death signal, driving the cell to destroy itself.[16] Fenbendazole executes a two-pronged attack: it inflicts direct oxidative damage while simultaneously activating the very signaling pathways that commands the cell to die.

Modulating Autophagy: The Cell's Recycling System

Autophagy is the cell's fundamental cleanup and recycling process, responsible for getting rid of damaged parts. Its role in cancer is complex. Sometimes it helps prevent cancer, but in established tumors, cancer cells hijack autophagy to survive stress and resist chemotherapy. Benzimidazoles, including fenbendazole, have been shown to interfere with this process.[17] By disrupting this critical survival system, fenbendazole can make cancer cells more vulnerable to other stresses, contributing to their death.

Inhibiting Angiogenesis: Cutting Off the Tumor's Supply Lines

A solid tumor cannot grow beyond the size of a pinhead without a blood supply. It achieves this through angiogenesis—the process of growing new blood vessels to deliver oxygen and nutrients.[18] Both fenbendazole and mebendazole are proven anti-angiogenic agents, meaning they interfere with a tumor's ability to create and maintain its own supply lines.[19, 20] By blocking angiogenesis, they effectively starve the tumor, restrict its growth, and prevent the spread of cancer cells through the bloodstream.

Modulating the Immune System: An Emerging Frontier

A new and exciting area of research is the potential for fenbendazole to modulate the immune system.[21] Cancer is notorious for creating an environment that suppresses the immune system, allowing it to hide from the body's natural defenses. Early evidence shows that fenbendazole may counteract these tactics.[22] It may alter the tumor environment to make it less hostile to immune cells or even enhance the activity of cancer-killing T cells. While more research is needed, the possibility that fenbendazole can help the immune system fight cancer adds another compelling dimension to its power, especially in the era of cancer immunotherapy.

These diverse mechanisms demonstrate the remarkably comprehensive nature of fenbendazole and mebendazole's anticancer activity. They launch a full-scale assault that targets cell division, metabolism, blood supply, stress responses, autophagy, and immune evasion. This multi-targeted profile makes it far more difficult for cancer to develop resistance compared to drugs that only hit a single target.

Considering all of the above, fenbendazole and mebendazole are compelling candidates as almost ideal multifaceted anticancer drugs with no harmful side effects.

Antiparasitic vs. Anticancer Doses of Fenbendazole and Mebendazole

Paracelsus, the father of toxicology, famously said, "Solely the dose determines that a thing is not a poison." This is often paraphrased as: the only difference between a medicine and a poison is the dose. A key question is whether the current doses of fenbendazole and mebendazole used to kill parasites are strong enough to kill cancer.

Inducing powerful, cell-killing effects against resilient cancer cells may require different drug concentrations than those used for parasites. However, this concern may be unfounded. As we will see, real-world evidence shows that self-treatment with standard, safe antiparasite dosages of fenbendazole has resulted in the clinical remission of various cancers with virtually no adverse side effects in humans.

The science shows us that the optimal doses required to disrupt microtubules, inhibit metabolism, induce massive oxidative stress, and suppress angiogenesis are clearly achieved with these standard dosing regimens. Researchers studying mebendazole for triple-negative breast cancer were deliberate in using these same physiological doses in their animal studies, which correspond to the 222 mg to 1000 mg per day that people are using to successfully self-treat their cancers.[23]

Encouragingly, a vast amount of data shows that fenbendazole and mebendazole have a remarkably wide margin of safety. They are exceptionally well-tolerated, even at doses far exceeding standard antiparasitic levels.[24] This is because cancer cells, with their high metabolic rate and dependency on specific metabolic pathways, are far more sensitive to these drugs than are healthy, lower metabolic rate cells.

Furthermore, fenbendazole is known to have better oral bioavailability than mebendazole, meaning more of it gets absorbed better into the body. This is one reason why people who self-treat their cancers often choose the more bioavailable, inexpensive, and over-the-counter fenbendazole.[25]

The antiparasitic drugs fenbendazole and mebendazole possess sophisticated and multipronged anticancer mechanisms. Their foundational activity disrupts the machinery of cell division and motility, and this is powerfully amplified by targeted assaults on cancer's core dependencies, including its unique metabolism, its need for a blood supply, and its ability to manage stress. The convergence of these multiple, validated mechanisms provides an exceptionally strong rationale for their use in treating cancer in humans.

The next chapter will present the wealth of scientific data showing the effectiveness of fenbendazole and mebendazole against a variety of cancers in more complex laboratory settings. This will set the stage for the powerful case reports detailing the stories of those who have successfully self-treated their own cancers with fenbendazole.

CHAPTER 3

The Science Is In: The Hard Evidence for Fenbendazole's War on Cancer

The proof that fenbendazole is a powerful anticancer agent isn't based on wishful thinking; it's built on a mountain of hard scientific evidence. This evidence comes from preclinical research—the foundational lab work that happens long before a drug is tested in humans. It includes studies in petri dishes (known as in vitro) and in living animals (in vivo).

This research is the bedrock of our understanding. It proves that fenbendazole and its relatives don't just work in a lab like we discussed in the previous chapter; they also deliver significant anticancer effects inside a living body. The data we will examine, from pioneers like Dr. Gregory Riggins and many others, is exactly why these drugs have ignited a firestorm of interest among scientists and patients alike.

This chapter will take you through that science to show you how researchers have proven that fenbendazole is a potent cancer killer. First, we'll look at the tools and methods scientists use for these experiments. Then, we'll dive into the groundbreaking studies that build the undeniable case for fenbendazole as a safe, effective cancer treatment.

But first, what led scientists to believe that antiparasitic drugs might kill cancer cells in the first place?

The Spark of an Idea: Connecting a Dewormer to Cancer

To understand why a simple deworming medicine like fenbendazole was ever considered a potential cancer treatment, we have to travel back to the early 2000s. The story isn't about a random guess; it's a brilliant piece of scientific detective work that connected two very different fields of study. Here's how the logic unfolded.

Step 1: The Double-Edged Sword of Chemotherapy

For decades, since the 1970s, one of the main strategies for fighting cancer has been to attack its ability to divide and multiply. To do this, scientists designed drugs that targeted microtubules.

Recall that microtubules are the internal scaffolding or highway system of a cell. They are crucial for giving a cell its shape, transporting vital materials, and, most importantly for this discussion, pulling the cell apart into two new cells during division (mitosis).

Cancer cells are characterized by their rapid, out-of-control division. So, the logic was simple: if you destroy the microtubules, you stop the cancer cells from multiplying. Drugs like Taxol (a taxane) and vincristine (a vinca alkaloid) were developed to do just this. They are powerful microtubule-targeting agents and have been cornerstone chemotherapy drugs for years.

But these treatments have a major drawback: they are blunt instruments. These drugs can't tell the difference between a cancerous cell and a healthy cell that also happens to divide quickly. They attack the microtubule scaffolding in any rapidly dividing cell. This "collateral damage" is why chemotherapy causes such severe side effects—it also harms the fast-growing cells in our hair follicles (hair loss), gut lining (nausea, diarrhea), and bone marrow (fatigue, infection risk). The very thing that makes these drugs effective, targeting rapidly dividing cancer cells, also makes them highly toxic to rapidly dividing healthy cells.

Step 2: A Clue from an Unlikely Place—Parasites

Meanwhile, in a completely different area of medicine, veterinarians and doctors were using fenbendazole and mebendazole to treat parasitic worms. These drugs were remarkably effective and, importantly, incredibly safe for the host—be it a dog, a sheep, or a human.

Scientists discovered that these dewormers worked by—you guessed it—attacking the microtubules of the parasite. They dismantled the worm's cellular scaffolding, starving it and leading to its death.

This led to a critical insight. Why were these drugs so deadly to the parasite but harmless to the person or animal they were treating? The answer was selectivity. The drug molecule was like a specific key. It fit perfectly into a "lock" on the parasite's tubulin (the protein that builds microtubules), but it didn't fit the lock on mammalian tubulin. This specific targeting was their magic bullet quality, allowing them to kill the invader while leaving the host's cells untouched.

Step 3: The Aha! Moment—Connecting the Dots

This is where the innovative leap occurred. In 2002, researcher Dr. Tapas Mukhopadhyay and his team connected these two separate ideas of cancer and parasites:[1]

- **Dot 1 (Cancer):** We have powerful microtubule-targeting chemo drugs, but they are too toxic because they are not selective. They are like an indiscriminate bomb.
- **Dot 2 (Parasites):** We have a microtubule-targeting deworming drug (mebendazole) that is extremely safe because it is highly selective. It is like a guided missile.

This sparked a brilliant question: Could the dewormers' selectivity also apply to cancer cells?

No one thought cancer cell tubulin was identical to parasite tubulin. But perhaps the tubulin in a cancer cell is different enough from the tubulin in a healthy human cell for mebendazole to work. Cancer cells are mutated, chaotic, and biochemically distinct. Could it be that their microtubule "locks" are slightly different or more vulnerable than healthy cells? Maybe the dewormer "key" wouldn't be a perfect fit like it was for the parasite, but perhaps it could still jam the cancer cell's lock enough to kill it while leaving healthy cells alone.

The incredible safety profile of these dewormers made the idea irresistible. For decades, millions of people had used them with few, if any, side effects. If they had even a modest effect against cancer, they could potentially offer a much better-tolerated treatment than the brutal chemotherapy regimens currently in use.

With this logical foundation, the theory was born: Mebendazole, and by extension its chemical sibling fenbendazole, might represent a safer, more targeted way to attack microtubules in cancer cells.

The goal was to see if this humble dewormer could inhibit cancer growth while sparing the patient the devastating side effects of conventional chemotherapy. It was a low-risk, high-reward idea. And so, researchers began pulling this old, safe medicine off the shelf to see if it held a hidden talent for fighting one of humanity's most feared diseases. This compelling chain of reasoning is what launched the scientific journey that we are exploring in this book.

One Family of Drugs, One Fight Against Cancer

Drugs like fenbendazole, mebendazole, and albendazole are all part of the same chemical family. They are so similar in structure and function that we can discuss them together and interchangeably. Their main attack strategy is to go after a protein called tubulin, which cancer cells desperately need to divide and grow. As we'll soon see, this is just one of many ways fenbendazole attacks cancer.

While there are minor differences—fenbendazole is generally absorbed better by the body and is superior at crossing the protective blood-brain barrier—their core cancer-killing abilities are nearly identical. Ironically, most lab research uses the human drug (mebendazole) on animals, while most human success stories, which you'll read about in the Case Report chapter later, use the animal drug (fenbendazole). This crossover further proves they work similarly against cancer.

Make no mistake: Fenbendazole is the star of this group for human use. It is easily absorbed when taken by mouth, it effectively reaches the brain, and it has an outstanding safety profile, plus it is very inexpensive and available over the counter. It would be a massive leap forward for science and cancer patients if any future clinical trials used safe, effective fenbendazole, the drug of choice for people who are already successfully self-treating their cancer.

A Survey of the Scientific Evidence: Fenbendazole's Winning Record Against Cancer

In vitro research is the first step. Scientists take cancer cells and grow them in controlled lab conditions, like flasks or petri dishes. This allows the researcher's to test the drug's power directly on the cancer cells, experiment with different doses, and uncover exactly how it works. Researchers use specific, well-known cancer cell lines, many of which date back to the 1950s, allowing their results to be compared with labs all over the world.

The first question scientists ask is simple: Does it kill cancer cells? This is called cytotoxicity. For fenbendazole and mebendazole, the answer is a resounding *yes*. These drugs have been tested against a huge variety of human cancer cell lines, including:

- **Glioblastoma:** Aggressive brain cancer cells were highly sensitive to mebendazole.[2, 3]
- **Breast Cancer:** Cells from common and aggressive triple-negative breast cancers were effectively killed by mebendazole and its relatives.[4, 5]

- **Non-Small Cell Lung Cancer (NSCLC):** A widely used lung cancer cell line was sensitive to both mebendazole and fenbendazole.[6]
- **Colon Cancer:** Colon cancer cells, even those resistant to standard chemotherapy, were stopped by mebendazole and fenbendazole.[7, 8]
- **Ovarian Cancer:** Fenbendazole proved its effectiveness against ovarian cancer cells.[9]
- **Prostate Cancer:** Researchers successfully used fenbendazole to target prostate cancer cells.[10]
- **Liver Cancer:** Fenbendazole triggered cell death in liver cancer cells.[11]
- **Melanoma:** Mebendazole was shown to be effective against aggressive skin cancer cells.[12, 13]

Fenbendazole and mebendazole are also lethal against blood cancers:

- **Leukemia:** Mebendazole is a potent killer of acute myeloid leukemia cells.[14, 15]
- **Lymphoma:** Fenbendazole has broad power against cancers like lymphoma, where it shatters the cell's internal structure and activates multiple kill signals.[16]

The results are stunningly consistent: fenbendazole and mebendazole kill cancer on contact in a dose-dependent way. This means the higher the dose, the more cancer cells die. The drugs stop cancer cells from multiplying and trigger their complete self-destruction.

Most importantly, the ultimate goal of any cancer treatment is to kill the cancer without harming the patient. This is called selectivity. Multiple studies have confirmed that fenbendazole and mebendazole are far more toxic to cancer cells than to healthy cells.[17] Research shows this is because cancer cells preferentially contain the very microtubule structures that these drugs destroy, making them uniquely vulnerable. This selectivity for cancer cell microtubules explains why fenbendazole has such a remarkable safety profile.[18] Safe, low doses of fenbendazole are all that's needed to kill a wide variety of cancer cells with little to no collateral damage to healthy cells. This means few, if any, side effects from their use as anticancer medicines.

Counting the Dead Cancer Cells Using Cell Viability Assays

To prove these drugs kill cancer, scientists need to count the dead cells using tests called cell viability assays. These tests measure the energy level of living cells—as cells die, the energy level plummets, which is what happens when cancer cells are exposed to fenbendazole.[19]

Through thousands of these tests, researchers have proven one simple fact: Fenbendazole and mebendazole kill cancer cells, lots of them.

How Fenbendazole Kills the Cancer Cell at the Cellular Level

It's not enough to know that fenbendazole works by counting the dead cancer cells; we need to know how it kills those cells. Scientists use advanced techniques to see what's happening inside the cancer cell as it dies and have confirmed that one of fenbendazole's primary weapons is its ability to disrupt microtubules.

Again, think of microtubules as the cell's internal skeleton and highway system. Recall that they are made of a protein called tubulin. Microtubules are essential for a cell to hold its shape, move things around internally, and—most critically—to divide and create more cancer cells.

Fenbendazole and mebendazole act like saboteurs. They bind to tubulin and prevent it from forming these essential structures.[20, 21] This sabotage triggers a two-pronged attack:

- **Cell Cycle Arrest:** Without a functional skeleton, the cancer cell cannot complete the division process. It gets stuck, typically in the G2/M phase of its life cycle, unable to replicate. This is like throwing a wrench into the machinery of cancer cell duplication.
- **Apoptosis (Programmed Cell Death):** A cell frozen in its cycle is a stressed cell. This stress triggers a self-destruct sequence called apoptosis. This is the body's natural way of eliminating damaged or unwanted cells. It is a "clean" death that doesn't cause inflammation, which further contributes to fenbendazole's lack of side effects.[22]

This dual-action attack—stopping replication and ordering self-destruction—shows just how powerfully fenbendazole dismantles cancer's survival strategy.

Targeting Cancer Stem Cells: Killing the Cells That Kill Us

This may be one of the most important discoveries about fenbendazole. Within every tumor, there is a small group of elite cells called cancer stem cells. These are like the "queen bees" of the tumor. They are responsible for driving tumor growth, spreading cancer to other organs (metastasis), and causing cancer to return after treatment. These cells are notoriously resistant to chemotherapy and radiation.

Incredibly, compelling in vitro evidence shows that fenbendazole and mebendazole hunt down and kill cancer stem cells. For example, one study showed that mebendazole shut down a key protein that gives breast cancer cells their "stemness," blocking their ability to form new tumors.[23]

This is an absolute game changer. It means fenbendazole may not only shrink tumors but also eliminate the very cells that cause long-term treatment failure when using traditional cancer drugs. By targeting these killer stem cells, fenbendazole may be able to stop cancer from ever coming back.

The evidence from these lab studies is irrefutable. Fenbendazole's ability to kill a broad range of cancers, its preference for cancer cells over healthy cells, its power to shut down cell division, and its potential to destroy cancer stem cells create an ironclad case for its use as a cancer treatment in humans.

In Vivo Studies: Proving Fenbendazole and Mebendazole Work in a Living System

Testing a drug in a petri dish is one thing. Proving it works in a living, breathing animal is the critical next step. These in vivo studies are essential to see if the drug can reach the tumor, shrink it, stop it from spreading, and do so safely. Success here moves a drug one step closer to human use.

Xenograft Models: Unleashing Fenbendazole on Human Tumors in Mice

A key experimental method of study is the xenograft model. Scientists implant human cancer cells into mice with weakened immune systems. The weak immune system prevents the mouse's body from rejecting the implanted experimental human tumor, allowing researchers to see how a drug affects a human cancer in a living mammal.

Across the board, these xenograft studies have been a stunning success.

- **Tumor Growth Is Obliterated:** Treating these mice with fenbendazole or mebendazole leads to dramatic reductions in tumor size and weight compared to untreated mice. This has been proven in the studies mentioned earlier for: glioblastoma (brain cancer), medulloblastoma (pediatric brain cancer), melanoma, lung cancer, colon cancer (even chemo-resistant types), breast cancer (especially aggressive triple-negative breast cancer), ovarian cancer, and liver cancer.
- **Longer Survival:** Shrinking tumors translates directly into longer life. In numerous studies, mice with deadly cancers like glioblastoma

and medulloblastoma lived significantly longer when treated with fenbendazole and mebendazole.

When researchers examined the tumors from treated mice, they found exactly what they saw in the petri dish: massive cancer cell death (apoptosis) and a dramatic halt in cell division. These findings were proof that fenbendazole and mebendazole kill cancer in living organisms.

These consistent victories in xenograft models provide powerful proof that fenbendazole can effectively crush human cancers in a living body.

Syngeneic Models: Proving It Works with an Active Immune System

The next step of experimental testing used mice with fully functional immune systems. These are called syngeneic models. They are crucial for seeing how a drug interacts with the body's own defenses. These models are useful because they show how the drug and the cancer are likely to behave in the real world when administered to a human patient. Studies using these models have also shown that fenbendazole effectively and dramatically shrinks tumors.

This research opens the door to another possibility: that fenbendazole might actually boost the immune system's own ability to fight cancer. How these drugs awaken and enhance the antitumor immune response is a hot area of ongoing research.

Inhibition of Metastasis: Stopping Cancer's Deadly Spread

Metastasis—the spread of cancer from its original location to vital organs—is what makes cancer so deadly. One of the most electrifying findings is that fenbendazole and mebendazole can block metastasis.

Studies in breast cancer and melanoma have shown that treatment drastically reduces the spread of cancer to the lungs and liver. This antimetastatic power likely comes from a combination of direct cell killing, stopping cancer cell migration, and cutting off the new blood supply that tumors need to grow and spread (the process of angiogenesis).

This ability to stop metastasis is a game-changing feature of fenbendazole's power as an anticancer treatment.

Pharmacokinetics, Safety, and Dosing

Animal studies are also used to figure out how the body processes the drug (pharmacokinetics) and to find the perfect dose—one that is lethal to cancer but safe for the host.

These studies confirmed that oral fenbendazole can reach high enough levels in the blood and in the tumor to be effective. While fenbendazole is already relatively well-absorbed, scientists are finding new ways to make it even better. One recent study found that formulations combining fenbendazole with common ingredients like cinnamic acid or salicylic acid dramatically improved its absorption.[24] Another team developed nanostructured lipid carriers to improve solubility and sustain drug release,[25] while a different group developed nanoparticles that delivered fenbendazole directly to ovarian tumors, making it even more potent.

Most importantly, these studies have repeatedly confirmed the incredible safety of fenbendazole and mebendazole. Even at doses much higher than those used for parasites, the drugs are remarkably well-tolerated, a fact supported by veterinary safety studies showing good tolerance in dogs even at elevated doses.[26] In a remarkable human case, one patient tolerated high-dose mebendazole daily for thirteen years for a parasitic infection, demonstrating its potential for long-term safety, although caution is always warranted when extrapolating from individual cases.[27] The Choi et al. (2021) study mentioned earlier in breast cancer models concluded that the drugs wiped out the cancer at doses that were completely nontoxic to the mice.

The consistent message from the in vivo studies is clear and consistent: Fenbendazole inhibits tumor growth, blocks metastasis, increases survival, and does it all with an outstanding safety profile. This provides an unshakable foundation for justifying its use in fighting cancer.

The Pioneers: The Scientists Who Built the Case for Fenbendazole and Mebendazole

The charge to bring fenbendazole and mebendazole into the cancer fight has been led by Dr. Gregory Riggins and his lab at Johns Hopkins University. Dr. Riggins is a champion of drug repurposing—the strategy of using safe, existing drugs for new purposes to get effective treatments to patients faster.[28] This approach leverages drugs with known safety profiles to bypass years of early-stage development, a strategy championed by researchers worldwide who see its potential and acknowledge its challenges.[29] His team's rigorous and focused research has been instrumental in proving these drugs work.

Dr. Riggins has tackled some of the deadliest cancers, including pediatric medulloblastoma and adult glioblastoma.[30] His lab's discovery that mebendazole could cross the blood-brain barrier and extend survival in mice with brain cancer was a landmark finding that helped ignite global interest in antiparasitics and cancer. The potential of these drugs for brain tumors continues to be a major focus of research.

His team's research has confirmed that microtubule disruption is a core weapon, but they've also uncovered others as well. They've shown that these drugs interfere with cancer cell growth signals, block the formation of new blood vessels that feed tumors (angiogenesis), and can even break down the protective physical barrier, known as stromas, that shield pancreatic tumors.[31]

Recognizing that the best cancer treatments often involve combinations of drugs, the Riggins lab has proven that fenbendazole and mebendazole work synergistically with standard cancer therapies. Their work showing that fenbendazole makes radiation therapy dramatically more effective against medulloblastoma is a prime example of this powerful synergistic strategy.[32, 33]

Dr. Riggins's high-impact research has built the scientific launchpad for using fenbendazole and mebendazole against cancer.

A Global Effort: Other Key Discoveries

In addition to Riggins, a worldwide community of other scientists has built on this foundation, replicating and extending this research and adding more layers of proof:

- **Starving the Cancer Cell:** Lucenda de Silva et al. (2023) showed that mebendazole throws cancer's metabolism into chaos, cutting off its energy supply and leading to cell death. This has since been supported by findings that benzimidazoles can directly inhibit key metabolic enzymes like hexokinase II, which cancer cells rely on for energy.[34]
- **Cutting Off the Blood Supply:** Multiple reviews and studies have confirmed that fenbendazole and mebendazole are potent anti-angiogenic agents, effectively starving tumors by preventing them from growing the new blood vessels they need to survive.[35]
- **Modulating Cellular Processes:** Researchers are also finding that these drugs interfere with other critical cell survival pathways. For example, in glioblastoma cells, mebendazole disrupts autophagy, a cellular recycling process that can help cancer cells survive stress.[36]
- **Conquering Aggressive Breast Cancer:** A 2021 study by Choi et al. proved mebendazole's power against triple-negative breast cancer (TNBC) and convincingly showed it could make radiation-resistant TNBC vulnerable to treatment again.

- **Boosting the Immune System:** A 2022 review gathered evidence suggesting these drugs can awaken the immune system to attack cancer, possibly by clearing out immunosuppressive cells from the tumor's neighborhood. Li et al. (2019) found that flubendazole blocked melanoma growth by affecting immune system modulation through programmed cell death mechanisms (PD-1).[37]
- **Shattering Pancreatic Cancer's Defenses:** In a major breakthrough from the Riggins lab, Williamson et al. (2021) showed that mebendazole can physically dismantle the dense, fibrous stroma shield that protects pancreatic tumors, making this notoriously difficult cancer vulnerable to attack.
- **Optimizing Delivery of Fenbendazole:** Recent studies are finding brilliant ways to make fenbendazole even more effective. A 2023 study encapsulated fenbendazole in nanoparticles, which dramatically improved its delivery and cancer-killing power in ovarian cancer models. A broad analysis of all the genes affected by fenbendazole in ovarian cancer confirmed its impact on cell cycle, apoptosis, and metabolism.[38] Another study mentioned earlier found that combining fenbendazole with simple organic acids, like the aspirin metabolite salicylic acid, could massively increase its availability to the body.

This global chorus of independent research all sings the same song: fenbendazole and mebendazole are multifaceted, powerful anticancer agents, and the case for their use is overwhelming.

The Power of Synergy: Making Marginal Treatments Great Again

Fenbendazole is a powerful weapon on its own. But when combined with traditional treatments like radiation and chemotherapy, it becomes a force multiplier. This is called synergy, where the combined effect is far greater than the sum of its parts. Think of it as 1 + 1 = 4. This strategy can make borderline treatments more effective, overcome resistance, and even allow for lower, safer doses of toxic conventional therapies.

Synergy with Radiation: A One-Two Punch

Radiation therapy works by damaging a cancer cell's DNA. Unfortunately, it also damages healthy cells' DNA as well, causing collateral damage and side effects.

Fenbendazole makes radiation work even better by:

- Holding Cancer Cells in Place: Fenbendazole arrests cancer cells in the G2/M phase of their life cycle—the exact phase when they are most vulnerable to radiation.[39] Fenbendazole holds the cell in place while radiation delivers the killing blow.
- Overcoming Resistance: By attacking the cell's structure (microtubules) instead of its DNA, fenbendazole provides a second, independent line of attack that cancer cells can't easily defend against. It has been shown to resensitize radiation-resistant breast cancers, making them treatable again.
- Better Tumor Control: Animal studies repeatedly show that combining fenbendazole or mebendazole with radiation leads to far greater tumor shrinkage and longer survival than either treatment alone. This has been proven in medulloblastoma, diffuse intrinsic pontine glioma, triple-negative breast cancer, and malignant meningioma.[40, 41]

Combining fenbendazole with radiation is a devastatingly effective strategy to make radiation great again without adding any adverse side effects.

Synergy with Chemotherapy: Breaking Down the Defenses

Chemotherapy is often limited by its toxicity and by the cancer's ability to develop resistance. Fenbendazole tackles both problems by:

- **Disabling Cancer's Shields:** Cancer cells can develop pumps on their surface to spit out chemotherapy drugs before they can work. Fenbendazole has been shown to disable these pumps, trapping the chemo inside the cancer cell where it can do its job.[42] It can also disrupt key survival signals like HIF-1 that cancer cells use to resist treatment in low-oxygen environments.[43]
- **Overcoming Resistance:** Fenbendazole has been proven to kill cancer cells that have become resistant to standard chemotherapies like 5-FU in colon cancer and temozolomide in brain cancer.[44]
- **Allowing for Lower Chemo Doses:** Because the combination is so effective, it may be possible to use lower doses of toxic chemotherapy, reducing side effects while achieving a better outcome. This has been demonstrated in studies on leukemia and glioma.[45] In fact, mebendazole

has been explored as a potentially less toxic partner or replacement for the microtubule-targeting chemotherapy drug vincristine.

Comprehensive studies have confirmed these synergistic pairings: fenbendazole with 5-FU in colon cancer, mebendazole with temozolomide in glioma, mebendazole with standard leukemia drugs, and fenbendazole with the metabolic drug dichloroacetate in lung cancer.

The evidence is clear: fenbendazole is a powerful partner that amplifies the effectiveness of conventional radiation and chemotherapy cancer treatments.

It's in the Genes: Fenbendazole Targets Cancer's Master Controls

Cancer is driven by broken genes called oncogenes—master control switches that are stuck in the "on" position, telling the cell to grow and divide endlessly. The most famous of these is the p53 gene. Fenbendazole has been shown to directly interfere with these broken master genetic controls.

Normally, the p53 gene is the "guardian of the genome." When a cell is damaged, p53 orders it to self-destruct by apoptosis.[46] But in most cancers, p53 is mutated and malfunctioning. This broken p53 gene not only fails to kill the cancer cell as it should but, unfortunately, instead can actively help it survive and resist treatment.[47]

Fenbendazole and mebendazole brilliantly overcome this problem in two clever ways:

- Fenbendazole and Mebendazole Activate Good p53: In cancer cells that still have a functional p53 gene, these drugs trigger a stress signal that activates p53, forcing the cancer cell to commit suicide.[48, 49]
- Fenbendazole and Mebendazole Kill Cancer Cells Without p53: Importantly, fenbendazole and mebendazole's effectiveness does not depend on p53. They have been shown to be potent killers of cancers that have a broken or missing p53 gene, like glioblastoma and medulloblastoma.

They do this by causing such catastrophic structural damage that the cancer cell dies anyway with or without the p53 gene. Fenbendazole and mebendazole essentially convert the p53 gene from a traitor back into a guardian.

This ability to kill cancer regardless of its p53 status gives fenbendazole and mebendazole an enormous advantage compared to traditional chemotherapeutic drugs against a wide range of aggressive tumors.

Beyond p53: Shutting Down Other Master Switches

The attack on cancer's command-and-control system doesn't stop there. Mebendazole has been shown to disrupt other key oncogenes, including:

- **MYC:** A master regulator of cell growth, MYC is a core driver of many cancers. Mebendazole has been shown to slash MYC protein levels in leukemia and medulloblastoma cells.[50]
- **Hedgehog/GLI1:** This pathway, hijacked by cancers like medulloblastoma and glioblastoma multiforme, is critical for tumor growth and cancer stem cell survival. Mebendazole has been identified as a direct inhibitor of this pathway.[51]
- **BCR-ABL:** The defining oncogene of chronic myeloid leukemia. Mebendazole inhibits its activity, even in cells resistant to standard targeted drugs.[52]
- **NRAS:** A common mutation in melanoma. Mebendazole is effective against NRAS-mutant melanoma, even in cells that have become resistant to targeted NRAS-inhibitor drugs.

Fenbendazole and mebendazole are not just simple microtubule disruptors. They are sophisticated, multi-targeting agents that dismantle cancer's core genetic programming. This broad attack helps explain their power against so many different cancers and their ability to overcome resistance.[53, 54]

A Foundation of Proof, a Future of Hope, and an Imperative to Act

The preclinical evidence is extensive, consistent, and compelling. Fenbendazole and mebendazole are powerful multimodal drugs that hit cancer cells at numerous vulnerable points simultaneously in an all-at-once barrage. Scientists worldwide have proven it repeatedly using a variety of methods as detailed above.

To be perfectly clear, the science shows that fenbendazole and mebendazole kill cancer using multiple, overlapping mechanisms, including:

Shattering the cancer cell's internal skeleton (microtubule disruption)
Starving the cell of sugar and cutting off its blood supply
Disabling the pumps that spit out chemotherapy drugs
Overriding the broken p53 "immortality" gene
Blocking cancer cell migration and metastasis
Triggering a self-destruct sequence (apoptosis)

This multifaceted attack is relentless, overpowering, and complete. The action of fenbendazole and mebendazole on a cancer cell is the very definition of overkill. It is important to point out that no other cancer drug has this multimodal power of fenbendazole or mebendazole.

Given all that we've covered so far, a compelling question comes to mind: If fenbendazole is such a great anticancer treatment, why doesn't my doctor know about it?

CHAPTER 4

Why Doesn't My Doctor Know About Fenbendazole?

The scientific data presented and the case reports ahead demonstrate that fenbendazole is a powerful tool against cancer. This leads to a crucial question: If fenbendazole is so effective, why doesn't my doctor know about it?

It's a fair question, and the answer is shocking. It points to a cover-up that has lasted for nearly fifty years. To understand what happened, we need to go back in time and understand the sequence of events that bring us to today.

Many people think the interest in drugs like fenbendazole and mebendazole is a recent trend, sparked by online stories and new scientific studies. But the truth is, the science justifying fenbendazole as a cure for cancer isn't new at all. In fact, much of what we celebrate today as a "new discovery" regarding fenbendazole was already proven, documented, and published at the dawn of the twenty-first century.

A groundbreaking study on the effects of mebendazole on cancer was published in 2002 in a top medical journal, *Clinical Cancer Research*. This paper, written by University of Texas researchers affiliated with the world-renowned MD Anderson Cancer Center, proved without a doubt that mebendazole had powerful cancer-killing abilities.[1] They convincingly showed that mebendazole killed cancer cells in lab dishes and in living animals.

This chapter will break down this 2002 study and then expose an even bigger secret—a smoking gun that proves this knowledge of this cancer curing drug existed decades earlier and was likely deliberately buried.

The Accidental Rediscovery: Proof That Mebendazole Kills Cancer

The study on mebendazole and cancer that inadvertently blew the lid off this whole thing was published in 2002 by scientists at University of Texas also affiliated with the MD Anderson Cancer Center. They were trying to solve a problem: the contemporary standard-of-care chemo drugs, like taxanes and vinca alkaloids, that affected cancer cell microtubules were incredibly toxic and ridden with side effects. They wondered if mebendazole, a deworming drug known to disrupt parasite microtubules as well, without harming the host, could be a safer alternative. They were right.

The researchers tested mebendazole on a variety of human cancer cells, including lung, ovarian, melanoma, and colon cancer. The results were stunning. Mebendazole stopped cancer cells cold, even at extremely low doses. It worked against a wide spectrum of cancers, including those resistant to other chemo drugs.

Next, they gave mebendazole to mice that had implanted human lung tumors. They gave one group mebendazole (orally, mixed in corn oil), another group the standard chemo drug paclitaxel (by injection), and a third group a placebo.

These comprehensive experiments provided irrefutable evidence for mebendazole's potent anticancer properties. They convincingly demonstrated:

- Broad-spectrum in vitro cytotoxicity against various human cancer cell lines at very low, nanomolar concentrations.
- Induction of apoptosis and G_2/M cell cycle arrest as key mechanisms of cell death.
- Direct inhibition of tubulin polymerization as the underlying molecular mechanism.
- Significant in vivo antitumor efficacy via oral administration in a human lung cancer xenograft model, comparable to paclitaxel.
- A remarkable lack of overt toxicity in vivo at therapeutically effective doses.

The study's authors concluded with a powerful statement: "Mebendazole elicits a potent cytotoxic effect on cancer cells. . . . Our results provide strong support for considering mebendazole as a potential anticancer agent that is likely to have a favorable therapeutic index because of its wide use in humans with relatively few side effects."

It is of paramount importance to recognize that these findings were published in the journal *Clinical Cancer Research* in 2002. This is not a fringe journal, nor were the findings ambiguous. The evidence was clear and compelling: a widely used, safe, off-patent, and inexpensive antiparasitic drug possessed significant, demonstrable anticancer capabilities. This predates the bulk of the contemporary (2015–2025) research and current widespread public interest in fenbendazole and mebendazole for cancer by well over a decade, if not closer to two.

They had scientifically proven that a cheap, safe deworming medicine, mebendazole, was a powerful, nontoxic cancer drug. They just didn't know they were twenty-six years late to the party.

The Smoking Gun Named Oncodazole

The story of fenbendazole/mebendazole and cancer doesn't start in 2002. It starts in 1976.

Almost fifty years ago, a drug that is nearly identical to fenbendazole was being studied for its effects on cancer. The scientists who discovered its power were so confident that they gave it a name that was impossible to misunderstand: Oncodazole.[2, 3, 4, 5, 6, 7]

In medicine, "onco" is the Greek root for tumor or mass. It's the root of the word "oncology," the study of cancer. Naming a drug "oncodazole" is like naming a new weapon the "tank-destroyer." There is no ambiguity of what the thing does based on its name.

The Latin phrase *res ipsa loquitor* means "the thing speaks for itself." A cancer drug named oncodazole speaks for itself.

In 1976, researchers published papers showing that oncodazole worked by disrupting critical structures inside cancer cells called microtubules (sound familiar?), killing them while leaving healthy cells unharmed.[8] This is the exact same mechanism celebrated as a new discovery for mebendazole twenty-six years later in 2002. As the famous baseball player Yogi Berra said, "It's déjà vu all over again."

So, what happened to oncodazole? Why didn't it become the cure for cancer in 1976?

It was suppressed. And the proof of this suppression is found in the very existence of that 2002 published research paper.

Proof of the Cover-Up of Oncodazole

Claiming that this knowledge was actively suppressed is a serious charge, but the evidence is written into the public record of science itself, embedded in three simple facts about how scientific research is published, in this instance the 2002 paper on mebendazole and cancer:

1. The *Authors* Didn't Know about Oncodazole. When the University of Texas/MD Anderson scientists published their mebendazole paper

Vol. 69, No. 2, 1976 BIOCHEMICAL AND BIOPHYSICAL RESEARCH COMMUNICATIONS

INTERACTION OF ONCODAZOLE (R 17934), A NEW ANTI-TUMORAL DRUG, WITH RAT BRAIN TUBULIN.

J. Hoebeke, G. Van Nijen and M. De Brabander*
Laboratory of Immunochemistry
*Laboratory of Oncology
Janssen Research Laboratories
B-2340 Beerse
Belgium

Received January 23, 1976

SUMMARY : Oncodazole (R 17934), methyl [5-(2-thienylcarbonyl)-1H-benzimidazol-2-yl] carbamate (I), a new synthetic drug with anti-tumoral activity, inhibits the polymerization of rat brain tubulin *in vitro*. It has no depolymerizing effect on preformed microtubules *in vitro*. Binding studies by means of molecular sieving and equilibrium dialysis indicates that the drug binds to purified rat brain tubulin in a mole to mole ratio. Finally the drug competitively inhibits colchicine binding to purified rat brain tubulin. From these results the conclusion may be drawn that oncodazole is a true microtubule inhibitor.

INTRODUCTION

Oncodazole (R 17934) (Fig. 1) has been shown to have anti-mitotic activity *in vitro* (1) and anti-tumoral activity *in vivo* (2, 3). On a cellular level the drug interferes with the structure and function of microtubules (1). The purpose of this study was to provide direct biochemical evidence that the drug acts on the tubulin molecule i.e. the protein subunit of the microtubular structure. Two properties which are common to all microtubule inhibitors were therefore investigated : their ability to inhibit the polymerization reaction of (4) and to bind on the tubulin molecule (5).

MATERIAL AND METHODS

Drugs and chemicals

Colchicine was purchased from Aldrich Europe, oncodazole (R 17934) is a product of Janssen Research Laboratories.

[^{3}H] Colchicine (3 Ci/mmol) was purchased from the Radiochemical Centre, Amerham, [^{14}C] Oncodazole (6.25 µCi/mg) was synthetized by the metabolic department of Janssen Research Laboratories.

Abbreviations used : EDTA : ethylene-diamino-tetra-acetic acid; GTP : guanosine-5'-triphosphate; Pipes : piperazine-N-N'-bis [2-ethane sulfonic acid]; EGTA : ethylene-glycol-bis (2-aminoethyl)-tetra-acetic acid in 2002, they claimed they were the first to report on the anticancer effects of this class of drugs. "Our results demonstrate for the first time the antitumor and antiangiogenetic effects of MZ (mebendazole) both in vitro and in vivo," p. 2963. Later in the discussion, they reiterate the claim stating, "The effect of MZ (mebendazole) as an antitumor agent has never been tested before," (page 2968).[9] To make such claims, they would have had to perform a thorough search of all previous scientific literature. They would have known that antiparasitic drugs fenbendazole, oncodazole, and mebendazole possessed similar chemical structure and anticancer mechanisms if the papers were available to be cited. The fact that they missed the 1976 oncodazole paper detailing its anticancer mechanisms means only one thing: that paper was nowhere to be found. It had been effectively erased from the scientific databases available at the time.

2. The *Expert Peer-Reviewers* Didn't Know about Oncodazole. Before a paper is published in a major journal like *Clinical Cancer Research*, it is sent to a panel of world-class experts for peer review. Their job is to find any flaws or mistakes. If the 1976 oncodazole research had been known, these expert reviewers would have immediately flagged the 2002 paper's multiple claims of originality as false. They didn't.
3. The *Entire Cancer Community* Didn't Know about Oncodazole. After publication, thousands of the world's top cancer researchers would have read the 2002 paper claiming that the antiparasitic mebendazole was also a novel anticancer agent. Not one of them stood up and said, "Wait a minute, this isn't new! These anticancer qualities were already proven in 1976 with another antiparasitic drug called oncodazole!"

The process of publishing a scientific paper is built on paranoid scholarship; scientists live in fear of being proven wrong. The fact that the authors, the expert reviewers, and the entire scientific community of expert readers all missed the 1976 oncodazole research points to an unavoidable conclusion: the knowledge of oncodazole, the antiparasitic with anticancer powers, had been deliberately and successfully buried.

A Crime Against Humanity

Why would anyone hide a cure for cancer? The answer, as it so often does, may come down to greed.

Imagine the excitement in that lab that discovered oncodazole in the early 1970s. They had discovered a safe, cheap, and effective cure for cancer. They did it! In their initial giddiness, they published their early work and gave the drug its telltale name: Oncodazole.

But that euphoria likely ended when someone with a calculator and no conscience realized the financial opportunity in what they had discovered. A cure is a one-time purchase. A treatment, especially a toxic one that requires other expensive drugs to manage its side effects, is a lifelong revenue stream. A patent on a drug lasts for only twenty years. After that, anyone can make a cheap, generic version, and the massive profits disappear.

But if the formula to make the drug is protected, not as a temporary patent, but as an eternal trade secret, like the developers of the formula for Coca-Cola did, it can be protected forever. The formula for Coke is not patented because that would require disclosure of the claim in the patent filing. The Coca-Cola formula is a trade secret and has been so since 1886, almost 140 years. It appears that's what happened to oncodazole as well. Treating oncodazole as a trade secret preserved its monetary value for almost fifty years—so far. Its immense, yet time-limited value as a cure was sacrificed for the far greater, longer-term, perhaps perpetual profits that its transformation into a cancer treatment could generate.

The Great Switcheroo: How the Cure Became a Poison

The plot gets even thicker. After oncodazole was buried and erased from the collective oncological awareness, its core mechanism—an antiparasitic drug that disrupts microtubules—appears to have been incorporated into or used to design subsequent cancer drugs. This pharmacological blueprint of fenbendazole (oncodazole) appears to have been used to understand and create some of the toxic, side-effect-ridden chemotherapy drugs that became the standard of care from the 1980s to today, like the taxanes (e.g., paclitaxel, docetaxel) and the vinca alkaloids (e.g., vincristine).[10, 11, 12]

But how was this not exposed until now? There was a classic switcheroo.

First, the smoking gun of the word oncodazole needed to be eliminated. Around 1984, just as the new toxic chemo drugs were being rolled out, the name "oncodazole" was quietly changed in the few remaining scientific contexts as references to "nocodazole" instead of oncodazole began to appear for no apparent reason (see Zimmerman, F. K., Mayer, V. W., & Scheel, I. [1984], for example).[13] This apparent meaningless name change from oncodazole to nocodazole in scientific papers helped erase oncodazole's original, obvious purpose. In fact, contemporary papers still refer to nocodazole as a microtubule inhibitor with promise that just didn't quite make it to the clinical trial stage.[14]

Second, the mechanism of the new toxic chemotherapy drugs was marketed as something entirely new even though it was not. The taxane drugs worked by stabilizing microtubules, locking them in place so the cell couldn't divide.[15] This was presented as a novel discovery in 1984 in an apparent attempt to disguise the fact that these drugs were likely based on oncodazole/fenbendazole's ability to destabilize and destroy those same microtubules. It was a half-truth. A dead cancer cell is a dead cancer cell. By advertising a specific cause of death, they ensured that's what other scientists would look for and find, distracting from the original, apparently superior mechanism attributed to oncodazole (fenbendazole).

The cover-up worked. Oncodazole faded into oblivion, and little pharma became Big Pharma apparently in part from the profits of these toxic, repurposed replacements of oncodazole/fenbendazole.

The Jig Is Up

So, how did we find the 1976 oncodazole paper if it was so effectively hidden from the world's top cancer experts in 2002?

In the 1970s and 1980s, scientific journals were only on paper. Hiding research could be as simple as tearing the pages out of the bound volumes in key medical libraries that scientists use, of which there is a limited number worldwide. But the architects of this cover-up could not have foreseen the internet. As old paper journals were digitized decades later, it is obvious they must have missed the one volume that ultimately was digitized. It only took one surviving copy of *Biochemical and Biophysical Research Communications* from 1976 to eventually be scanned and uploaded to the internet, to inadvertently expose the entire deception. Because the 1976 oncodazole paper is discoverable now, and apparently was not in 2002 as evidenced by its lack of citation by the 2002 article essentially replicating its effects as described in 1976, indicates that the article appeared, disappeared, and then reappeared as described.

The efforts to suppress oncodazole/fenbendazole as a cancer cure were effective for nearly fifty years. But that is over now.

It should now be clear:

- Fenbendazole, or oncodazole, a drug nearly identical to it, was known to be a cancer cure as far back as 1976, likely 1971 coincident with the development of fenbendazole.

- This knowledge and awareness of this cancer cure was actively suppressed.
- The mechanism of fenbendazole/oncodazole was likely pirated and repurposed to create the toxic, expensive, and far less effective chemotherapy drugs that have been the standard of care for many cancers for decades.
- This deception continues today, as many modern "miracle" drugs still rely on fenbendazole-like agents to do the heavy lifting.[16, 17]
- Since 1975, approximately 25,000,000 American citizens have died from cancer.[18] Hundreds of millions worldwide. Many of them suffered and died needlessly.
- The pain inflicted on families and loved ones is unimaginable.

Who have you lost to cancer since 1976?

I lost my mother, Agnes, in 2003 to cervical cancer, and my dad, Bill, in 2017 to renal cancer. I also lost my father-in-law, Philip, in 2020 to bladder cancer, and, later that same year, my good friend and neighbor George to glioblastoma.

Why Your Doctor Doesn't Know About Fenbendazole

Your doctor doesn't know about fenbendazole because they, too, were victims of this deception. They would have eagerly used fenbendazole to treat their patients, friends, and family—and themselves—had they known! The information was kept from the scientific and medical communities for generations. But it cannot be hidden any longer.

Timeline of the Cover-Up of Fenbendazole/Oncodazole as a Cancer Cure and Its Rediscovery

- **1971:** Fenbendazole is first synthesized.
- **1971–1974:** A drug based on fenbendazole is discovered to have potent anticancer properties.
- **1976:** This drug is named oncodazole, and its cancer-killing mechanism of microtubule disruption virtually identical to that of fenbendazole appears in a publication.
- **1976–1983:** Toxic chemo drugs based on microtubule disruption are developed and refined.

- **~1984:** The name oncodazole is changed to nocodazole for no apparent reason.
- **1984–2002:** Knowledge of oncodazole is effectively erased from the scientific mainstream, evidenced by the 2002 mebendazole paper claiming primacy.
- **2002:** Researchers at MD Anderson Cancer Center rediscover that mebendazole is a potent, nontoxic cancer-killing drug.
- **2009–2025:** Grassroots movements and a new wave of scientific interest bring fenbendazole back into the spotlight, confirming what was known regarding its anticancer actions dating back to 1976.

Note: Mukhopadhyay et al.'s (2002) research was conducted by University of Texas scientists in conjunction with a major cancer center, which may be surprising. A little background information on how some experiments are conceived, funded, and performed in most academic research facilities is useful. All experiments try to extend the existing knowledge base. Since public money is usually used to conduct the studies, the results are shared freely with others through publication in scientific journals. (Note: this is in contrast to private research institutions like pharmaceutical or medical device manufacturers that may elect to keep their discoveries proprietary.) New ideas usually are not fundable until pilot studies confirm those new ideas, which then justify financial support. Ideas are cheap, but results are expensive. Therefore, pilot studies are typically funded by in-house institutional money, "extra" funds from current extramurally funded projects or from "dark" money like a private investor or, in rare instances, the investigator's own pocket. This work-around solves the chicken-or-egg problem regarding ideas and funding. The sources of the money that fund published research is usually listed in the published works. Mukhopadhyay et al.'s (2002)1 funding for their mebendazole study came from several sources, most interestingly from tobacco settlement funds in the late 1990s divvied up by the Texas legislature and sent to various investigators. This source of dark money may partially explain how these investigators could get away with conducting this type of anticancer research right from inside MD Anderson Cancer Center.

At the risk of redundancy, it needs to be said again that fenbendazole and mebendazole kill cancer cells using multiple, complementary, and overlapping mechanisms including microtubule disruption, glucose uptake inhibition/angiogenesis, disruption of molecular mimicry, disruption of the tumor microenvironment, disabling P-glycoprotein efflux pumps, disabling p53 oncogene rescue, blocking migration, p38 MAPK intracellular destruction, mitotic catastrophe, and triggering apoptosis. This multifaceted attack unleashed on the cancer cell by fenbendazole and mebendazole is unrelenting, overpowering, and complete. Keep in mind the cancer cell only needs to be killed once. Fenbendazole and mebendazole actions on cancer cells are the very definition of overkill.

In contrast to the multimodal actions of fenbendazole, standard-of-care chemotherapy drugs appear to be single-action agents. They attack the cancer cell using one line of attack: microtubule stabilization. Because the cancer cell has multiple defense mechanisms, these drugs are easily defeated. The cancer cell adapts and the drugs are no longer effective. We'll discuss the advantages of multimodal fenbendazole as a cancer treatment vs. unimodal traditional chemotherapies in chapter 12.

So far, most of what we've covered has been the basic science explaining how fenbendazole kills cancer to showing how fenbendazole kills cancer in experimental animal models. That's all great. However, the burning question is: How effective is fenbendazole on cancer in humans? Before we get to those inspiring case reports we need to briefly cover one reason why the people in the case reports were able to survive and cure their cancers with fenbendazole when traditional treatments using standard-of-care drugs failed. That is because fenbendazole kills the cancer stem cells that are created by those traditional treatments.

CHAPTER 5

Cancer Stem Cells: How Fenbendazole Annihilates the Roots of Malignancy

The biggest challenge in fighting cancer isn't just shrinking tumors. It's destroying the treacherous cells that cause cancer to spread and come back: cancer stem cells.[1, 2] Standard treatments like chemotherapy, while able to shrink the main tumor, often fail to kill these stubborn cells. This leads to the cancer returning and, ultimately, the treatment failing.[3, 4] When they say "treatment failure," that means the patient dies.

However, a new understanding of these cancer stem cells, combined with drugs like fenbendazole and mebendazole, offers incredible hope.[5] These affordable and easy-to-get medications have shown a remarkable ability to destroy cancer stem cells and stop cancer from spreading, suggesting they can fundamentally change how we fight this disease.[6, 7] As you will read in the next chapter, many people who successfully treated their own cancer with fenbendazole had already gone through rounds of chemotherapy and radiation without success. Their cancers had likely transformed into a deadly, treatment-resistant stage driven by cancer stem cells. This chapter is essential to understanding how and why fenbendazole saved their lives when modern medicine failed and had given up.

The Cancer Stem Cell Threat: Architects of Death

Understand this: cancer is not one single disease. A tumor is a chaotic environment, constantly changing and evolving. This process naturally creates stronger, deadlier types of cancer cells.[8] This is like a Darwinian survival-of-the-fittest process inside the body, producing a dangerous mix of original cancer cells, treatment-resistant cells, and the most lethal of all: cancer stem cells.[9]

Tragically, conventional chemotherapy often makes this worse. It kills the weaker cancer cells but leaves the toughest ones behind, including cancer stem cells. This actually helps the most dangerous cells take over.[10] Cancer stem cells are unique because they have two deadly abilities: they can start new tumors, and they can spread throughout the body to create new colonies (metastasis).[11] These are the cells that travel to distant organs like the lungs, liver, and brain, forming new tumors that are immune to standard treatments. This is what leads to organ failure and death.[12] The complex, evolving tumors filled with cancer stem cells are responsible for the vast majority of cancer deaths.

Bluntly put, cancer stem cells are the cancer cells that kill us.

Most standard cancer treatments can be effective against the first wave of cancer cells.[13] But their greatest failing is that they are completely ineffective against cancer stem cells and the resistant clones they create. To make matters worse, until very recently, there were no drugs on the horizon that could specifically target and kill this deadly population of cells.

Enter Fenbendazole and Mebendazole: Destroying Cancer Stem Cell Strongholds

This gap in treatment creates a perfect opportunity for safe, proven drugs like fenbendazole and its close chemical cousin, mebendazole, to be repurposed to attack these resistant cancer stem cells. Groundbreaking research, again from Dr. Gregory Riggins's laboratory at Johns Hopkins University, provides clear proof that these drugs destroy cancer stem cells.

Triple-Negative Breast Cancer

Seminal studies using human breast cancer cells in mice show that mebendazole, at oral doses easily achievable in humans, completely wipes out breast cancer, including the notoriously aggressive triple-negative breast cancer (TNBC). Just as importantly, mebendazole treatment dramatically reduced or even eliminated the spread of these cancer cells to other organs. This is a monumental finding, given that breast cancer kills over 500,000 women worldwide every year, and it is the cancer stem cells that are doing the killing.[14]

Breast cancers are classified by whether they have receptors for hormones (estrogen [ER], progesterone [PR]) or a protein called HER2.[15] While there are targeted therapies for cancers with these receptors, TNBC has none of them (it is ER-, PR-, and HER2-). This makes it exceptionally difficult to treat and gives it a very poor prognosis. The prognosis is poor because of the limitations of existing standard-of-care drugs. TNBC is known for its aggression and its tendency to spread to the bones, brain, liver, and lungs, making it a perfect test for any new therapy designed to stop metastasis and kill cancer stem cells.[16]

A 2022 study by Joe et al. investigated mebendazole's effect on TNBC using models both in lab dishes and in live animals. Their findings were crystal clear: mebendazole didn't just prevent TNBC from starting, it wiped out existing TNBC tumors. Even more good news, it drastically reduced the spread of cancer to the lungs and completely blocked it from spreading to the liver. These experiments demonstrate that mebendazole prevents and destroys TNBC cells while also shutting down their ability to spread to new locations.

How does it do this? The researchers discovered that mebendazole dramatically reduces the expression of a protein called Integrin β4 (ITGβ4), which is a key marker found on cancer stem cells that helps them metastasize.[17] This is strong evidence that mebendazole directly attacks the metastatic process by targeting cancer stem cells.

The Multifaceted Mebendazole Assault on Triple-Negative Breast Cancer Stem Cells

The Joe et al. (2022) experiments prove that benzimidazoles like mebendazole (and by strong inference, fenbendazole) launch a multipronged attack against cancer stem cells by:

1. **Directly Killing Aggressive Cancer Cells:** Mebendazole powerfully kills TNBC cells at doses that are comparable to those used to treat parasites in humans—doses that are known to be safe.
2. **Stopping Cancer Cells from Moving:** Lab experiments show that mebendazole severely cripples the ability of TNBC cells to move, which is the first step in metastasis. The treated cancer cells could barely move or spread.
3. **Halting Cell Division and Forcing Cancer Cells to Self-Destruct:** Mebendazole stops TNBC cells from dividing (arresting them in the G2/M phase of the cell cycle) and forces them to undergo programmed cell death (apoptosis) within seventy-two hours. This is a direct attack on the cancer's ability to replicate and survive.
4. **Shrinking Tumors and Blocking Metastasis in Live Models:** In mouse models, oral doses of mebendazole dramatically shrank implanted human TNBC tumors. Most importantly, it significantly

reduced the spread to the lungs and prevented all spread to the liver. Giving the drug orally is key, as this is exactly how human patients would take it themselves.

5. **Targeting the Cancer Stem Cell "Signature":** Most importantly, researchers identified a specific mechanism for how mebendazole stops metastasis: by shutting down Integrin β4 (ITGβ4), a cellular marker for cancer stem cells. They found mebendazole decreases the ITGβ4 marker, which is known to be elevated on cancer stem cell populations. They also showed it reduced other cancer stem cell markers (CD44 and CD24). These findings show that mebendazole directly targets and disrupts the growth and spread of cancer stem cells. The ability to target ITGβ4 is particularly exciting, as this protein identifies a highly metastatic type of cancer cell that behaves like a stem cell.

In a powerful confirmation of these findings, another independent lab found that mebendazole also reduced the spread of TNBC cells to the brain.[18] Furthermore, research on other cancers, like the brain cancer glioblastoma, shows mebendazole can shut down other critical pathways that cancer stem cells need to survive, such as the Wnt and Hedgehog signaling pathways.[19, 20] This shows that mebendazole is a powerful anticancer stem cell agent that works against a variety of cancers through multiple, redundant mechanisms.

In a study examining different type of cancer another lab has found similar effects of fenbendazole killing cancer stem cells in animal models of ovarian cancer. They found a dual-targeting mechanism of fenbendazole where it not only kills the bulk of ovarian cancer cells but also specifically inhibits the growth and self-renewal of cancer stem cells.[21] Collectively, these experiments show that both fenbendazole and mebendazole are effective at killing cancer stem cells in a variety of cancers.

Glioblastoma: Mebendazole Is More Effective than the Standard-of-Care Drug

In 2017, De Witt et al. investigated repurposing mebendazole for treating deadly brain tumors, especially glioblastoma. A key focus of this research was on mebendazole's effect on brain cancer stem cells. These are the cells within the tumor responsible for starting it, fueling its growth, and making it resistant to chemotherapy and radiation. Targeting these brain cancer stem cells is absolutely essential to achieve a cure for glioblastoma patients.[22]

The study's experiments proved that mebendazole is a powerful weapon against this lethal cell population. They showed mebendazole could stop the growth of "neurospheres," which are balls of brain cancer stem cells grown in the lab—a direct indicator that it disrupts their ability to reproduce and spread. In live mouse models where human glioblastoma cells were implanted in the brain, mebendazole powerfully inhibited tumor growth and led to longer survival. Because these tumors are driven by brain cancer stem cells, the success of the drug is a strong indicator that it effectively targets this deadly stem cell population.[23]

Based on these incredible findings, De Witt and his colleagues argued for replacing the current standard-of-care drug, vincristine, with mebendazole. Their reasoning was simple and powerful:

- First, mebendazole was just as effective, if not more effective, than vincristine at killing glioblastoma cells.
- Second, mebendazole has a far better safety profile. Vincristine is known for causing severe side effects, including nerve damage. Mebendazole has been used safely for decades as an antiparasitic drug, even in children, with few, if any, side effects.
- Third, they found that mebendazole did cross the blood-brain barrier in their experiments, a critical requirement for any drug meant to treat brain cancer.

The authors concluded that mebendazole represents a safer, cheaper, and more effective alternative to vincristine for treating brain tumors. In light of our discussion regarding the likely genesis of some chemotherapy drugs as side-effect-ridden variants of fenbendazole analogues in the previous chapter, the irony is thickened by De Witt et al.'s (2017) request that mebendazole replace vincristine as the standard of care for glioblastoma.

Fenbendazole: The Readily Available, Functional Equivalent to Mebendazole

While much of this rigorous scientific research focuses on mebendazole, we cannot ignore the overwhelming success reported by people self-treating with fenbendazole, which is much easier to obtain (see chapter 6).[24] Given that the two drugs have nearly identical chemical structures and work in many of the same ways—by disrupting microtubules, the cell's internal skeleton—it is scientifically sound to conclude that fenbendazole has the same anticancer and anti–cancer stem cell powers.[25] The mountain of case report evidence for fenbendazole in the next chapter, combined with the hard scientific data for mebendazole, builds a compelling case.

Implications: Rethinking Cancer Treatment

The stunning findings from the Joe et al. (2022) and DeWitt et al. (2017) studies demolish old dogmas. The ability of mebendazole to destroy triple-negative breast cancer—a cancer defined by its lack of targets—suggests that it, or its analogue fenbendazole, should be immediately considered for any patient with TNBC. It should come as no surprise that the upcoming case reports from women who self-treated their TNBC with fenbendazole are resounding successes.

Furthermore, the powerful antimetastatic and cancer stem cell–killing effects documented in these studies raise urgent questions for doctors and patients. Shouldn't every newly diagnosed breast cancer, ovarian and glioblastoma patient, especially those with high-risk cancers like TNBC, be considered for immediate adjuvant therapy with safe and inexpensive mebendazole or fenbendazole? This would prevent the formation of tiny, hidden metastases and wipe out any remaining cancer stem cells. The evidence strongly suggests this approach demands immediate and serious consideration.

The fact that mebendazole also makes radiation therapy more effective against TNBC only strengthens the case for immediately integrating it into standard care.[26] The researchers in the Joe et al. study deliberately used mebendazole doses that match those used for treating parasites—the same doses (e.g., 222–888 mg/day) commonly used by people self-treating with fenbendazole. This confirms that these lab results can be translated to real-world use today. Their finding that the drug worked better for animals when taken with a high-fat meal (sesame oil) also aligns with studies showing this improves absorption, offering a practical tip for anyone using fenbendazole.[27]

Unleashing the Power of Fenbendazole Against Cancer's Deadly Root

The evidence is overwhelming: benzimidazoles, specifically mebendazole and fenbendazole, have a remarkable power to target and destroy cancer cells, including the elusive and deadly cancer stem cells that fuel recurrence and metastasis. They strike at the very root of the cancer, offering a real chance against cancers deemed "untreatable" by conventional medicine.

In a stunning irony, fenbendazole and mebendazole not only kill cancer cells but also destroy the very cancer stem cells that standard treatments can leave behind, or even create! Fenbendazole and mebendazole kill the cancer cells that kill people, and they also kill the cancer cells caused by the failures of traditional treatments. It is important to appreciate that fenbendazole kills cancer stem cells because it will help explain how the people who self-treated their cancers, as described in the next chapter, some of whose case reports were published in a peer-reviewed journal, were able to save themselves using fenbendazole when traditional medicine could not.

The path forward is clear and urgent. We must rapidly optimize the use of fenbendazole and mebendazole in oncology. We need to determine the best doses, delivery methods, and treatment combinations to maximize their power. We already possess agents that can fundamentally change the outcome of cancer by eliminating the very cells that make it so deadly. What we need now is the institutional courage and unwavering political will to turn this knowledge into lifesaving action for the millions of people with cancer who cannot afford to wait.

The basic scientists, whose work has been presented here, have done the heavy lifting regarding fenbendazole and cancer, and they deserve to see the fruits of that labor applied to eradicate cancer in humans. However, the medical establishment must not dillydally in this endeavor lest they be passive observers to this evolving modern medical miracle. Intrepid cancer patients, many of whom exhausted traditional treatments and were given up for dead by their doctors, have proceeded, based in large part on the overwhelming scientific evidence described above, and applied that knowledge to successfully self-treat their cancers with fenbendazole. Based on the overwhelming number of anticancer actions of fenbendazole described above, it should come as no surprise that these people have not only survived but thrived and have lived to tell their stories. Rather than our reading of their fighting a courageous battle against cancer in their obituaries, we will read their heartfelt, transformational stories of how they defeated their cancers by self-treating with fenbendazole. Their courageous, inspiring, and actionable experiences are genuine acts of generosity, caring, and love for people they've never met who may be facing the same dire situation they once were.

Next, we will present the incredible case reports from those who did not wait. These were terminally ill cancer patients who decided to self-treat their cancers with safe, inexpensive, and readily available fenbendazole. Many of them had already exhausted all standard-of-care options and were told to get their affairs in order. They were likely in the grip of lethal cancer stem cells, likely made worse by the very standard of care cancer treatments they had received. Fortunately, they knew that fenbendazole was highly likely to cure their cancers. They were right!

CHAPTER 6

Demonstrating Fenbendazole's Power as a Cancer Treatment through Human Case Reports

The study of fenbendazole as an anticancer agent now shifts from its biochemical mechanisms and preclinical animal data to the most important evidence: human case reports. These reports from individuals self-treating their cancer are important for understanding the medication's real-world potential and justifying further research. We may be past needing clinical trials for simple proof of concept; instead, future trials should focus on optimizing fenbendazole treatment by determining ideal dosing, improving bioavailability, and exploring synergistic combinations, all while using a revamped process that facilitates rather than hinders its integration into mainstream care.

The Power of Case Reports in Medicine

Case reports are a cornerstone of medical progress, providing real-world evidence that identifies novel outcomes, sparks hypotheses, and guides future research. Their power is proven by history: the first description of AIDS emerged from a 1981 case report, and the recognition of thalidomide's devastating effects stemmed from case observations.[1, 2] These examples show how case reports are often the first to identify new diseases or cures.

Case reports are also indispensable educational tools. They provide patient-centered narratives that can quickly disseminate novel clinical information, such as rare adverse drug reactions, long before larger studies are completed.[3] While sometimes criticized for lacking the rigor of controlled trials, the unique strength of case reports is hypothesis generation. They do not necessarily prove causality but demand it be investigated, as when fenbendazole use is followed by cancer remission in these case reports here. A well-known example of this process is the experiment by Barry Marshall on himself where he discovered that *H. pylori* bacteria was a cause of stomach cancer.[4]

The following case reports are from the Substack publication *Fenbendazole Can Cure Cancer*, which was started shortly after my mother-in-law eradicated her terminal cancer within a few months with fenbendazole. These case reports were submitted by the individual affected by cancer or by a loved one that assisted them with their treatments. As you'll see, the range of cancers that fenbendazole eradicates is broad and varied. Each case report was initially submitted as an email and then follow-up questions were answered to the best of the respondent's memory and ability. Except in several instances, the author was not a medical professional.

The case reports presented here were selected based on their detail and relative completeness. They are but a handful of the hundreds of additional case reports, from all corners of the world—all documenting success in eradicating cancer—submitted that did not rise to a standard of completeness for publication. Some of those "incomplete" case reports are available on the *Fenbendazole Can Cure Cancer* Substack for reference.

A further note regarding how case report material is submitted and prepared. We receive comments or emails that usually start out with something to the effect of "Hey, it worked for me!" Some initial contacts can have more detail but most don't. From there, we ask for more details in a follow-up, and if the person responds and it seems like an interesting case, we will ask if they'd like to help prepare an anonymous case report of their experiences for publication on the Substack. This can take the form of back-and-forth emails or a phone interview in some instances. Keep in mind that the people submitting this information have just come through a hellish time and they may not have kept detailed records or remember everything to the extent and detail that we would all ideally like to know. With those limitations and caveats, we feel that the case reports we have compiled are excellent in their level of detail and heartfelt effort expended by the former cancer patient in an effort to help others who might benefit from their experiences. Finally, the following case reports have been edited for brevity and relevance. All of the original content, including potentially lifesaving comments from readers on each case report, are available on the *Fenbendazole Can Cure Cancer* Substack, https://fenbendazole.substack.com.

Collectively, all of these case reports appear to rise to a new status, something similar to a community trial. These intrepid people, who chose to self-treat their cancers with fenbendazole, are absolute heroes to the rest of us, as they have paved the way and bridged the gap between basic science and clinical application, giving us the confidence to state that fenbendazole can cure cancer.

Joe Tippens: The First Case Report of Fenbendazole Curing Cancer

Before we dive into new case reports we need a little history lesson. A quick internet search finds the case report of a man named Joe Tippens, who in 2017 eradicated his incurable metastatic lung cancer with fenbendazole, after he was given up for dead by the medical community (this situation—being given up for dead because traditional medicine failed— turns out to be a quite common experience among the human cases reported next). While there may be other unknown "Joe Tippens" out there who predate the person we're referencing now, we are confident in designating Joe Tippens as the father of the practical application of fenbendazole to treat human cancers. He is, at a minimum, the first person we could find who documented his experiences with fenbendazole. A better way to say it is that Joe Tippens is a true hero to those who have self-treated their cancers and subsequently saved themselves and loved ones with fenbendazole.

The story of Joe Tippens is a must-know for those interested in the power of repurposed drugs. Joe was diagnosed with incurable, advanced small cell lung cancer and was given a 1 percent chance of survival and three or so months to live. Joe was interviewed by Dr. David Williams in 2019 for his *Alternatives for the Health Conscious Individual* newsletter.[5] Here is that interview:

> In the fall of 2016, Joe was leaving the US to start a new job in Zurich, Switzerland. Two days prior to his flight, he was experiencing what he thought was simple congestion. He stopped at a neighborhood clinic for a prescription. However, a routine chest X-ray revealed a mass in his left lung the size of a fist. This led to a diagnosis of small-cell lung cancer and within a few days, the start of intensive chemo and radiation therapy at MD Anderson. As Joe put it, "The radiation turned my esophagus into fried bacon." He couldn't eat or swallow anything. Rather than agree to a feeding tube, he decided to "live off his fat stores" and use an IV to keep his body hydrated. After eight weeks, his weight dropped from 200 pounds to 105.
>
> After completing chemo and radiation in January 2017, Joe was scheduled for another PET scan. It revealed the therapies had indeed stopped the growth in his left lung. But it also showed that the cancer had spread to his neck, right lung, stomach, liver, bladder, pancreas, and tailbone. In his words, "The PET scan lit up like a Christmas tree."

As I mentioned, the odds of curing small-cell lung cancer aren't good to begin with, and when it has spread to that many locations, it is considered incurable . . . less than one percent cure rate with an average life expectancy of three months. That's when doctors told Joe they wanted to put him in clinical trial—not one that would save his life, but one that might extend it by a year or so. He obviously agreed.

Many of these types of cancer studies are not designed to test for a possible cure, but rather to see if a drug can either improve quality of life during a patient's last days or possibly extend remaining time. Typically, these studies are only approved for patients whose cases are considered hopeless and there's nothing more that can be done. In Joe's case, this was one of those studies.

With little hope left, Joe returned home to Oklahoma. Two days later, he contacted his friend, a large animal veterinarian, who had posted a story online about a scientist working for Merck pharmaceuticals in the veterinary division.

The scientist happened to be testing the effects of their existing products on mice that had various cancers. That's when she discovered that one of their dog products (a dewormer) was 100 percent effective. This same scientist had stage 4 brain cancer and, like Joe, was also given three months to live. She started taking the dog dewormer and six weeks later, she was clear of the cancer.

On January 15, 2017, without informing the oncologists at MD Anderson, Joe started taking the same dewormer while continuing on the experimental drug.

Every quarter since he began this treatment, Joe goes to MD Anderson for a PET scan. May 2017 was three months after having the PET scan that lit up like a Christmas tree, with cancer from "head to tail." The May scan came back all clear. There was no sign of residual tumors, no recurrent tumors, and no signs of metastasis. The oncologists were totally mystified. Joe suspected it was the dewormer but decided that it wasn't the right time to tell them. At that point, he couldn't be 100 percent certain whether it was the dewormer working or the clinical trial drug they were giving him. He certainly didn't want them to take him off the trial drug if it was responsible for clearing the tumors. The clinical trial ended in September 2017, and he was scheduled for another PET scan. That scan was also all clear, without any sign of cancer.

> Since the clinical trial had ended and getting kicked off was no longer a concern, he decided it was time to come clean and tell the oncologists about using the dewormer. But before telling them, he wanted to know how many people were in the same clinical trial as he was, and how many of them had responded positively to the experimental drug. He was told 1,100 patients were in the same trial and taking the exact same medication as Joe. However, Joe was the only person whose cancer had gone into remission. It obviously wasn't a result of the experimental drug. That's when Joe told them about taking the dewormer. They were shocked. But their reply was even more shocking. Here is their conversation with Joe, as he relayed it to me: "We've known for decades that the anthelmintic class of drugs could have possible efficacy against cancer. In fact in the 1980s and 1990s there was an anthelmintic drug called Levamisole that was used on colon cancer." Joe said, "Doc, if you have known for decades, why hasn't more research been done on it?" He replied, "Probably because of money. All of these drugs are far off patent and nobody is going to spend a gazillion dollars to repurpose them for cancer, only to have generic competition the next day."

With Joe Tippens's story as a starting point, the stage is set to venture into other examples of the power of fenbendazole to cure cancer without any adverse side effects.

The first case report (Metastatic Breast Cancer) is of my mother-in-law. Her courage and determination to try an approach that was nontraditional was the seminal act that led to further connecting the dots regarding the science and discoveries on fenbendazole and cancer and uncovering and documenting how truly effective it was in eradicating the cancers of many others similarly affected. The following case report of her experiences is the genesis of the idea that fenbendazole can cure cancer, while the following more than twenty case reports compellingly reinforced, extended, and confirmed that idea.

CASE REPORT 1: METASTATIC BREAST CANCER, AGE EIGHTY-THREE

Remission of Stage 4 Metastatic Breast Cancer Following Fenbendazole Administration after Refusing All Traditional Treatment

On October 30, 2021, an eighty-three-year-old female, RGR, went to the emergency room with symptoms subsequently identified as an intestinal obstruction. During the diagnostic workup, positron emission tomography (PET) scans and blood tests confirmed the presence of metastatic breast cancer. Tumors were identified in the lungs, liver, and bones (spine, ribs, pelvis). She had a history of estrogen-dependent breast cancer diagnosed eleven years prior, which had been treated with surgery and adjuvant therapy, resulting in remission. Annual follow-ups at Moffitt Cancer Center had previously indicated no recurrence, with an "all-clear" report issued most recently in 2019.

Hospital Course and Initial Management

My mother-in-law was hospitalized for approximately three weeks, including one week in the intensive care unit (ICU), for management of the intestinal obstruction. Treatment included nasogastric tube decompression, and oral intake was prohibited. Intravenous fluids were administered with restricted glucose content due to the metastatic cancer diagnosis. The obstruction resolved without surgical intervention, though surgery had been considered high-risk by the gastroenterology team. RGR's condition significantly deteriorated during hospitalization, necessitating the administration of last rites. Following stabilization and resolution of the obstruction, she requested discharge. The oncology team offered a palliative approach, stating that the cancer was incurable but treatment might extend life for an indeterminate duration. She declined all conventional oncological treatments, including chemotherapy and radiation, and was discharged home with hospice care. At discharge, she was significantly weakened, requiring a walker and in-home assistance.

Alternative Therapy Initiation: Fenbendazole

Following discharge, RGR commenced treatment with fenbendazole, an over-the-counter benzimidazole anthelmintic agent, on November 22, 2021. Her immediate family was presented with the rationale for considering fenbendazole based on anecdotal reports and preclinical studies suggesting potential anticancer activity. As presented earlier, fenbendazole is reported to exert anticancer effects through several mechanisms, including disruption of microtubule polymerization, interference with glucose metabolism, and upregulation of the p53 tumor suppressor gene. Studies suggest it selectively targets cancer cells. Fenbendazole has demonstrated cytotoxic effects against human cancer cell lines in vitro and in vivo. Prior to administration, close family members ingested fenbendazole for three days to assess tolerability, reporting no adverse effects. RGR initiated fenbendazole at a dose of 222 mg orally once daily, mixed with yogurt administered by her husband. A copy of the letter justifying trying fenbendazole that I sent to her children, my in-laws, is on the Substack https://fenbendazole.substack.com

Clinical Course and Monitoring

Within two weeks of initiating fenbendazole, notable improvements in RGR's strength, appetite, and overall appearance were observed. After four weeks, hospice care was discontinued as she regained functional independence, including ambulation without assistance, and began to gain weight.

On December 28, 2021, RGR consulted with an oncologist. While continuing to refuse systemic chemotherapy or primary radiation, she consented to receive intramuscular injections of fulvestrant, an estrogen receptor antagonist. Fulvestrant limits the growth of estrogen-dependent tumors but is not typically considered curative or directly responsible for rapid tumor marker decline. She continued daily fenbendazole concurrently.

On January 10, 2022, RGR received targeted palliative radiation therapy to two metastatic lesions in the spine causing significant pain. Pain relief was achieved rapidly, within days. Subsequently, the treating radiologist noted an unusually rapid response to radiation, consistent with reports suggesting fenbendazole may potentiate conventional therapies.

Tumor marker CA 27.29, specific for metastatic breast cancer, was monitored. The initial level on November 22, 2021 (near discharge), was 316 U/mL (normal <38 U/mL). On January 20, 2022, the level had decreased to 131 U/mL. A follow-up PET scan on April 20, 2022, confirmed the absence of abnormal metabolic activity indicative of active cancer, corroborating the declining tumor marker trend and observed clinical improvement.

Subsequent CA 27.29 levels continued to decline:

- May 4, 2022: 47 U/mL (PET scan confirmed no evidence of disease)
- July 20, 2022: 37 U/mL (normal range)

There were no reported adverse side effects attributable to fenbendazole throughout the treatment period.

Treatment Adjustments and Long-Term Follow-Up

Daily fenbendazole (222 mg) was discontinued on July 28, 2022, after eight months of continuous use. Coincident with fulvestrant administration, transient elevations in liver enzymes (ALT and AST) were noted; these normalized by August 20, 2022.

Subsequent CA 27.29 levels remained within or near the normal range for the next eight months:

- August 20, 2022: 33.3 U/mL
- September 21, 2022: 30 U/mL
- December 4, 2022: 29.9 U/mL (fenbendazole restarted, dosed every other day)
- January 4, 2023: 27.9 U/mL (fenbendazole increased to daily)
- February 1, 2023: 27.5 U/mL (fenbendazole reduced to three times weekly)
- February 27, 2023: 26.8 U/mL (fenbendazole continued three times weekly)

By June 2023, she was no longer receiving active cancer treatment and transitioned to surveillance monitoring every three to six months. There were no abnormalities in her blood work. Fulvestrant injections were discontinued due to reported discomfort.

A CT scan of the chest, abdomen, and pelvis performed on January 22, 2025, revealed no evidence of recurrent disease.

Outcome

My mother-in-law, now eighty-seven years old and over four years post-diagnosis of widely metastatic stage 4 breast cancer, remains in complete remission with no evidence of disease confirmed by diagnostic serial imaging. This outcome was achieved after declining standard chemotherapy and radiation and utilizing daily fenbendazole for eight months, alongside palliative targeted radiation to spinal lesions and concurrent fulvestrant injections (later discontinued). Complete remission was achieved within several months of daily fenbendazole treatment (222 mg per day). She experienced no side effects attributed to fenbendazole. She continues periodic monitoring and continues to take fenbendazole daily.

Summary

An eighty-three-year-old female with biopsy-proven stage 4 metastatic breast cancer involving multiple organs and bones declined conventional systemic therapy. RGR initiated treatment with oral fenbendazole 222 mg daily in yogurt. Concurrent therapies included fulvestrant injections and targeted palliative radiation to two spinal lesions. Complete clinical, biochemical (CA 27.29 normalization), and radiological (PET/CT) remission was achieved and maintained.

Fenbendazole administration was well-tolerated without any reported adverse effects. The transient elevation in AST/ALT in July 2022 were either due to fulvestrant or an interaction between fenbendazole and fulvestrant. Fenbendazole alone did not result in any liver enzyme fluctuations. She continues to take fenbendazole. She is fortunate to have an oncologist who is encouraging her to "keep doing what you're doing" and will provide periodic diagnostic tests to monitor her condition. FYI, the fulvestrant injections caused much discomfort and would probably be avoided in the future. Fulvestrant is not associated with dramatic remissive outcomes like this and was very unlikely to have played a significant role (personal communication, oncologist). This case highlights an unexpected complete and total remission associated with the use of fenbendazole in advanced malignancy.

Note: RGR's case report was published in the peer-reviewed journal *Case Reports in Oncology* by Makis, M., Baghli, I. & Martinez, P. (2025). Fenbendazole as an Anticancer Agent? A Case Series of Self-Administration in Three Patients. *Case Reports in Oncology*, 18 (1), 856–863. https://doi.org/10.1159/000546362.[6]

CASE REPORT 2: BRAF-POSITIVE MALIGNANT MELANOMA, STAGE 4, AGE SIXTY-THREE, MALE

Conquering BRAF+ Melanoma: The Power of Fenbendazole

According to Johns Hopkins Medicine, BRAF is a gene found on chromosome seven that encodes a protein also called BRAF. This protein plays a role in cell growth by sending signals inside the cell that promote, among other functions, cell division. When there is a mutation in the BRAF gene, it creates an abnormal protein that sends erroneous signals that lead to uncontrolled cell growth and cancer. When a person has BRAF-positive melanoma, it means their cancer may grow more aggressively. In 40–50 percent of the patients with advanced melanoma, BRAF gene mutations are present. Interestingly, the BRAF gene mutation is most likely not inherited, which means that an environmental factor probably led to the mutation.

The following case report is from a sixty-three-year-old man, JF, who was initially diagnosed with BRAF-positive malignant melanoma in 2020. Chemotherapy put him into remission but the cancer came back in 2023, which is when he tried a different approach using fenbendazole. This case report is in JF's own words.

> In July 2020 I had noticed a growth on my hip. It was biopsied and was determined to be a BRAF mutation-positive melanoma which had spread to some of my lymph nodes. My oncologist recommended chemotherapy, tafinlar, which I took for a year and it worked as I was put into remission.
>
> Fast-forward to late August 2023: I had a PET scan that showed that the cancer had returned with metastases to my lower abdomen, back next to my spine, leg, and four tumors in my ureter. I had follow-up biopsies that confirmed that the DNA in the tumors were the BRAF-positive melanoma cells that had returned and had spread.
>
> In December 2023 the tumors had disrupted my ureter, causing problems with urination, so I had surgery to remove that tumor. My oncologist wanted me to hold off on scheduled immunotherapy treatments with Opdivo (nivolumab) until I had recovered from the effects of the surgery. My oncologist also stated that nivolumab was by no means a cure of any kind but that it might give me some more time.
>
> A few days later my wife heard about fenbendazole and the *Fenbendazole Can Cure Cancer* Substack through a friend of a friend.

I was able to track that person down and he was kind enough to speak with me. He was very encouraging and, because my doctor said that immunotherapy was no cure and I had a traditional treatment-free window ahead of me while recovering, so while I was skeptical of fenbendazole there was really no reason not to give fenbendazole a shot.

I started taking fenbendazole 222 mg once or twice per day around mid-December 2023. As you can see from the graph of the blood tumor markers (which measures the amount of the tumor's DNA in the blood) for my cancer, that before I started any fenbendazole treatments, that on November 29 it was 123.37. Less than seven weeks later, on January 17, 2024, it had dropped to 0.38 and about a month later on February 21, 2024 it was 0, zero!

In that time period I did have two immunotherapy treatments but those are not the likely cause of my cancer disappearing for two reasons. First, my oncologist said immunotherapy wouldn't cure me, just give me more time, maybe. And, two, last week when my oncologist came in to the room to tell me about the February 21 blood test she said "I don't know how to tell you this but there is no evidence of cancer. Nothing. This just doesn't happen after only two treatments." Of course she knows nothing about fenben because I didn't tell her I was taking it.

—JF, Ozark, Missouri, March 7, 2024

Q: How old are you? Weight? How do you feel?
A: Sixty-three years old, 232 pounds when this started. About 170 pounds now and gaining my weight back, which is good. I feel wonderful!
Q: What brand of fenbendazole were you taking? And how many times per day? Any side effects?
A: It is TheLife brand of fenbendazole, and my wife bought it on Amazon. I took 222 mg once or twice a day. There were no side effects from the fenben. FYI I saw the health insurance bill for the immunotherapy drug, Opdivo, it was $72,000. My wife spent $60 on the fenbendazole, which is what worked!
Q: Are you still taking fenbendazole?
A: Yes. I take 222 mg once per day.

Doing really well. Gained my weight back, working out daily, walking. No issues. Still take fenbendazole daily (222 mg). I'm talking to everyone and anyone that will listen regarding fenbendazole. I can't tell you how many people I have shared this with, 60–70 at least. I appreciate you and everything you are doing to help me and others. I will share this until the end! —JF, May 3, 2025.

Summary

Congratulations to JF for taking matters into his own hands and having a tremendous outcome. We wish him the best going forward and are greatly appreciative of his sharing his experiences so that others faced with similar circumstances may benefit.

BRAF mutations are not restricted to melanomas alone. Again, according to Johns Hopkins, the cancers associated with the BRAF gene mutation are not specific to one part of the body or a certain cell type and include hairy cell leukemias, non-Hodgkin's lymphomas, thyroid cancer, ovarian cancer, lung adenocarcinoma, colorectal cancer, and certain brain cancers, including glioblastoma, pilocytic astrocytoma, and pediatric low-grade glioma.

In this case report, a very aggressive BRAF-positive variant of melanoma appears to have been completely eradicated by fenbendazole. This report is yet another example of fenbendazole eradicating purported "aggressive" forms of untreatable cancers, including triple-negative breast cancers, as we've previously detailed in prior case reports. These results in humans should not be surprising given the wealth of preclinical animal data on fenbendazole and mebendazole presented earlier. In fact, the only surprise is related to the dismal outcomes of traditional treatments compared to those observed with fenbendazole.

JF's remission was rapid. Roughly 2.5 months after starting fenbendazole, his blood tumor markers went from 123 to 0.38 to 0. He remains cancer-free.

Because JF did receive another treatment, there could be alternative explanations for his tremendous outcome. First, JF did receive two doses of immunotherapy (nivolumab). It is a possibility that that protocol was effective for him in eradicating his BRAF-positive melanoma. Unique individual differences aside, such an outcome would be highly unlikely given the published data on nivolumab as well as JF's oncologist's expectations and surprise at his complete remission.

Second, it is possible that there was an interaction between the two doses of nivolumab, and fenbendazole resulting in a synergistic effect that eradicated the cancer. If this is what happened it is a major discovery, supported by the preclinical data, to be further investigated.

Third, fenbendazole alone was the effective anticancer agent that eradicated the BRAF-positive melanoma cells. Based on the references previously cited throughout this book examining fenbendazole/mebendazole's role in cancer treatment, fenbendazole is both necessary and sufficient to achieve the results in experimental preclinical models of cancer that JF obtained in his own self-treatment cancer clinical trial.

Finally, according to Johns Hopkins again, the BRAF gene mutation is most likely caused by an environmental factor that led to the mutation, presuming that the factor responsible for the mutation can be eliminated or avoided, the possibility of a true "one-and-done" cure for BRAF-positive cancers using fenbendazole, or a synergistic combination, may be at hand.

Note: JF's case report was published in the peer-reviewed journal *Case Reports in Oncology*, Makis, M., Baghli, I. & Martinez, P. (2025). "Fenbendazole as an Anticancer Agent? A Case Series of Self-Administration in Three Patients." *Case Reports in Oncology*, 18 (1), 856–863. https://doi.org/10.1159/000546362.[7]

CASE REPORT 3: METASTATIC PROSTATE CANCER, AGE SEVENTY-FIVE.

Near-Complete Regression of Metastatic Prostate Cancer Following Multimodal Therapy Including Fenbendazole: Possible Synergistic Effect of Fenbendazole with Traditional ADT

This report details the experiences of a seventy-five-year-old, 205-pound man (BK) diagnosed with recurrent, metastatic prostate cancer (stage 4) approximately ten years after initial surgical treatment for localized disease. His initial postoperative prostate-specific antigen (PSA) level remained undetectable (<0.01 ng/mL) for eighteen months post-surgery before beginning a slow but steady rise, signaling biochemical recurrence.

In December 2021, BK was formally diagnosed with stage 4 metastatic prostate cancer. At this time, his PSA level was 6 ng/mL.

Imaging confirmed widespread metastatic disease. A computed tomography (CT) scan in December 2021 revealed prominent left periaortic lymph nodes (representative node 0.8 cm, noted as new) and multiple sclerotic densities in the lumbar spine, sacrum, and pelvis, consistent with osseous metastases.

Bone scan (December 2021): Showed "intense radiotracer uptake" in the right T12 vertebral body/pedicle (correlating with CT sclerosis) and the right humeral head, highly suspicious for metastatic disease.

Treatment Course

In December 2021, BK commenced standard-of-care androgen deprivation therapy (ADT) and bone health management[3]: Orgovyx (relugolix), Erleada (apalutamide), and Xgeva (denosumab).

Concurrently, BK initiated and maintained a self-directed adjunctive regimen comprising repurposed drugs and supplements, many used intermittently since his initial diagnosis:

Vitamins/Minerals: Vitamin D3 (5,000–10,000 IU/day, adjusted per lab results), vitamin K complex (K1 1500 mcg, K2-MK4 1000 mcg, K2-MK7 100 mcg), magnesium (400 mg/day), boron (3 mg/day).

Supplements: Melatonin (increased from 1–3 mg/night pre-metastasis to 10–40 mg/night post-diagnosis), berberine (500 mg TID with meals), high-absorption curcumin with BioPerine, artemisinin (400 mg/day), low-dose lithium (5 mg/day), and liposomal vitamin C (intermittently).

Repurposed Drugs: Cimetidine (400–800 mg/night, sometimes alternated with omeprazole), loratadine (10 mg/day).

Approximately October–November 2023 (around twenty-two to twenty-three months after starting ADT), BK added fenbendazole to this regimen. Fenbendazole dosing: Initially 444 mg/day (222 mg BID), taken daily for approximately two or three months leading up to the January 2024 scans. Subsequently reduced to 222–300 mg once daily, most days.

Outcomes and Follow-up

- PSA Response: Within thirty days of initiating ADT and the adjunctive regimen (by January 2022), BK's PSA dropped from 6 ng/mL to undetectable levels (<0.05 ng/mL). This undetectable status was maintained for over two years (as of early 2024).
- One-Year Follow-up Imaging (December 2022):
  Bone Scan: Uptake in the right T12 pedicle was described as "subtle" (previously "intense"). Uptake in the proximal right humerus was "less conspicuous than on prior study".
  CT Scan: No problematic lymph nodes mentioned. Described as "Stable bony metastatic disease" involving lower thoracic spine, lumbar spine, and bony pelvis (sacrum no longer mentioned)
- Two-Year Follow-up Imaging (January 2024):
  Bone Scan: Showed a "prominent decrease" in uptake at the right T12 vertebral body focus. The right humerus lesion was no longer mentioned. No new uptake was visualized.
  CT Scan: No pathologically enlarged lymph nodes noted. Scattered osseous sclerotic foci were described as "similar to prior CT scan dated 12/2/2022" and "likely representing prior metastatic disease." Impression: Unchanged osseous sclerotic lesions; no significant interval change.
- PSMA PET/CT Scan (September 2024): The vast majority of previously noted sclerotic bone lesions showed no abnormal radiopharmaceutical accumulation. A single focus in the cervicothoracic spine demonstrated low-level uptake (SUV max 5.0), interpreted as equivocal (potentially inflammatory/arthritic vs. low-level metastatic). No abnormal uptake was seen in lymph nodes or soft tissues.

Side Effects: BK reported significant side effects consistent with ADT (e.g., fatigue). No adverse effects were specifically attributed to fenbendazole. Liver function tests remained within normal limits, even slightly low, throughout the treatment period, including after the addition of fenbendazole. There were no side effects attributable to fenbendazole.

This case report illustrates a significant and sustained response to fenbendazole and other treatments in a seventy-five-year-old male with recurrent, widespread metastatic prostate cancer. BK achieved a rapid PSA decline to undetectable levels within thirty days of starting treatment, maintained for over two years, alongside progressive radiographic regression of metastatic disease over the same period, culminating in a near-complete metabolic response on the most recent PSMA PET/CT imaging.

BK's therapeutic regimen was complex, combining standard ADT (relugolix, apalutamide) and a bone-protective agent (denosumab) with an extensive, patient-directed protocol of supplements and repurposed drugs. Fenbendazole was introduced approximately twenty-two or twenty-three months into this multimodal treatment. While continued radiographic improvement was noted on scans performed two or three months after starting fenbendazole, it is impossible to definitively isolate the contribution of fenbendazole from the ongoing effects of ADT and the numerous other adjunctive agents, however see Q&A at end for BK's ideas on what actually worked and why. On another note, the addition of fenbendazole may have had synergistic potentiating effects on the actions of the ADT treatments, or vice versa, leading to the observed near-complete remission.

The residual sclerotic lesions seen on CT, described as "likely representing prior metastatic disease," coupled with the lack of significant uptake on bone scan and PSMA PET/CT, may indicate treated, metabolically inactive disease or bone remodeling, see chapter 11 for discussion of bone remodeling, bone flare, and cancer. The low SUV max (5.0) of the single equivocal focus on PSMA PET/CT further supports minimal active malignancy. The phenomenon of "bone flare" or active bone remodeling after treatment can sometimes mimic active disease, although this is less likely with low PSMA uptake.

While the specific contribution of fenbendazole cannot be quantified in this particular case, the overall positive outcome in the context of multimodal therapy, including repurposed agents, is noteworthy. The case furthermore suggests interesting potential synergistic effects with traditional treatments and highlights BK's proactive approach, achieving a durable response beyond initial expectations.

Importantly, BK experienced no detectable toxicity, particularly hepatotoxicity, attributable to fenbendazole, despite concurrent use of multiple agents.

Follow-up questions and answers from BK:

Q: How much fenbendazole were you taking? And how many times per day?
A: Honestly, I have been all over the place. As a retired anesthesia provider (CRNA), I have thirty-six years of thinking in terms of mg/kg for every med that I ever pushed into an IV. Since I weigh a bit over 200 pounds, and Joe Tippens (at 105–115 pounds) used 222 mg per day, three days on/four off, I started with 222 mg twice a day, for a total of 444 mg/day. But, I did seven days a week, except when I would forget or it was inconvenient. I was trying to have this much fenbendazole added to my normal repurposed drug/supplement cocktail for at least a month before my two-year scans (two years since stage 4 diagnosis) which were due about last Thanksgiving. The scans got delayed until this last January. So, I had more like three or four months of FenBen in me by the time of my scans and my next PSA. More recently, I have reduced to between 222 mg and 300 mg once per day, most days.
Q: Did you notice any side effects that might be attributable to the fenbendazole?
A: Zero so far. My liver enzymes (measured every three months) are actually on the low side, and did not increase even 1 percent—some may have even decreased a bit- since starting FenBen. I have plenty of drug side effects, but they were all present long before I started FenBen due to the two prescription drugs I am still on, Orgovix and Erleada, which wipe out my testosterone. Which sort of wipes me out. If I ever get to 100 percent NED—rather than the 95 percent or so per my last scans—I'm really going to push my docs to get me off of these drugs, which they want me on for life. But FenBen did not add anything to their unwanted side effects. But unless my PSA begins to increase—it has been undetectable for over two years—I probably won't have any more scans until a year passes.
Q: You mentioned you were taking other supplements?
A: I do remember, surprisingly, because the list is long. I have been taking many of the supplements from the time of my original stage 3 diagnosis and surgery ten years ago, or even before: [NL]
1: Vitamin D 5K to 10K per day (depending on lab results) with Life Extension K2 M4 1000 mcg, K2 M7 100 mcg and K1 1500 mcg/day.

Magnesium 400 mg/day, boron 3 mg/day. (Mainly for bone health and antiviral and general health, but also for possible anticancer). Mainly, trying to reduce the chance of the anti-testosterone drugs they are giving me from thinning my bones. Along with their prescription drug Xgeva, seems to be working.
2: Low-dose lithium supplement 5 mg/day(for brain health, but lately has also shown some anticancer traits).
3: Melatonin 1 to 3 mg per night X 20+ years, but raised to 10 to 40 mg per night once I got my stage 4 diagnosis.
4: The following were started a month or so before my stage 4 diagnosis 2 years and 3 months ago:

Artemisinin 400 mg per day
Loratidine 10 mg per day
Cimetidine 400 to 800 mg per night, sometimes alternated with omeprazole (both anti-heartburn drugs that have shown strong anticancer effects)
Berberine 500 mg per meal (as a "natural" substitute for prescription Metformin)
High-absorption curcumin (with BioPerine).
Berberine and curcumin I had taken on and off before and after the first cancer diagnoses in Nov 2013. But I got more consistent with them after my relapse/stage 4 diagnosis.
Sometimes, Liposomal vitamin C, particularly when concerned about viruses

I really wanted to take thymoquinone/black seed, but it was so nasty I just took it for a few days.

Most recently, starting about five months ago, I added fenbendazole to the above. I got in a couple of months use before my last (the two-year) scans, which had very much improved from the already much improved one-year scans.

Since my stage 4 diagnoses two years, three months ago, I have been on the prescription drugs Orgovix, Erleada, and Xgeva. I very much hope to get off of these expensive, side-effect-riddled drugs.

Q: That's a lot. What do you think was the most important in your experience?

A: I think all of my drug/supplement cocktails have helped, but I have a feeling that the fenbendazole has helped the most in the shortest time. But I can't prove it. In fact, I can't prove that all of my improvement did not simply come from the drugs (Erleada/Orgovix). However, my research indicates that is unlikely, both in degree and duration. For example, one study showed "PSA90 response is defined as the patient's earliest attainment of ≥90 percent decline in PSA relative to their baseline PSA at treatment initiation. At nine months and by the end of follow-up, 70.4 percent of patients treated with ERLEADA® achieved PSA90 and 62.5 percent for enzalutamide (HR=1.49; p=0.024). The median time to PSA90 response was 3.1 months for patients treated with ERLEADA® and to 5.2 months for enzalutamide.

I had a 99.3 percent drop (from PSA 6 to <.05 ng/ml) in thirty days, and have remained <.05 for twenty-seven months. In addition to my scan improvements, I believe that adds up to a much greater response than normally seen with these drugs alone. "Median treatment duration was nearly three times longer for patients treated with ERLEADA® plus ADT (33 months) compared with the those treated with placebo plus ADT (12 months)." What does that mean? I think it means that the treatment had stopped working by thirty-three months at median. I am at twenty-seven months. So, time will tell. Also, these drugs I am on had "a 52% reduced risk of radiographic progression (HR=0.48; 95% CI, 0.39–0.60; P<0.0001) for patients in the ERLEADA® plus ADT group vs. placebo plus ADT group after 22.7 months of median follow-up." What I cannot yet find out: did any of these patients have actual lasting radiographic regression, for two years straight? If so, what percentage? I would love to know, because I have had exactly that evidence. Is that normally seen with these drugs? I suspect not. I think it is the repurposed drugs, particularly FenBen.

Note: at the time of this writing, BK is at forty months, and still NED.

BK's case report was published in the peer-reviewed journal *Case Reports in Oncology* Makis, M., Baghli, I. & Martinez, P. (2025). Fenbendazole as an Anticancer Agent? A Case Series of Self-Administration in Three Patients. *Case Reports in Oncology*, 18 (1), 856–63. https://doi.org/10.1159/000546362.[8]

CASE REPORT 4: AGGRESSIVE METASTATIC SQUAMOUS CELL ESOPHAGEAL CANCER, AGE SEVENTY-FOUR, MALE

Remission of Metastatic Squamous Cell Esophageal Cancer Following a Multimodal Approach Incorporating Fenbendazole

This case report details the experience of a seventy-four-year-old male diagnosed with metastatic squamous cell esophageal cancer, a malignancy recognized for its aggressive clinical course and poor five-year survival rates. Presented from the perspective of his wife, Barbara S., this account documents the integration of fenbendazole into his treatment regimen alongside conventional therapies. While a single case study, it provides valuable observational data regarding the potential utility of fenbendazole and the significance of proactive intervention in managing aggressive cancers.

Clinical Presentation and Initial Management

In the summer of 2021, the patient presented with dysphagia. Diagnostic evaluation revealed a growth subsequently identified via biopsy as squamous cell esophageal cancer. Further staging confirmed metastasis to a single lymph node, establishing a stage 3 diagnosis. Given the aggressive nature of squamous cell esophageal cancer and evidence of metastasis, the prognosis was inherently challenging.

Immediately following diagnosis, the patient and his wife initiated treatment with the "Joe Tippens protocol," a regimen recognized within online patient communities involving fenbendazole (three days on, four days off), vitamin E, CBD oil, and curcumin. This self-directed fenbendazole administration commenced prior to any conventional treatment and continued for approximately thirty days. This early, independent intervention with fenbendazole represents a significant deviation from standard oncological practice.

Conventional Therapy and Subsequent Fenbendazole Use

Following consultation with their doctors, the patient underwent standard-of-care treatment consisting of weekly chemotherapy and daily radiation therapy (five days per week) for seven weeks. During this period, fenbendazole administration was intentionally discontinued to focus solely on conventional medical treatments.

Immediately upon completion of the final chemotherapy and radiation session, the patient resumed fenbendazole at a daily dose of 222 mg. This continuous, lower dosage marked a change from the initial pulsed protocol.

Treatment Response and Follow-Up

Four weeks after completing chemo-radiation and resuming fenbendazole, follow-up imaging revealed no evidence of disease. However, persistent esophageal wall thickening was noted on the scan, prompting continued monitoring. Rather than proceeding directly to invasive endoscopic evaluation, the decision was made to continue fenbendazole treatment and observe the clinical course.

A subsequent scan three months later confirmed the persistence of esophageal wall thickening. Most importantly, biopsies obtained during endoscopy at this time showed no evidence of malignant cells. Based on these findings, the patient and his wife elected to continue fenbendazole indefinitely at 222 mg daily. Barbara S. affirmed their commitment: "We will remain on fenbendazole forever (222 mg/day every day)."

Barbara S.'s Perspective and Additional Details

Treatment attribution: Barbara S. attributes the successful outcome primarily to fenbendazole. She bases this conclusion on the reported surprise of the oncology team regarding the complete response and their initial recommendation for esophagectomy and partial gastrectomy, suggesting a lack of confidence that chemo-radiation alone would suffice. The prevention of further metastasis following the initial diagnosis is also interpreted as a potential effect of the early fenbendazole intervention.

- **Side Effects:** The patient reportedly experienced no adverse effects attributable to fenbendazole. Liver enzyme levels remained within normal limits throughout the treatment period involving fenbendazole.
- **Product Specifics:** The fenbendazole product used was the "Happy Healing" brand, obtained as a veterinary formulation.
- **Vaccination Status:** Had not received COVID-19 vaccinations or boosters.
- **Physician Communication:** The oncology team was informed their patient was taking unspecified "supplements" necessitating liver function monitoring. Fenbendazole was not specifically named, and the oncologist reportedly did not request further details.

This case report highlights several pertinent aspects warranting consideration:

1. **Early Intervention:** The proactive initiation of fenbendazole immediately post-diagnosis, preceding conventional therapy, represents a notable aspect of this case. This interval provided a window for fenbendazole monotherapy, potentially influencing the initial tumor burden or metastatic potential prior to standard treatment commencement.
2. **Context of Standard Treatment Efficacy:** The reported recommendation for surgery even after planned chemo-radiation underscores the clinical challenges and sometimes guarded prognosis associated with standard treatments for locally advanced squamous cell esophageal cancer, thereby contextualizing the search for adjunctive or alternative therapies.
3. **Fenbendazole Safety Profile:** The absence of any reported side effects and maintenance of normal liver function aligns with existing literature suggesting a favorable safety profile for fenbendazole, particularly in contrast to the known toxicities of conventional chemotherapy and radiation.[2]
4. **Low-Dose Fenbendazole Activity:** The achievement and maintenance of remission while utilizing a continuous low dose (222 mg/day) of fenbendazole provides observational data relevant to dosage optimization studies. This finding indicates that clinically relevant anticancer activity may occur at doses significantly lower than those used in some preclinical models or other anecdotal reports.
5. **Multimodal Therapeutic Strategy:** This case involved sequential and potentially synergistic application of fenbendazole and conventional therapies. While fenbendazole was used initially alone and then resumed post-conventional treatment, the possibility exists that it sensitized remaining cells to chemo-radiation or targeted residual disease resistant to standard therapy. Determining the precise interplay requires further investigation.

This case report contributes to the growing body of anecdotal and preliminary evidence suggesting potential anticancer activity for fenbendazole. The observed remission of metastatic squamous cell esophageal cancer, following a treatment course incorporating fenbendazole both before and after conventional therapy, is noteworthy.

CASE REPORT 5: METASTATIC PROSTATE CANCER (ADENOCARCINOMA), AGE SEVENTY-SEVEN

The following case report, as shared by his son, DY, details the story of a seventy-seven-year-old man's battle with metastatic prostatic adenocarcinoma, a particularly challenging form of prostate cancer that is among the most common cancers among men in the United States and is a leading cause of cancer death. The report also highlights how informed decision-making and a willingness to consider all available options can make a world of difference to the overall outcome, even for diseases that are generally considered to be untreatable. It is presented here to further demonstrate the potential of fenbendazole, as well as the value of a multimodal approach to cancer treatment. The case report also includes a discussion of some of the other factors that are also present in the person's health journey.

This account, as is often the case, begins with a concerning diagnosis. In November 2017, he underwent an abdominal ultrasound after complaining of difficulty with urination, which is often a key sign of a prostate issue. That ultrasound detected an echogenic structure on his left kidney, which, after further testing was determined to be an angiomyolipoma, which is a benign tumor of the kidneys. However, this was not the only finding, and a subsequent CT scan in January 2018, showed that there were masses in the left periaortic lymph node, in the right external iliac lymph node, the right inguinal lymph node, the left external iliac lymph node, and the left posterior perirectal node. The CT scan also revealed a mass in his prostate and bladder. A biopsy of the left pelvic lymph node, after the CT scan, revealed the devastating news that the tumors were metastatic prostatic adenocarcinoma. His cancer was determined to be stage 4, with a five-year survival rate of only 30 percent, and which carries with it a very poor long-term prognosis. It is clear that by the time the tumor was discovered, it had already metastasized to many different regions of the body, and that, therefore, this would be a challenging case for medical treatment.

After consulting with his oncologist, in February 2018, he began treatment with Lupron injections to halt the production of testosterone. This hormone therapy treatment is used to suppress the hormone testosterone, which is one of the drivers for prostate cancer growth, and is often a first line of defense against this disease. This was done every three months. His treatment was then supplemented with the addition of Zytiga (abiraterone) and prednisone, which were added in July 2018, to further decrease testosterone production in the adrenal glands. It is commonly understood that these medications are often only effective for eighteen to twenty-four months, after which, the tumors often develop resistance, which is referred to as castration-resistant prostate cancer, and at this point, the prognosis for survival drops drastically.

The family was aware of the limitations of the current treatment paradigm and were working under the assumption that their loved one had, at best, only two to four years left to live. Given these predictions, they were committed to exploring every possible avenue for treatment, in an effort to both extend his life, and also to improve his overall quality of life. This understanding drove the decision to look beyond conventional medical protocols and to find new ways of thinking about cancer treatment.

Driven by a deep desire to help his father, the author of this report began to research alternative treatments for prostate cancer and, in doing so, came upon the story of Joe Tippens. This then, lead to the discovery of a paper detailing the mechanisms of action of fenbendazole, in its ability to disrupt microtubules and induce cell death. While the idea of treating cancer with a dewormer seemed, at first, far-fetched, the family was nonetheless intrigued by the logic, and also the growing amount of data to support its potential. They recognized that there was no significant risk to trying this novel approach to treatment, and, given the dire prognosis, they determined that there was truly nothing left to lose.

In February 2019, in an attempt to find more specific treatment options for his father, the author of this report also arranged a consultation at Memorial Sloan Kettering. The oncologists at MSK recommended radiation therapy for the treatment of specific tumors, suggesting the use of image-guided, intensity-modulated radiation therapy. Then, during one of these meetings, with the oncologist at Memorial Sloan Kettering, the author of the case report showed the oncologist a copy of the NIH paper on fenbendazole, asking for his opinion. The oncologist acknowledged the interesting nature of the research, but stated that it was not standard of care and, therefore, could not be incorporated into their treatment protocol. This was a significant hurdle to overcome, as it highlights the limitations of the current approach to medical care, which is often unwilling to incorporate innovative or unconventional approaches.

Despite these limitations, the patient received a total of twenty-six radiation treatments at Memorial Sloan Kettering from March to May 2019. It was after all of these treatments were completed, and in June 2019, that he began the "Joe Tippens Protocol," which involved three days of fenbendazole (Panacur-C 222 mg) per week, with four days off, along with daily use of vitamin E, CBD oil and curcumin, as is commonly recommended in online reports from other people who have been using fenbendazole. He continued to take the traditional medications (Lupron, Zytiga, and prednisone), that had been prescribed by his physicians, and, therefore, this approach involved the combination of both conventional and alternative methods.

He also began a regular monitoring program, looking at the progression of his disease through the monitoring of PSA, or prostate specific antigen. As PSA levels increase, the probability of prostate cancer also increases. A PSA reading above 10 indicates a high likelihood of the presence of prostate cancer, while a PSA reading below 4 is generally considered within normal limits. It is also important to note that in this case, the PSA levels and the overall tumor size had responded somewhat to the initial Lupron and Zytiga treatments, which is what would be expected. However, it was noted that the PSA levels did not reach normal ranges until the fenbendazole was also added, at which point it dropped below 1 and has remained in that range ever since.

Based on the results of these studies, and the specific data on PSA levels and tumor sizes, it is thought that the fenbendazole was not only effective at reducing the tumor burden, but it may also be preventing the cancer from returning.

When asked about the various treatment options, and the multiple factors involved, DY noted, that, while the initial conventional hormone and radiation treatments were effective at lowering his father's PSA levels and reducing tumor size, he believed that "my father's continued use of the Joe Tippens fenbendazole protocol has kept his cancer in remission after the likely effectiveness of Lupron and Zytiga have worn off." This is another example of a patient who has taken charge of their own health care and who is, therefore, best equipped to understand the subtleties of the interactions of various medications and treatments that have been used.

DY notes that the fenbendazole protocol has maintained his father's remission after the likely effective period of Lupron and Zytiga had passed.

In a follow-up interview, it was noted:

- **Side Effects:** No side effects from the use of fenbendazole were reported, and he also noted that his father works out daily, doesn't get sick, and is still enjoying spending quality time with his family and grandchildren, which, again, highlights the safety profile of the drug.
- **Medical Disclosure:** The oncologist was not specifically informed about the use of fenbendazole, though the patient had mentioned

that he was taking supplements that required liver monitoring. This was also a conscious choice of the family, due to some concerns about a negative response by the oncologists, as well as a concern that the oncologist would request that he stop the fenbendazole treatment.

- **Vaccination Status:** He also noted that his father had unfortunately received two COVID-19 vaccinations and also two boosters, which, he said had him "worry and keep an eye out for Turbo Cancer."

The major take-home message from this case study is that fenbendazole, when added to a traditional treatment regimen, has the potential to dramatically improve overall outcomes. And also, that when a person takes control of their own health-care decisions and combines their knowledge of traditional treatments with a holistic view of new and emerging therapies, that they may well be able to dramatically alter the course of their disease.

The experience described here highlights a number of concepts that are emerging in the discussion surrounding the use of fenbendazole:

- **The Importance of Early Action:** The rapid start of fenbendazole, in combination with standard treatments, is an important factor in achieving the best possible outcome, especially when dealing with fast-growing cancers. It is, often, in these aggressive cancers where patients will benefit most from immediate, proactive approaches to treatment.
- **Limited Traditional Efficacy:** This case, as with many others, highlights the shortcomings of traditional cancer treatments, particularly in the longer term, as well as the need for new and innovative treatment options. Chemotherapy and radiation, while clearly beneficial in some cases, also have major limitations that make their long-term efficacy quite difficult to achieve.
- **The Safety of Fenbendazole:** Once again, the safety profile of fenbendazole was demonstrated to be exceptional. The fact that there were no side effects noted is extremely promising, and this also highlights the potential of the drug to be used as a long-term option, with fewer unwanted consequences.
- **Low-Dose Effectiveness:** The dose that was used in this case report (222 mg three times a week), while different from other reported cases, was still effective, and this further highlights the potential for smaller, more targeted doses, to generate positive therapeutic effects. The fact

that such a low dose is effective means that higher doses may also be effective for even more challenging cancers.

- **Synergistic Effects:** This case also hints at a possible synergistic action between fenbendazole and the radiation therapy, further emphasizing the importance of using a combination therapy approach, when considering all of the options for cancer treatment.

CASE REPORT 6: METASTATIC RENAL CELL CARCINOMA, AGE SIXTY-THREE, MALE

The following case report presents the compelling story of a sixty-three-year-old man, JC, diagnosed with metastatic renal cell carcinoma (kidney cancer), an aggressive malignancy that had spread to multiple organs. His journey is particularly remarkable due to his quick recovery following the use of fenbendazole as a monotherapy, after having failed traditional treatment options. This case report is also exceptional as it has been the subject of a published case study in *Clinical Oncology and Case Reports*[9] and offers invaluable insights into the potential of fenbendazole in targeting even the most aggressive forms of cancer.

As JC reported, in April 2019, he received a devastating diagnosis of stage 4 kidney cancer that had spread to his inferior vena cava (IVC), the right atrium of his heart, both lungs, pancreas, hip, and spine. His prognosis was considered terminal, and he was given only six months to live. This initial diagnosis was extremely challenging, given the extent of his disease, and the number of organs that were involved, which, by itself, limited the possibilities of surgical intervention. The standard of care for his cancer called for immunotherapy, and, therefore, he began treatment with a combination of cabozantinib and nivolumab, a combination that has proven effective in some other cases. However, he was only able to tolerate three half doses of the immunotherapy before the treatment had to be terminated due to severe side effects, including a serious rash and colitis. The treatment, while promising in concept, was clearly not going to be a sustainable option for this particular person. After exhausting that option, the only available recourse was for supportive, or palliative, care, which would only seek to manage the symptoms, rather than try to attack the root of the problem. He had been given a prognosis of approximately six months to live, and at that time, he felt he had nothing to lose by trying something completely different.

The story shifted when JC sought out information regarding new and different types of cancer treatment, and he discovered information about the use of fenbendazole for treating cancer. He began his treatment in the first week of August 2019, with a dose of 222 mg of fenbendazole, and notably, with no other additional vitamins or supplements, and also with no CBD oil or other natural treatments. He chose to start with just fenbendazole as a monotherapy, in order to better understand its effects. He also made the decision to use a schedule of three days on and four days off, which is different from what other patients had used, and it is likely that this cycle had a role in the outcome.

Remarkably, after only two months, in the second week of October 2019, MRI scans at Stanford clearly showed that his largest tumor, in his left kidney, was gone. Furthermore, his other tumors had also shrunk considerably. After the initial results, further testing was done in January 2020, when Stanford MRI scans revealed that there was no evidence of disease. All of the cancer was gone. At that time, he was still taking fenbendazole, using the original three days on, four days off schedule, and still used only fenbendazole, with no other vitamins or supplements. He noted that he is living proof of fenbendazole's effect as a monotherapy, and, that the medication itself is all that was required to eradicate his disease.

JC also emphasized that "Fenbendazole is extremely safe to take, even every day. I've never had any elevated liver enzymes." He was specifically addressing any concerns about the potential for liver toxicity, an area that is often highlighted as a risk factor for medications. He, in contrast to this, highlighted his experience as proof that fenbendazole has an extremely high safety margin, even with long-term use.

These remarkable results did not go unnoticed by his doctors, and it is of significance that, unlike many other cases described so far, that his oncologists at Stanford were not only aware of his use of fenbendazole but also decided to write up his case and publish it in a medical journal.[10] This unusual step further highlights the significance of this case and the overall efficacy of the treatment.

Currently, and as of the writing of this report, JC is still using fenbendazole, taking a 222 mg dose daily, for three days each week, and then having four days off before the next dose, and his cancer remains in remission. The case study published by his doctors also further supports the findings of other case reports in this series that fenbendazole has the ability to treat and eradicate cancer, particularly when aggressive treatment is initiated. His ongoing treatment plan is also a key piece of evidence to suggest that even at a relatively low dosage, the drug has a positive and protective effect.

JC continues to take fenbendazole (222 mg daily, three days on/four days off). His cancer remains in remission.

Several key takeaways can be identified from this specific case report:

- **The Power of Monotherapy:** JC used only fenbendazole, without any other supportive or complementary therapies, and still had a complete eradication of all detectable cancer cells. This outcome strongly indicates that fenbendazole can, indeed, be effective as a monotherapy, and that it is also able to act on its own, without the need for other medications or approaches.

- **Low Doses Can Be Effective:** The fact that JC's cancer responded to only 222 mg per day is very important, especially considering that some others have been using higher dosages. His experience suggests that lower doses of fenbendazole can still be very effective in eradicating cancer. This is also important to note as it could allow for more therapeutic dosing strategies where drugs may be more effective when used at lower doses for longer periods of time.
- **Speed of Treatment Response:** The fact that it took only two months to reduce tumor size, and only five months to completely eliminate all cancer, is also noteworthy. The speed of tumor regression highlights how powerful and effective fenbendazole can be at directly targeting cancer cells. The timeline here suggests a rapid rate of action that is not often observed in other forms of cancer treatment.
- **Confirmation from Medical Professionals:** It is also highly significant that his doctors decided to write and publish a case report about his experience (Chiang et al., 2021), using his name, in a peer-reviewed medical journal. This is an extremely unusual step, and one that shows the potential importance of fenbendazole as a treatment for cancer. The fact that his doctors were sufficiently impressed with his outcome that they wrote up his story in a formal, public manner is a major endorsement, and this data cannot be ignored. Moreover, three more of the case reports presented here were also published in a prestigious medical journal.
- **The Importance of a Positive Perspective:** JC was motivated to take an active role in his care, and he approached his cancer with hope and determination. It is important to highlight the need for people to have a positive mindset and to participate in their health journey, as this type of attitude has been correlated with improved outcomes in multiple diseases.

In summary, this case report provides a compelling and very clear example of the power of fenbendazole and its ability to provide effective, and less toxic, therapy to those affected by cancer. It is also important to highlight the ongoing work that needs to be done to further evaluate the overall utility of this medication, as well as to determine the optimal dose and combination strategies that will ultimately lead to the best possible outcomes for patients. The case of JC also provides a strong message for those who are in the early stages of cancer treatment and highlights that even a terminal diagnosis may not be an absolute death sentence. The goal of all of these case studies is to provide evidence that there are, indeed, new ways of approaching the disease and that, through scientific rigor, and also, with a willingness to look beyond traditional models, better treatments are possible.

CASE REPORT 7: METASTATIC MELANOMA, AGE FIFTY-EIGHT, MALE

The case of Chris, a fifty-eight-year-old man diagnosed with metastatic melanoma, provides a powerful example of the potential for early intervention using fenbendazole, and it highlights the importance of sharing information with loved ones in an effort to inspire new treatment approaches. Melanoma, while it only accounts for a small percentage of all cancers, is an aggressive type of skin cancer that often has the potential to metastasize and is therefore associated with a relatively high rate of cancer-related mortality. The American Cancer Society estimates that in 2022, nearly 100,000 cases of melanoma were diagnosed in the United States, with nearly 8,000 people expected to die of the disease. What makes melanoma so challenging is its propensity to spread throughout the body, and that treatment, in many cases, becomes challenging once that spread has begun. It is these types of metastatic cancers that may benefit most from novel approaches, including the use of fenbendazole.

In July 2022, Chris was diagnosed with melanoma that had spread to his lymph nodes, and he also had a noticeable growth under his right arm. His case, therefore, was considered to be high risk, and it prompted the family to begin researching ways to target and treat his disease.

In August 2022, the malignant tumor and the affected lymph nodes were surgically removed. However, even after surgery, the risk of recurrence was high, given the known aggressive nature of the disease, and therefore he began treatment with 444 mg per day of fenbendazole, which he started taking only one week after his surgical procedure. The logic was that the surgery would remove the existing tumors, and that the fenbendazole would target any remaining cancer cells and also act as a preventative treatment, to avoid the reoccurrence of his disease. This approach shows a strong consideration of the need to be proactive in all aspects of treatment.

In September 2022, Chris had brain and full-body scans, and they revealed that there was no longer any evidence of cancer in his body. This is a key aspect of this case, as it highlights the fast-acting nature of the treatment and the capacity for fenbendazole to have an impact in such a short period of time. He decided to continue taking the fenbendazole, at a maintenance dose of 444 mg per day, and scheduled his next scan for December 2022. At the time of this writing Chris remains cancer-free.

In a follow-up interview, Chris's cousin, LP, provided the following information:

- **No Other Treatments:** He did not take any other treatments beyond the initial surgery. By this point, he had already obtained a clear result using just fenbendazole alone, and there was no clear reason for additional treatments. It was also known that any further treatments would be unlikely to prevent cancer recurrence, especially in light of the well-known difficulties associated with treating metastatic melanoma. The family decided that it was best to rely on the observed efficacy of the fenbendazole rather than to subject him to other medical procedures.
- **Lack of Side Effects:** The patient reported having no side effects from the fenbendazole, which is consistent with other case reports that have been discussed. He used the brand of fenbendazole that was purchased from "FenBen Labs," demonstrating that commercially available veterinary products are a useful way to access the medication.
- **Personal Advocacy:** LP was instrumental in sharing the information about fenbendazole with her cousin, highlighting the importance of public awareness and the role of patient advocacy in exploring new treatment options. It was because of her knowledge, and sharing of that information, that her cousin was able to access this new therapeutic approach and ultimately eradicate his cancer.

The fact that he was completely cancer-free by the time of his December 2022 scan, only a few months after he was first diagnosed, and after undergoing surgery, is also a notable achievement, and this outcome highlights the potential power of early intervention when using fenbendazole. He also continued to use the same approach of a single 444 mg dose per day, which is consistent with the data that suggests that a lower dose is often sufficient to generate a therapeutic benefit.

Chris, and his family, did not have time to wait for weeks or months to determine the efficacy of the treatment, and it was, therefore, important that the fenbendazole worked quickly. Only a couple of months after the initial dose of fenbendazole, he was declared cancer-free, and that is a testament to its rapid action. Also, the combination of the surgery and the quick introduction of fenbendazole was a key component of his treatment approach.

By the time of the December 21, 2022, scan results, Chris was reported to be cancer-free, and his cousin excitedly announced, "My cousin, Chris, who has melanoma and has been taking FenBen for several months, just received the results from his latest scans and he is cancer free!!!!! Yahooooooo!!!!!" Almost three years since the original diagnosis, Chris remains cancer-free.

This report provides yet another example of a patient who was diagnosed with cancer, who sought out information for a treatment that they believed could work, and who ultimately had a very positive outcome.

The overall message of this report, as is the case with the other reports in this book, is to emphasize the key aspects of this type of patient-directed health care:

- **Rapid Action:** The importance of acting quickly upon diagnosis and using therapies that can generate a rapid response to the tumors.
- **Fenbendazole as a Monotherapy:** This case demonstrates the potential of fenbendazole as a stand-alone treatment, and it is particularly remarkable that no other interventions, beyond surgery, were required for complete cancer eradication.
- **Importance of Patient Advocacy:** The role that a supportive relative played in informing the patient about fenbendazole highlights the need for the sharing of information and the importance of a strong support network when dealing with a cancer diagnosis.
- **A Call for Early Treatment:** Given that metastasis is a clear indicator of more severe and life-threatening cancers, it is highly beneficial that fenbendazole was initiated as soon as possible after his initial diagnosis. This strategy is a major factor in improving cancer treatment outcomes.
- **A Strong Safety Profile:** It is also important that no adverse effects were reported during the use of fenbendazole, which further highlights its very strong safety profile and reinforces the view that this medication has the potential for widespread use.

In conclusion, this case highlights how quickly fenbendazole was able to target and eradicate metastatic melanoma. It also shows the power of patient-led treatments and taking immediate action to address the underlying mechanisms of disease. This serves as yet another example of the potential of fenbendazole in the fight against cancer.

CASE REPORT 8: PLASMACYTOID UROTHELIAL (BLADDER) CANCER, AGE FIFTY-FOUR, MALE

A Rare Cancer Vanquished: Fenbendazole and the Power of Self-Advocacy

This case report details the remarkable journey of MS, a fifty-four-year-old man diagnosed with plasmacytoid urothelial cancer, a rare and aggressive form of bladder cancer, which is known for its poor response to conventional treatments and its poor prognosis for long-term survival. MS's story, like those of others who have been discussed in this book, is one of hope and determination, where he took control of his own health-care decisions, using a combination of research, determination, and, ultimately, fenbendazole. This particular case is an example of a complete remission using only fenbendazole, after a diagnosis that was, essentially, a death sentence. The fact that he was able to obtain a full and complete remission so quickly using fenbendazole provides additional supporting data for its value in the treatment of cancer.

As MS reported, on April 22, 2022, he was diagnosed with plasmacytoid urothelial cancer, a rare variant of bladder cancer, after having two tumors removed from his bladder and then biopsied. This specific type of cancer is extremely rare; it accounts for only 1–3 percent of all urothelial cancers and is also highly aggressive. He was informed by his physician that this cancer type was known to be unresponsive to both chemotherapy and radiation, and that his available options were, essentially, limited to bladder removal, with a high level of uncertainty as to the overall benefits. Given that this is also a form of cancer that has a very aggressive metastatic nature, this meant that the only option that was being proposed would likely not lead to a cure. He noted that, when he asked about his prognosis, he was given a very vague estimate of his remaining time to live; "maybe a year, maybe six months," with the final outcome being described as "between me and God!"

This prognosis, and the lack of available treatment options, was a devastating blow to MS, but it also served as a powerful motivator. He described this experience of having a death sentence written down on his medical reports as a "difficult time," and that, initially, it caused him to feel a great deal of despair. As he notes, he has been in recovery from alcoholism for ten years, as of April 2, 2022, and, therefore, he was motivated to continue in his fight to overcome the disease. Given the situation, and a lack of available treatment options, MS refused to accept his fate, and this inspired him to take action. He said he "thought that there must be something I could do" and that he "prayed to God for direction."

His first impulse was to contact MD Anderson Cancer Center, and he considered donating his body to them for the purpose of research. However, he was frustrated when he learned that the institution wanted a large amount of money, up front, for his body to be used for research purposes. This unexpected barrier angered him and fueled his determination to look further into new methods of treatment. His decision to take charge of his own care was prompted by his realization that he could no longer rely solely on the opinions and recommendations of the traditional medical establishment, and that he had to look beyond the mainstream. This is, all too often, the situation that many cancer patients find themselves in, and it underscores the importance of patients seeking out new and innovative approaches to treatment.

Driven by his frustration, and by the knowledge that conventional medicine offered him very little, MS began researching new cancer treatment options, that included some that were not commonly being used or discussed by traditional cancer specialists. While doing so, he came across information about fenbendazole, an antiparasitic medication, that, based on reports that he found on the internet, "seemed to work for lots of others." He was impressed by the ability of fenbendazole to kill cancer cells, with no apparent negative side effects and, therefore, he decided to give it a try.

His treatment regimen started in late April 2022, when he began taking 444 mg of fenbendazole per day (222 mg in the morning and 222 mg in the afternoon). By July 19, 2022, he had been on this protocol for approximately three months, at which time he underwent new CT scans and PET scans to evaluate his progress. The results were nothing short of miraculous. His doctor reported that the cancer "didn't spread, and he didn't see any tumors or cancer in my bladder! Also he couldn't see any cancer anywhere in my body!!!"

Timeline:

- April 22, 2022: MS is formally diagnosed with plasmacytoid urothelial cancer based on biopsy results.
- Late April 2022: MS starts self-treating with fenbendazole (444 mg per day: 222 mg a.m., 222 mg p.m.).
- July 19, 2022: MS undergoes follow-up CT and PET scans (after approximately three months on fenbendazole). Scans show no evidence of cancer spread, no visible tumors in the bladder, and no cancer anywhere in the body (reported as a complete remission).
- Post–July 19, 2022: MS continues taking fenbendazole daily (444 mg/day).

MS remains on fenbendazole treatment every day, and, additionally, he has also changed his diet, incorporating more lean protein (fish and chicken) while avoiding red meat. He also drinks hot lemon juice daily, and also eats plenty of fruits and berries, and takes other vitamins, which, he says, he believes are important to his overall health and also to his recovery from cancer. He also credits his faith in God as playing an equally important role in his overall health and well-being.

MS's key takeaway from his experience was that "if it healed me then maybe it can heal them too." This belief, which he obtained from his own treatment, may well be useful to others as well. His words are intended to offer hope to those who are suffering from this terrible disease, while also acknowledging the need for everyone to be proactive in their own health care.

When asked further questions about his treatment, MS shared the following:

- **Ongoing Dosage:** He continues to take 444 mg of fenbendazole per day.
- **Lack of Side Effects:** As is now a recurring theme with the use of fenbendazole, he also did not experience any side effects, highlighting the overall safety of the drug, even when taken for extended periods of time.
- **Absence of Other Treatments:** Other than surgery to remove the tumors for biopsy, MS did not use any other type of cancer treatment. This is a very significant observation, because it means that his recovery can be primarily attributed to the fenbendazole alone.
- **Physician Knowledge:** He indicated that he did not initially disclose his use of fenbendazole to his physician, but he did later discuss the fact that it was only the use of fenbendazole that eradicated his cancer.

The story of MS is not just one of hope, but also it serves as an important call for people to take control of their health care and to explore all available treatment options, including those that may be outside conventional medicine. His experience highlights the importance of challenging existing paradigms and seeking out innovative new approaches to care in order to obtain the best results and also to promote the best overall quality of life.

His rapid and complete remission from a very aggressive and typically fatal cancer cannot be ignored and should be seen as yet another powerful piece of data in the rapidly evolving puzzle of fenbendazole and its role in the treatment of cancer. It is a reminder that hope should never be abandoned, and also that an open mind, combined with well-informed action, can be the keys to unlocking previously unknown potential.

CASE REPORT 9: METASTATIC RECTAL CANCER, AGE SIXTY-NINE, MALE.

A Multipronged Assault on Metastatic Rectal Cancer—Fenbendazole, Ivermectin, and Determination

The following case report details the journey of WM, a sixty-nine-year-old man diagnosed with stage 3 rectal cancer that had metastasized to the adjacent lymph nodes and tissues. His story provides a powerful example of a patient who took control of his own care and who sought a multipronged approach by combining a variety of treatments including surgery, chemotherapy, radiation, fenbendazole, and ivermectin, with a positive and noteworthy outcome. This case is notable for the combination of therapies that were chosen, as well as for the specific dosages that were used, and it also highlights the importance of WM's determination to be proactive in his own health.

Colorectal cancer, as has been well documented, is a major public health issue. It is the third most common type of cancer in the United States. In 2023, the American Cancer Society estimated that there would be 106,970 new cases of colon cancer and 46,050 new cases of rectal cancer diagnosed in the United States. While overall colorectal cancer incidence rates have declined in older adults since the 1980s, data shows that these rates are actually increasing in individuals who are under the age of fifty, which highlights the need for an awareness of how this disease can affect a much younger population. The data also shows that it will also remain a leading cause of cancer-related death for both men and women, and it is estimated that colorectal cancer will account for 52,550 deaths in the United States during 2023. These numbers emphasize the importance of finding new and effective treatment options for these specific types of cancers.

WM was diagnosed with stage 3 rectal cancer in July 2023, with a tumor that was five cm x three cm, located near his anus. Further testing showed that the tumor had penetrated the outer wall of the rectum, and it had also spread to an adjacent lymph node in his pelvic region, which was also enlarged and measured approximately 2 cm. At this point, he was experiencing a significant amount of pain and nerve irritation due to the tumor's growth and location. Faced with this challenging diagnosis, WM began researching different treatment approaches, which eventually led him to discover information about the Joe Tippens Protocol and a variety of other supplements with reputed anticancer properties. His immediate action, upon hearing the diagnosis, demonstrates the powerful role of patient agency in the treatment of cancer.

WM immediately implemented a multipronged approach, which involved:

- **Fenbendazole:** He started with a daily dose of 450 mg of fenbendazole, which he had acquired as an over-the-counter medication for animal use.
- **Ivermectin:** WM also added 48 mg of ivermectin, which he had acquired from overseas sources, and which is another well-known medication for treating parasitic infections, and, more recently, for treating various forms of cancer.
- **Curcumin:** He was also taking 1200 mg of curcumin twice per day.
- **Multivitamins and Vitamin D3:** A daily multivitamin, along with 3 gel caps of vitamin D3, was also added to his daily routine.
- **CBD oil:** WM also initially used CBD oil at 24 ml per day, but this was later switched to olive oil.

This specific combination of treatments, which combined medications designed to act directly on tumors with others that may have a supportive role in the function of the immune system, demonstrates the value of understanding all available options.

In September 2023, WM began a six-week course of chemotherapy and radiation therapy. Three weeks after the end of these traditional medical therapies, he had his first follow-up scans. His medical team acknowledged that this testing may have been done too early, as they noted that radiation therapy often continues to have an effect for about six weeks after treatment is discontinued. It is also important to note that he had only been on the fenbendazole protocol for approximately four months, which is also a relatively short time frame.

Nonetheless, the results were extremely positive, and MRI readings revealed that his tumors had shrunk significantly, with the remaining tissue being described by his radiologist as a "scab" and no evidence of disease was observed in any other part of his body. This rapid response, particularly given the extent of the original tumors, was quite remarkable. WM's doctors, though happy with the result, still felt that some residual cancer cells may remain, and that standard protocol recommended that he also undergo follow-up chemotherapy, which he agreed to undergo in the coming months.

WM is symptom-free, and he is no longer experiencing the pain, nerve irritation, or the bleeding that he had been experiencing prior to his new protocol. This clear improvement in his health and well-being further demonstrates that he is responding well to this treatment. WM also noted that he is "feeling better than I have in some time," and that he is "quite confident the fenbendazole has helped shrink the enlarged lymph node and prevented any other metastasis from forming." This feeling of hope and optimism is a recurring theme when people use these alternative approaches, and it also highlights the psychological benefits that can be experienced.

This case describes a man with locally advanced rectal cancer who experienced a significant positive response following concurrent treatment with standard neoadjuvant chemoradiation and a self-administered regimen of complementary therapies, including fenbendazole, ivermectin, curcumin, and vitamin supplements. The follow-up MRI demonstrated a marked reduction in the primary tumor and resolution of nodal involvement.

This case report is an interesting example of the use of multiple treatment strategies to fight cancer. In his initial steps, WM elected to start multiple different treatments at the same time to give himself the best chance to eradicate his cancer. He used fenbendazole, curcumin, ivermectin, and vitamin supplements, in addition to chemotherapy and radiation, and, while it is impossible to determine what exactly eradicated the cancer, it is highly likely, based on the weight of the previous case reports here, that fenbendazole was the active agent.

CASE REPORT 10: INOPERABLE METASTATIC ESOPHAGEAL CANCER, AGE SIXTY-SIX, MALE.

Overcoming a Death Sentence—A Story of Metastatic Esophageal Cancer and the Power of Self-Directed Treatment

This case report details the extraordinary experience of AR, a sixty-six-year-old man diagnosed with stage 4 metastatic esophageal adenocarcinoma, a cancer known for its aggressive behavior and its poor response to traditional medical interventions. This case is particularly noteworthy, because, unlike many other reports, the medical establishment was aware of AR's status, and had, essentially, given up on providing any treatment options beyond palliative care. This highlights the importance of looking beyond conventional methods and exploring other, novel approaches to treatment, and also demonstrates the power of taking an active role in one's own health-care decisions. AR's story, while anecdotal, adds further data to the growing body of knowledge supporting the need for more research into the use of fenbendazole for cancer.

In the summer of 2021, AR began experiencing difficulties with swallowing, which led him to seek out medical care. What was initially thought to be a minor issue was soon revealed to be a serious and life-threatening illness. An initial biopsy confirmed a diagnosis of squamous cell esophageal cancer, and subsequent testing revealed that the tumor was a massive eighteen cm, and that it had also metastasized to one of his lungs, as well as to the lymph nodes in that region. The cancer had also enveloped the arteries and veins of the area, which made surgical removal an impossibility, and also meant that treatment options were severely limited. The oncologist team, recognizing the dire situation, concluded that his cancer was far too advanced for radiation or chemotherapy to be effective, and his only remaining option was palliative chemotherapy. It is essential to highlight that palliative chemotherapy is not a treatment designed to eradicate cancer, but rather, it is a method designed to treat symptoms and improve the quality of life for the remaining time the patient has left. He was, therefore, given a death sentence with no other viable treatment options being offered.

Despite this extremely grim prognosis, and the belief from his doctors that he had very little time to live, AR chose to not simply give up. He decided to actively engage in his own health-care decisions, and to explore all available options for treatment. In his own words, he described that he "started doing my own research," because he "was given up on." This initial action demonstrates his determination to pursue all possible options, and it is also a powerful endorsement for the use of self-education in the face of a life-threatening illness. This search for new information led him to discover a number of compounds with suspected anticancer properties, and based on that research, he put together a treatment protocol that combined both established and experimental agents, all at the same time.

- **A Multifaceted Treatment Protocol:** The treatment plan he created included multiple different strategies to attack his cancer and was based on combining treatments with different mechanisms of action.
- **Fenbendazole:** He started on a daily dose of 222 mg of fenbendazole (Panacur-C), once per day.
- **Shiaqga Rapid Immune Recovery:** He also used 2 ml of Shiaqga Rapid Immune Recovery (a blend of mushroom, frankincense, black cumin, and lemon), twice daily.
- **Multigenics Intensive Care multivitamin:** He included a daily multivitamin, that specifically did not contain any iron.
- **Calcium, Vitamin D3, Potassium, Vitamin B12:** He also took 400 mg of calcium twice per day, 1000 IU of vitamin D3 twice per day, 99 mg of potassium twice per day, and 5000 mg of vitamin B12 once per day, all for general health.
- **Curcumin:** He also took 600 mg of curcumin (Theracumin HP), twice per day.
- **Milk Thistle Extract:** He supplemented with 1000 mg of milk thistle extract, once per day, to help with liver detoxification.
- **CBD Oil:** He also used 33 mg of CBD (Recepta Relief 33 Fresh Berry CBD) once per day.

He followed this protocol for approximately fourteen months, and after about three months, he noted a significant improvement in his overall well-being. He specifically noted that "it was easier to swallow which made life so much more normal," and that the tumors appeared to be shrinking, which then enabled his body to start to function more normally.

By April 2022, AR was declared to be cancer-free, with "no evidence of disease." This incredible result was confirmed by another set of scans, in November 2022. He also stated that at that point, he had been cancer-free for eight months and that his recovery was ongoing. He went on to exclaim, "*Thank you, Jesus!*" His strong faith also served as a key point in his approach to dealing with cancer and highlighted that treatment is not just physical, but is also highly emotional, and, at times, spiritual.

Currently, he continues to take a single 222 mg packet of fenbendazole every day, in addition to the curcumin, milk thistle, potassium, and also, of course, his faith in God. In addition to taking these medications, he also stated "Proverbs 17:22 tells us, 'A merry heart doeth good like a medicine; but a broken spirit drieth the bones.' Prayer and laughter (good attitude) were essential in my recovery!"

During a follow-up interview, he answered some additional questions:

- **Side Effects:** He specifically reported that he did not experience any side effects from the various substances he was taking.
- **Rationale for Specific Supplements:** When questioned about the inclusion of certain substances, such as potassium, which are not usually associated with anticancer effects, AR noted that "those other things like potassium and calcium I took for heart health, B12 for energy, vitamin D for bones, and the milk thistle as a liver detox agent. Fenbendazole is what killed the cancer." This statement emphasizes his belief that fenbendazole was the primary therapeutic agent and that the others were only used to improve his overall well-being.
- **Communication with His Doctors:** After he started to see some initial benefits, AR contacted his oncologist and informed him that he was taking fenbendazole and other supplements. However, AR reported that he did not receive any response from them.
- **Treatment Timeline:** When asked about the timing of the various treatments, AR noted that he started fenbendazole in July or August 2022, and by April 2023, he was declared cancer-free, and a follow-up scan in November also showed that he was clear. AR stated that he began to feel better only a few months after starting the fenbendazole, and this is very consistent with other case reports that have been collected, that suggest that fenbendazole acts rapidly.
- **Vaccination Status:** It is also important to note that AR specifically reported that he did not receive any COVID-19 vaccines or boosters, another key data point that must be considered when analyzing the overall trends in health and illness.
- **The Importance of Improved Health:** Finally, AR also noted that, for him, it was the improved swallowing ability that was the first key indicator that treatment was, indeed, working, as he was no longer experiencing the intense discomfort that was associated with his cancer

> progression, and this allowed him to start living a more normal and comfortable life.

This case report is a compelling example of how, even when faced with a terminal diagnosis, individuals can still take steps to improve their own health outcome. It is a story that encompasses self-education, hope, and determination and it is an excellent reminder that the human spirit, combined with science and a strong commitment to well-being, can do the seemingly impossible.

This case is also important to consider from a scientific perspective. Given the terminal prognosis, AR's case is a remarkable example of how a combination of readily available substances, but most notably the use of fenbendazole, resulted in the complete remission of his cancer. As was discussed earlier, in the summary of this case report, the average survival time for patients with inoperable esophageal cancer may only be a few months, while the five-year survival rate, even when the standard therapies of chemotherapy, radiation, and surgery are employed, is typically only around 8–20 percent. This is further complicated by the fact that tumor size is also a significant predictor of a poor outcome, and AR's 18-cm tumor was unusually large. Yet, despite all of these factors, AR is not only still alive, but, according to all available diagnostics, he is also completely cancer-free.

AR's ability to overcome the odds and to eradicate a disease that, by most metrics, was considered to be a death sentence, is a testament to the power of self-directed treatments, and also to the promise of drugs such as fenbendazole. It is clear that AR may not have survived if he had not done his own research and found new and different ways of approaching the challenges presented by his cancer diagnosis.

CASE REPORT 11: TRIPLE-NEGATIVE BREAST CANCER STAGE 3, AGE FORTY-FIVE

Conquering Triple-Negative Breast Cancer: Fenbendazole's Solo Act

The following case report details the inspiring journey of LKT, a woman who was faced with a devastating diagnosis of stage 3 triple-negative breast cancer (TNBC), which, as is well-known, is one of the most aggressive and challenging forms of breast cancer to treat. Her case is noteworthy, because it showcases the potential for fenbendazole, when used as a monotherapy, to not only halt the spread of aggressive malignancies, but to completely eradicate the disease. This story is particularly meaningful as it offers a glimmer of hope for individuals facing TNBC, a disease for which traditional therapies often fall short. It also serves to highlight the need for more research in this specific area.

For context, as reported by the Cleveland Clinic, triple-negative breast cancer is an especially dangerous form of invasive breast cancer, accounting for approximately 15 percent of all invasive breast cancer cases. Unlike most breast cancers, which have receptors for hormones, such as estrogen and progesterone, the cancer cells that constitute TNBC do not. This lack of receptors means that standard hormonal therapies, which target these receptors, are ineffective, and for this reason, the prognosis for TNBC is often very poor, compared to other forms of breast cancer. Receptors are molecules on the surface of cells that determine what substances can attach to cells and affect what the cells do. The lack of these receptors in TNBC makes them invisible to hormonal treatments.

LKT, a forty-five-year-old woman (145 pounds, 5'6"), first noticed changes in the skin of her breast, as well as some pain in the area, in October 2022. She was diagnosed with stage 3 triple-negative breast cancer after undergoing a mammogram, CT scan, and biopsy. The cancer had already metastasized to the surrounding lymph nodes, and was causing the skin on her breast to discolor, indicating an advanced and aggressive stage of the disease. After consulting with physicians and considering her options, she made the courageous decision to use fenbendazole, and, therefore, to engage in her own independent and proactive treatment approach.

Her treatment plan involved taking Safe-Guard (fenbendazole), starting with the three days on, four days off protocol, as had been used by Joe Tippens. She continued on this regimen for the first seven weeks, using a dosage of one box of Safe-Guard per week (each box contains three packets). She then increased the dosage to a box and a half per week (approximately five packets of 222 mg each), and remained on this increased dosage for seven additional weeks. In total, she was on the fenbendazole protocol for only fourteen weeks. At that time, she was very pleasantly surprised.

It was at around eleven weeks that LKT first noticed positive changes, which she describes as her skin clearing up, with a disappearance of the small spots on her breast that may accompany breast cancer. Throughout this entire time she did not experience any noticeable side effects, a significant benefit when compared to the often debilitating side effects of chemotherapy.

However, the biggest and most important achievement, came after only sixteen weeks of fenbendazole use, when LKT received confirmation that there was no longer any evidence of cancer in her body, and that she was completely cancer-free. As of the writing of this report, approximately sixteen months later, LKT remains cancer-free, and also, symptom-free.

It is clear from her story that her consistent approach and the quick action that she took are what lead to her highly successful results. In her own words, her key recommendation was to "take fenben, and don't stop. At least not until it's gone." She also states that her current results are that "I've been cancer-free for almost 16 months. Best of wishes to all of you!"

In her correspondence with the authors, LKT also shared additional pertinent information:

- **Lack of Side Effects:** She reported that she did not experience any side effects from the use of fenbendazole.
- **Lack of Other Treatment:** No other cancer treatments, beyond the use of fenbendazole, were used. This lack of other interventions helps to support the fact that it was, indeed, the fenbendazole that had caused the successful eradication of the disease.
- **Physician Not Involved:** She reported that she did not inform her doctor of her use of fenbendazole, highlighting her level of control over her health care decisions.
- **Vaccination Status:** LKT did not receive any of the COVID-19 vaccines or boosters.

LKT's experience is nothing short of remarkable, as she was able to overcome a very aggressive form of cancer using a safe and simple medication. Another important factor was that she never gave up hope.

This case supports the theory that has been posed previously in this book, which is that fenbendazole appears to be a safe, accessible, and effective option to combat aggressive types of cancer. So far, all of these case reports have very similar trends, which suggests that the underlying reasons that they were successful are due to the common factor of fenbendazole use.

Previous chapters presented preclinical evidence (petri dish, animal experiments) suggesting that fenbendazole would likely be effective in treating human TNBC. Particularly encouraging were the findings that fenbendazole was very effective in reducing or eliminating cancer stem cells that appear to be involved in metastatic spread and chemotherapeutic resistance (Joe et al., 2022). Furthermore, triple-negative breast cancer is aggressive and often leads to bone, brain, liver, and lung metastases. Because of the tendency of triple-negative breast cancer to metastasize, Joe et al. (2022) thought it would be a useful type of cancer to test whether mebendazole (fenbendazole) would be safe and effective in preventing metastases in animal models.

As a review, using a variety of in vitro and in vivo models, Joe et al. (2022) showed that mebendazole prevented the development of triple-negative breast cancer and eradicated previously established triple-negative breast cancer and also reduced distant lung metastasis while preventing liver metastasis. Furthermore, mebendazole treatment led to a dramatic reduction in the cellular marker, Integrin β4 (ITGβ4), which is linked to the development of cancer stem cells in distant locations (this finding is related to the development of metastases). Even though these data were primarily animal data they would likely be applicable to humans, and it looks like they may very well be.

In the present case report LKT's experiences definitely appear to validate the usefulness of fenbendazole in treating metastatic TNBC in humans. Treating is an understatement, to say the least, as it appears LKT eradicated her triple-negative breast cancer with fenbendazole in about sixteen weeks. It is important to point out that LKT did not do any other traditional treatments, just fenbendazole.

LKT used a relatively conservative dosing amount of fenbendazole. She took 222 mg of fenbendazole per day for three consecutive days for the first seven weeks. She then increased to five 222 mg packets per week for seven weeks. At the eleven-week juncture was when LKT noticed the "spots," skin discoloration, disappearing on her breast (skin metastases are a secondary breast cancer that forms on or just below the surface of the skin and can be visible). At about sixteen weeks, LKT received confirmation of what she suspected from observing the skin lesions disappear earlier, she was now cancer-free. Some three years later, LKT is symptom- and cancer-free.

LKT's experience is an amazing outcome. While there is always the possibility of unappreciated individual differences or other as-yet-unidentified factors that may determine or contribute to dramatic outcomes like this, LKT's result, combined with the basic preclinical science reviewed in our previous chapters supports the notion that fenbendazole can cure cancer.

CASE REPORT 12: SIGMOID COLON ADENOCARCINOMA (STAGE 2), AGE SEVENTY, FEMALE

Steering Clear of Chemotherapy: A Case of Sigmoid Colon Adenocarcinoma Treated with Fenbendazole and Ivermectin

This case report, as reported by SJ, details a highly personalized, and ultimately successful, approach to the treatment of stage 2 sigmoid colon adenocarcinoma in a seventy-year-old female through the use of fenbendazole and ivermectin, and with a purposeful avoidance of traditional chemotherapy. Colorectal cancer, which includes both colon and rectal cancers, continues to be a major health concern, with the American Cancer Society estimating approximately 150,000 new cases each year, and with over 50,000 annual deaths attributed to these cancers in the United States alone.

SJ's case is particularly significant because it also involved the successful treatment of cancer without the need for what some view as toxic and harmful chemotherapy, and, while surgery was involved, this case report serves to provide support to the notion that an integrative approach can be both effective and safe.

SJ's initial diagnosis of was sigmoid colon cancer, stage 2; well-differentiated adenocarcinoma of the colon mucosa, on January 10, 2023. She underwent initial treatment by a surgeon, who performed an emergency surgery in order to establish a stoma, which would bypass the affected region of the digestive tract, and, at the time, it was considered to be a lifesaving measure. However, a troubling prognosis had been provided by the initial surgeon, who believed that the cancer had already metastasized to the kidneys, likely giving SJ very little time to live. Later tests revealed that this assessment was not accurate, but, at the time, this dire prediction may have impacted many of the decisions that were subsequently made by both SJ and her family.

Fortunately, a second surgeon, located in another city, agreed to take the SJ's case, and, in a subsequent surgery performed in February, removed the tumor, along with several surrounding lymph nodes in order to prevent any potential future metastasis. While this approach proved to be successful in removing the known tumor burden, the medical team still recommended several chemotherapy treatments, as a preventative measure to address any small pockets of cancer cells that may still be present in the body. At this point, the family became doubtful, and, based on all that they had learned, were hesitant to start such an invasive and harmful treatment, especially when considering the possibility that the cancer had been fully removed with the surgical procedure. Given her strong reservations, the oncologist agreed that it was fine to not pursue chemotherapy. The family saw this to be the best possible outcome. With this being settled, the family began exploring other potential measures that they could take to best protect this patient's health.

It was at this point, a month after surgery, that SJ began the alternative protocol that would now become their primary approach to maintaining her long-term health. On March 9, 2023, she began a regimen that included ivermectin at 6–12 mg three days per week, as well as quercetin, twice daily. This combination was easily accessible, and was readily available, given that quercetin, is also another over-the-counter remedy.

Then, in April 2023, SJ was able to add fenbendazole into the treatment protocol. They transitioned away from the initial treatments with quercetin and ivermectin, and instead, relied on fenbendazole, as well as the other remedies as part of a comprehensive approach. Their overall approach to health was becoming more fully realized.

In addition to her previous supplements, she began taking on a daily basis:

1. Turmeric Root Extract at 600 mg twice daily.
2. Berberine 500 mg twice daily.
3. Quercetin 500 mg twice daily.
4. FenBen Labs brand fenbendazole at 222 mg once daily.

When asked about it, SJ noted that they were careful to take the fenbendazole and ivermectin a few hours apart from the dose of quercetin, as they learned from the medical community that there was a potential that those medications would have some interactions that would reduce their efficacy.

Also in April, SJ transitioned away from the previously used supplements and, instead, added Pathway 2, as prescribed by the company Ultra Botanica, while continuing to take the berberine. It was after using these medications that there was a notable improvement in SJ's overall condition.

Starting in July 2023, SJ also added back ivermectin to her regimen, using a dose of 6–12 mg twice per week for several months, in addition to her other daily medications, highlighting her overall commitment to this alternative therapeutic approach.

On August 17, 2023, new tests showed that everything looked good and the treatment has worked. SJ takes only quercetin and fenbendazole every day. During her course of treatment, it was also noted that berberine was stopped due to the potential for a blood-thinning effect, and turmeric was also briefly stopped.

To better understand her situation, SJ was also asked more questions and provided the following additional details:

- **Age, Weight, Sex:** The patient is a seventy-year-old female, and her weight was 70 kg (154 pounds), with a height of 158 centimeters.
- **Cancer Type:** The diagnosis was "Sigmoid colon cancer, stage II; well-differentiated adenocarcinoma of the colon mucosa," measuring 10mm x 40mm.
- **Physician Prognosis:** She also shared that the first surgeon, who performed the emergency surgery, had a very poor prognosis for this patient. The surgeon "thought that there were metastasis to kidneys, and did not give more than 3 weeks of prognosis," clearly highlighting the dire circumstances and that, from their viewpoint, the situation was very grim, and she was close to death. Thankfully, a surgeon from a different city removed tumor and surrounding lymph nodes (February 10, 2023) to prevent future metastasis, and, while he did not provide any prognosis, had recommended at least a few chemotherapy treatments. However, after evaluation, their oncologist stated they "would not advise or force patient to do chemo against their wishes," stating that she "decided there are fewer risks with this path vs. chemotherapy," which was seen as nothing but harmful with nothing good to come of it.
- **Treatment Timing:** As of March 9, 2023 (approximately one month after surgery to remove the tumor), she began treatment with ivermectin, as well as with quercetin. Starting in March, approximately a few weeks after the surgery, she then added the fenbendazole into the treatment regimen.
- **Current Treatment Plan:** She currently continues to take a regimen that includes a single dose of 222 mg fenbendazole every day.

SJ was also asked about the impact that this treatment had, what the diagnostics had reported, and how she felt overall. She replied that these tests "are needed for the next round of reconstructive surgery to remove/close stoma and remove gall bladder; then another surgery is needed to fix an abdominal hernia."

With those test results in hand, her health team reported:

"CT scan on Aug. 17, 2023 was clear and colonoscopy on Sept. 26, 2023 had no findings." The data showed that her cancer was resolved after approximately six months on these medications. There were further recommendations to deal with related issues, but there was no longer a focus on further treating or eliminating cancer. These results highlight the success of the therapies that were utilized.

Regarding the communication between the family and the medical team, SJ elected not to share information regarding the use of fenbendazole. As SJ reported, "No, since we know their opinion already." This is a statement that summarizes one of the ongoing challenges with using alternative approaches to care, as there is often resistance from the established medical community.

Perhaps most tellingly was a quote from another, previous, patient at this hospital, in similar circumstances, who simply shook his head "no" to advise their family member of not doing chemotherapy. He stated that "he has seen a male patient, who did well with the surgery, was on his way to recovery, then did a few rounds of chemotherapy, and did not live more than 10+ months after." The medical team was seen, therefore, as only able to offer harmful treatments, so it became clear that they were in the best place, using the approaches that the patient felt most comfortable with.

During this experience, SJ noted that it "is good some people have courage to speak and share their experiences." She has also noted that when they tell others about the positive benefits of fenbendazole, they tend to not believe her. She has also found that many of those who are already on chemotherapy will not consider any other approach to treatment.

What is striking from this case are the rapid and very positive effects that occurred with the use of fenbendazole and ivermectin. To emphasize, this individual elected to treat their own colorectal cancer, rather than receive a standard chemotherapy regimen. With the success of ivermectin and fenbendazole, we can now see the impact a two-pronged attack has on the growth of cancer cells, and these may require more studies to analyze the interaction of the various medications on tumor cell dynamics, in order to better refine these methods.

Finally, it should also be noted that conventional chemotherapy was not used by SJ to achieve remission. She also noted that she had no discernable side effects from either ivermectin or fenbendazole.

CASE REPORT 13: NON-SMALL CELL LUNG CANCER (NSCLC), STAGE 4, AGE FIFTY-FOUR, FEMALE

Positive Experience with Concurrent Fenbendazole and Pembrolizumab for Metastatic Non-Small Cell Lung Cancer

This case report concerns a fifty-four-year-old female KC, 5'8", 145 pounds, diagnosed with adenocarcinoma, non-small cell lung cancer (NSCLC) with metastatic spread to liver. She was diagnosed in early 2024 and was given a prognosis of one or two years if she did not do any treatment. KC opted for immunotherapy along with self-treatment with fenbendazole. She initiated treatment with pembrolizumab (an immunotherapy agent). Concurrently, KC began self-administering fenbendazole (222 mg for four consecutive days followed by three days off). Fenbendazole was taken with a "fatty snack" (including either olive oil, butter, yogurt, or peanut butter) to enhance absorption. KC also reported taking ivermectin intermittently, "if I and when I could get my hands on some I take it, usually 12 mg tablets," also consumed with a fatty snack.

No other cancer treatments were reported before starting pembrolizumab and the concurrent fenbendazole protocol.

KC first noticed an effect attributed to the regimen after approximately six months of concurrent pembrolizumab and fenbendazole use. KC felt better overall, less pressure in chest. KC reported that pulmonary tumors shrank and liver tumors were absent.

Diagnostic tests, PET, CT, or MRI results confirming shrinkage were used to observe the tumor shrinkage and resolution of hepatic tumors.

Other than fatigue, KC reported experiencing no noticeable side effects that they could attribute specifically to fenbendazole.

Like many of the others in these case reports, KC stated they did not inform her treating physician about the use of fenbendazole. KC reports continuing the fenbendazole regimen, alongside ongoing pembrolizumab therapy.

KC reported not receiving any COVID-19 vaccinations or boosters prior to the cancer diagnosis.

KC encourages others to consider fenbendazole "Give it a go, it's safe."

When sharing her experience with others regarding fenbendazole, KC reports encountering reactions ranging from mild interest to disbelief. "They think I'm nuts."

This case report describes a fifty-four-year-old female with metastatic NSCLC who experienced tumor shrinkage at approximately six months while receiving standard-of-care immunotherapy (pembrolizumab) concurrently with a self-administered, off-label regimen including fenbendazole and intermittent ivermectin. Her six-month incomplete response compared to other case reports described here may be due to underdosing of fenbendazole as many others used more aggressive dosing protocols compared to KC's, four days of one 222 mg dose, followed by three days of no fenbendazole.

KC attributes the positive outcome, in large part, to the fenbendazole regimen. However, a critical confounding factor is the simultaneous use of pembrolizumab, an established immunotherapy agent known to induce significant tumor responses and improve survival in a subset of patients with NSCLC. It is impossible to isolate the effect of fenbendazole (or ivermectin) from the known therapeutic effects of pembrolizumab in this scenario, however there may have been synergistic effects as commented on in earlier chapters.

On May 3, 2025, her response to a follow-up inquiry regarding her present state of health was, "I'm good thanks. I feel great! I have no new updates."

CASE REPORT 14: AMELANOTIC MELANOMA, AGE SIXTY-EIGHT, MALE

This case report details the experience of a sixty-eight-year-old, health-conscious male, BK, of European descent with a significant family history of heart disease, though he himself has managed his cardiac health well (nine stents, quadruple bypass in 2008, no issues for over five years) through a vegan lifestyle, regular exercise, and supplementation. He is currently on no prescribed medications except baby aspirin.

In the summer of 2023, BK noticed a persistent red pimple on his forehead, which was subsequently diagnosed as Amelanotic Melanoma (4.2mm thick, Clark Level V). Concurrently, BK had squamous cell carcinoma spots on his right arm and a spot on his chest.

Upon diagnosis, and prior to surgery for the melanoma, BK commenced self-treatment with oral fenbendazole (222 mg daily, starting around November 10, 2023) and topical ivermectin paste on the skin lesions. He did not disclose the fenbendazole use to his medical team.

In December 2023, BK underwent wide excision surgery for the forehead melanoma and a biopsy of seven lymph nodes. The surgical margins were clear, and all lymph nodes were negative for cancer. A previously excised spot on his chest also returned a negative biopsy.

Following the successful melanoma surgery, oncologists recommended radiation therapy as a precautionary measure, which BK declined. A PET scan in early February 2024 showed no new areas of concern, apart from the known squamous lesion on his arm.

As of August 2024, BK continues to manage the SCC on his upper right arm with oral fenbendazole, topical ivermectin, and additional supplements including quercetin, nigella sativa (black seed oil), and soursop tea, alongside sensible sunlight exposure. He reports the squamous cell carcinoma has not worsened but has not resolved. BK remains steadfast in his decision to refuse radiation and is skeptical of conventional treatments for his arm squamous cell carcinoma, preferring his alternative regimen.

CASE REPORT 15: HER2-/+ BREAST CANCER, AGE FORTY-SIX

Triumph over Breast Cancer Using Fenbendazole, No Traditional Treatments

This report chronicles the decisive and successful journey of JD, who, upon receiving a diagnosis of stage 1 HER2 negative breast cancer on September 11, 2023, resolutely chose a natural healing path. This decision was powerfully informed by prior experience, including the loss of her mother to lung cancer treated conventionally and her own history with misdiagnosed symptoms, fortifying her conviction in alternative methodologies.

Inspired by a holistic nurse practitioner (NPR) within her church community—who herself had conquered a similar, stage 2b cancer naturally— JD immediately embarked on a comprehensive natural protocol. Initially, in mid-September 2023, she commenced with 222 mg of fenbendazole for three days, followed by three days of ivermectin (12 mg), repeating this cycle for two weeks. Subsequently, under her NPR's guidance, the fenbendazole dosage was systematically escalated to a target of 2000 mg daily. This was meticulously administered by dividing the powdered and ground tablet forms into three equal parts, mixed with high-quality olive oil, and consumed throughout the day.

Concurrently, a strategic suite of supplements was integrated to optimize cellular health and support the body's innate healing capacities. This included nano minerals, magnesium, potassium, Relyte minerals, and Pico Silver (a nano silver) to bolster mitochondrial function. Liver support was provided through liver nutrients and TUDCA, alongside iodine. Furthermore, commencing in October 2023, JD proactively incorporated regular electric lymph node treatments to enhance detoxification and immune response.

In February 2024, the protocol was further refined with the addition of THC-free CBD oil, chosen for its potential to synergize with fenbendazole and enhance its efficacy. Throughout this period, JD committed to significant dietary modifications, which contributed to a notable twenty-five-pound weight loss and a profound improvement in overall well-being.

Eight months later, in May 2024, a 3-D topography scan revealed the complete resolution of the cancer. JD reports feeling the best she has in years, a testament not only to the eradication of the disease but also to the holistic revitalization achieved through her protocol. This outcome stands in stark contrast to the initial conventional prognosis, which offered only a 50–60 percent chance of survival and cautioned that her specific cancer type often demonstrates limited responsiveness to chemotherapy over time.

JD expresses immense gratitude for the individuals who guided her toward this natural approach, affirming her love for the journey and the empowerment that came with her choice. She remains unwavering in her commitment to this protocol, planning to continue it for another six months to a year, eventually tapering the fenbendazole to a maintenance dose for ongoing cancer and parasite prevention.

Case Summary

This report details the case of a woman diagnosed with stage 1 HER2 negative breast cancer in September 2023 who, driven by personal conviction and prior experiences, elected a comprehensive natural treatment regimen. This protocol, centered on a progressive fenbendazole dosage reaching 2000 mg daily, was augmented by targeted supplementation (including nano minerals, silver, CBD oil, and liver support), dietary modifications, and electric lymph node treatments. Eight months post-diagnosis, in May 2024, a 3-D topography scan demonstrated complete cancer resolution, an outcome JD confidently attributes to her chosen natural healing journey. She reports a significant enhancement in her overall well-being.

CASE REPORT 16: STAGE 4 NRAS-VARIANT METASTATIC MELANOMA, AGE SIXTY-NINE, MALE

Complete Response to Fenbendazole and Subsequent Immunotherapy

This report details the case of a sixty-nine-year-old male, PC, with a thirty-five-year history of surgically managed malignant melanomas. Eighteen months prior to his metastatic diagnosis, a lesion on his leg was reportedly missed, leading to widespread disease. In January 2023, he was diagnosed with stage 4 metastatic melanoma involving the clavicle, aorta, abdomen, leg, mediastinal lymph nodes, and a suspicious brain lesion. PC initiated treatment with fenbendazole (222 mg once per day). Over the following months, imaging showed significant resolution of several metastatic sites, though some activity persisted. After a transient elevation in liver enzymes that normalized with continued fenbendazole use (and a dose increase to 444 mg per day in June 2024), he achieved a further reduction in tumor activity. Immunotherapy (nivolumab/relatlimab) was subsequently introduced. Despite experiencing immunotherapy-related colitis, follow-up scans in January 2025 indicated a complete metabolic response. As of May 2025, PC remains cancer-free and in good health.

PC is feeling well (a box of birds, according to his wife), active (gym, swimming), and has been cancer-free for approximately seven or eight months. Immunotherapy-related side effects have resolved.

This case report describes a sixty-nine-year-old male with a history of malignant melanoma who developed stage 4 metastatic disease. He initiated treatment with fenbendazole, an anthelmintic agent with purported anticancer properties, and demonstrated a significant partial response over approximately 1.5 years, with resolution of several metastatic sites and reduction in activity of others. Subsequently, combination immunotherapy (nivolumab/relatlimab) was introduced, and PC achieved a complete metabolic response. He remains disease-free as of May 2025, though he experienced significant immunotherapy-related gastrointestinal toxicity that has since resolved.

Potential Synergistic Effects of Fenbendazole with Immunotherapy

The substantial tumor reduction achieved with fenbendazole monotherapy prior to immunotherapy is noteworthy. Fenbendazole exerts its anticancer effects through mechanisms like microtubule disruption, glucose metabolism interference, and p53 stabilization. It is plausible that by reducing tumor burden and potentially altering the tumor microenvironment (e.g., by inducing immunogenic cell death and exposing tumor neoantigens), fenbendazole may have "primed" the remaining tumor, making it more susceptible to the effects of checkpoint inhibitors like nivolumab and relatlimab. Immunotherapies rely on a functioning immune system and the presence of recognizable tumor antigens. A reduced, less aggressive tumor mass might allow for a more effective immune response when checkpoint inhibition is applied. Fenbendazole, by potentially increasing tumor cell stress and death, could enhance the presentation of antigens to the immune system, thereby potentiating the action of immunotherapy. On the other hand, tumor resolution was largely achieved before starting immunotherapy, indicating that fenbendazole did the heavy lifting in this instance. Finally, it is important to exercise caution with immunotherapy, as its potent activation of the immune system can lead to severe immune-related adverse events, as seen with PC's gastrointestinal distress.

Transient Elevation of Liver Enzymes with Fenbendazole

PC experienced a transient elevation in ALT and AST liver enzymes, which normalized despite continued (and even increased from 222 mg to 444 mg per day) fenbendazole use. This phenomenon has been anecdotally reported in many of the other case reports, either explicitly noted or relayed privately. One hypothesis is that as fenbendazole exerts its cytotoxic effects on cancer cells, the resulting cell death and breakdown products place an increased metabolic load on the liver, which is responsible for detoxification and clearance. This increased workload could manifest as a temporary elevation in liver enzymes. The subsequent normalization of these enzymes, even with ongoing fenbendazole treatment, coincided with a further reduction in tumor burden in this case. This observation supports the idea that the elevation might be related to the liver processing by-products of tumor lysis rather than any direct hepatotoxicity from fenbendazole at these doses, especially since the enzymes returned to normal limits as the overall disease responded to treatment. Further research is needed to substantiate this hypothesis and to clearly differentiate between transient, tumor-lysis-related enzyme elevations and potential transient drug-induced alterations in liver function.

CASE REPORT 17: TRIPLE-NEGATIVE BREAST CANCER, AGE SIXTY-FIVE

Registered Nurse's Triumph over Incurable Triple-Negative Breast Cancer Utilizing an Integrative Approach

TR is a registered nurse with firsthand experience of both the conventional medical system and the profound potential of patient-driven, integrative care. This report details her journey navigating a diagnosis of triple-negative breast cancer (TNBC), a path TR chose to walk with a blend of mandated oncological treatments and a robust, self-researched complementary regimen.

The morning of May 23, 2023, was a seismic shock: TR awoke to a distinct, hard, chicken cutlet–sized mass in her right breast. Having previously endured a hysterectomy for a melon-sized uterine tumor and the subsequent years of debilitating side effects from internal and external radiation—chronic diarrhea, pervasive weakness, and internal atrophy—TR was no stranger to the body's capacity for disease, nor to the harsh realities of conventional treatments. That prior experience, where TR felt vulnerable and followed traditional advice to her detriment, fortified her resolve to approach this new challenge with greater agency and a broader perspective.

TR's diagnosis was confirmed: triple-negative breast cancer. Scans and biopsies identified five distinct masses, with six biopsies returning malignant. The oncological team was unequivocal: infusions of chemotherapy and immunotherapy were the sole recommended path, and they strongly advised against any supplements or non-prescribed drugs, citing potential interference. TR understood their position, yet she made a calculated decision. TR would undergo their prescribed infusions, but she would not relinquish her autonomy or the potential benefits of a meticulously researched integrative strategy. TR chose to discreetly incorporate a comprehensive protocol.

TR's self-directed adjunctive therapies commenced immediately alongside the conventional treatments and included:

- Fenbendazole (222 mg daily)
- Ivermectin equine paste
- Mebendazole (100 mg daily)
- Astaxanthin (Valasta)
- Methylene blue drops
- Bitter apricot seeds
- Red light therapy (NIR LED, twice weekly)

Further bolstering this, TR consulted a functional MD—a former surgeon and also a pharmacist—who understood the multifaceted mechanisms of repurposed drugs. He additionally prescribed:

- Metformin ER (500 mg daily)
- Sildenafil (20 mg, 3x daily)
- Melatonin (10 mg daily)
- Naltrexone (4.5 mg daily)

For six arduous months, TR endured a regimen of four chemotherapy drugs and Keytruda infusions. The side effects were severe, impacting nearly every facet of her well-being, short of mortality. Upon completion of this six-month cycle, TR ceased the conventional infusions. She continued her entire supplementary and repurposed medication protocol, alongside daily bone broth, comprehensive vitamins, minerals, and additional vitamin D.

The transformation was palpable. After six months TR could no longer detect any lumps in her breast. As a courtesy, she attended a final appointment with her surgical oncologist. Her examination of her right breast yielded nothing. In a telling moment, she even asked to examine TR's left breast, seemingly unsure which side had harbored the extensive cancer. When pressed for a comment, the oncologist conceded the results were "very impressive." Yet, her immediate follow-up was to discuss surgical options, while also stating she had never witnessed such a complete response to chemotherapeutic drugs and Keytruda in TNBC. TR found her lack of inquiry into her adjunctive treatments and her adherence to a rigid protocol deeply disheartening.

Today, TR is thriving. Her blood work is optimal, and her cancer markers are negative. She continues her full regimen of supplements and repurposed medications, including daily fenbendazole. She is no longer perceived as a "cancer patient" by herself and others. TR's experience has solidified her belief in a holistic approach: a positive mindset, a nourishing diet, a supportive environment, strong faith, and, well-researched, intelligently applied treatments that extend beyond the conventional.

This case details the experience of TR, a registered nurse, who, following a diagnosis of multifocal triple-negative breast cancer in May 2023, undertook a conventional six-month course of chemotherapy and Keytruda. Concurrently, and with conviction born from prior negative experiences with standard treatments, she implemented a comprehensive integrative protocol including fenbendazole, other anthelmintics, supplements, and repurposed medications.

Upon cessation of conventional therapy, she achieved a complete clinical and biochemical remission. Her oncologist acknowledged the "very impressive" outcome, noting its rarity for TNBC treated with chemotherapy and Keytruda alone, which strongly suggests that adjunctive therapies, potentially with fenbendazole playing a key synergistic role, may significantly enhance the efficacy of traditional oncological treatments, leading to outcomes not typically observed.

CASE REPORT 18: GLIOBLASTOMA MULTIFORME, AGE SIXTY-ONE, MALE

This report details the extraordinary journey of SM, a sixty-one-year-old male, as reported by his sister MM, a patient who defied the typically grim death sentence prognosis of glioblastoma multiforme through a combination of conventional and determined, patient-led adjunctive therapies, most critical of which was fenbendazole.

Timeline of Diagnoses, Treatments, and Outcomes

February 1, 2023: SM received the diagnosis of glioblastoma multiforme. Comprehensive imaging, including PET, CT, and MRI scans, painted a clear, albeit bleak, picture. This diagnosis was unequivocally confirmed by biopsy of resected tissue following an urgent neurosurgical intervention aimed at debulking the tumor mass—a procedure carefully balanced to maximize tumor removal while preserving vital neurological function. SM then embarked on the standard-of-care pathway, which included chemotherapy with Avastin (bevacizumab) and a rigorous course of radiation treatments.

September 7, 2023: A Formidable Resurgence

Despite aggressive conventional treatment, the glioblastoma multiforme returned with alarming ferocity. Imaging revealed the cancer had "cauliflowered," spreading insidiously throughout his brain. The clinical impact was severe: SM lost the use of his left side, rendering him unable to perform basic self-care activities such as dressing himself. The prognosis, at this juncture, was exceptionally poor.

September 14, 2023: A Bold New Direction, Fenbendazole to the Rescue

Faced with a seemingly insurmountable challenge, SM and his support system made a pivotal decision. He began a daily regimen of 1000 mg of fenbendazole paste, cycled twenty-five days on and five days off. This was complemented by a carefully selected suite of supplements:

- Tagamet (cimetidine): 600 mg twice per day
- AHCC (mushroom derivatives): 500 mg three times per day
- Curcumin: 400 mg three times per day
- Annatto: 300 mg three times per day

SM continued to receive Avastin (zerobev) concurrently.

October 18, 2023: A Stunning Reversal Just Thirty-Four Days Later

A mere month after initiating the fenbendazole-centric protocol, an MRI delivered astonishing news. All new tumor manifestations had vanished, and the established, original tumor mass was visibly necrosing—dying from the inside out. This rapid and profound response strongly indicated that the adjunctive therapies, particularly fenbendazole, were having a decisive impact, effectively reversing the aggressive disease progression within weeks.

December 2023: Reinforcing the Arsenal

Buoyed by these incredible results, SM further augmented his regimen with the addition of ivermectin. He steadfastly maintained his fenbendazole and supplemental protocol.

December 2024: Defying All Expectations

Fast-forward to one year later, SM's treating oncologist, thoroughly astounded by the sustained and dramatic improvement, declared him "cancer-free for all intents and purposes." This assessment was particularly remarkable given that the oncologist acknowledged the conventional chemotherapy SM had received would typically have left a patient in his situation severely debilitated, unable to be left alone, and certainly not capable of independent living.

In stark contrast, SM was not merely surviving; he was thriving—driving, hunting, fishing, gardening, and actively making precious memories, basically living his normal life. His vitality stood as a testament to a recovery that can only be described as miraculous. SM and his support network attribute this outcome to divine intervention, coupled with their proactive use of fenbendazole.

May 8, 2025: Official Confirmation of Remission

SM was officially pronounced "for all intents and purposes" cancer-free, solidifying his extraordinary outcome.

Upon revealing his full adjunctive treatment regimen to his oncologist, the physician was quiet. When presented with a scientific paper with the title concerning mebendazole (a similar benzimidazole anthelmintic) and brain cancers by the family, the oncologist became notably reserved upon seeing the word "mebendazole." When asked about him prescribing mebendazole, he declined, citing the electronic prescribing system, which was interpreted as an inability or unwillingness to prescribe a non-standard-of-care treatment. Most importantly, SM's oncologist admitted, "He's never had a success story like SM's and has never been able to do a referral for another surgery or treatment because the cancer is so aggressive." This statement underscores the grim reality that, typically, his glioblastoma multiforme patients succumbed to the disease so rapidly that further interventions were not afforded the opportunity. SM began his brain cancer journey alongside approximately fifty other individuals facing the same diagnosis; he is the sole survivor of that group.

In our discussions with MM we asked her how her brother initially reacted to her suggestion of incorporating fenbendazole into his treatment. She said, "He's a country boy that thought I was an idiot for asking him to take dog dewormer for brain cancer, until he was like, "I have nothing to lose—I'll be dead in a month." It does sound insane unless you've read documentation and read the testimonies, but here we are, one of those success stories!" MM said.

Finally, MM commented, "I don't envy the position you are in because so many people are crying out for help. It's heartbreaking. I thank you for putting the information out there for us to decipher and choose for ourselves. I think my brother has helped six more people become cancer-free now because of his story. Thank you from the bottom of my heart."

SM was diagnosed with glioblastoma multiforme in February 2023, undergoing surgery, Avastin, and radiation. Following an aggressive recurrence in September 2023 that left him significantly impaired, he initiated a daily regimen of 1,000 mg fenbendazole, cimetidine, AHCC, curcumin, and annatto, while continuing Avastin. Astonishingly, an MRI just one month later, in October 2023, showed all new tumors gone and the original tumor dying. Ivermectin was added in December 2023. By December 2024, his oncologist declared him essentially cancer-free, a status officially affirmed in May 2025. Throughout this period, SM maintained an excellent quality of life, a profound deviation from the expected trajectory of glioblastoma multiforme.

Glioblastoma multiforme carries a notoriously dismal prognosis. It is the most common and aggressive primary malignant brain tumor in adults. Even with multimodal standard-of-care treatment—typically involving surgical resection, followed by concurrent radiation therapy and chemotherapy (temozolomide, though Avastin is used in recurrence). Recurrence is virtually inevitable and often rapid, with subsequent treatments offering diminishing returns.

SM's experience of being alive, thriving, and deemed "cancer-free for all intents and purposes" nearly two years post-diagnosis, especially after a severe, function-impairing recurrence, is exceptionally rare. Survival beyond two years is uncommon, and achieving a state of no detectable disease with such a high quality of life after such aggressive recurrence falls into the category of an outlier event within the established medical understanding of glioblastoma multiforme. The vast majority of patients, sadly, do not survive this long, nor do they maintain the ability to drive, hunt, and garden. The oncologist's candid admission of never having a comparable success story and the tragic fate of SM's initial patient cohort powerfully contextualize the rarity of this outcome. The dramatic and rapid tumor regression observed one month after the introduction of fenbendazole presents a compelling temporal correlation that warrants serious consideration.

Glioblastoma multiforme was present before fenbendazole introduction despite traditional standard-of-care treatments. Glioblastoma multiforme was eradicated thirty-four days after introduction of 1000 mg fenbendazole per day.

Finally, thank you to MM for her heartwarming comments. SM and MM are spreading their knowledge and paying their gratitude forward by spreading the word about fenbendazole and cancer to others. Based on personal experience, the gratification received when someone tells us that fenbendazole cured their cancer is beyond words. You have to give that knowledge to receive the gift of that profound experience, and it truly is a gift, as you will never be the same again.

CASE REPORT 19: BLADDER CANCER, AGE SEVENTY-FOUR, FEMALE.

Five Weeks of Fenbendazole Eradicates Bladder Cancer

In September 2021, TS, a seventy-four-year-old woman, was confronted with a diagnosis of bladder cancer. This determination followed six months of persistent urinary tract infections, which ultimately led to the discovery of a tumor, subsequently confirmed by biopsy. Her initial treatment phase was robust: a stent was placed to facilitate tumor removal without compromising the right kidney or bladder, followed by six weekly immunotherapeutic Bacillus Calmette-Guérin treatments administered in her urologist's office. This protocol, described as a new treatment with a high success rate for localized cancer, involved no chemotherapy and no radiation. While the stent surgery was particularly challenging, TS adhered to the treatment, even maintaining activities like yoga.

Following this initial intervention, TS embraced a proactive approach to her health. She immersed herself in anticancer diets, continued exercise, and focused on stress reduction. For nearly two years, regular quarterly cystoscopies delivered reassuring news: she remained cancer-free. No other cancer treatments were administered during this period.

However, on August 17, 2023, a routine cystoscopy revealed a new lesion—a visible spot on the monitor that signaled to both TS and her surgeon the cancer's return. Subsequent biopsies confirmed this recurrence.

This critical juncture marked a decisive shift in TS's approach. Dissatisfied with conventional options for the recurrence, she embarked on intensive personal research. Her investigation led her to information regarding fenbendazole, including accounts of its success in other cancer cases, such as a Joe Tippens story with lung cancer, and the *Fenbendazole Can Cure Cancer* Substack. Supported by friends adept at navigating medical journals, she explored the potential of antiparasitic compounds in oncology. Armed with this knowledge, near the end of August 2023, TS made a resolute decision: she commenced a self-directed protocol of fenbendazole, taking 444 mg daily. This became her singular, targeted anticancer intervention for the recurrence, pursued alongside her established anticancer diet. She sought no other conventional treatments.

The biopsy surgery for the newly identified lesion was performed on October 5, 2023. On that same day, TS, accompanied by a friend, received the pathology results. The findings were nothing short of extraordinary: There was no cancer. After approximately five weeks of exclusively using fenbendazole as her active anticancer agent, the malignancy had vanished. Her surgeon was visibly stunned, admitting that the negative result was so unexpected he had requested the lab repeat the tests, as he had personally seen the lesion. TS then shared her regimen: the fenbendazole, alongside Chinese mushrooms (which she had also incorporated), her anticancer diet, and steadfast prayer. Her physician, trained in Western medicine, acknowledged her experience and supported her continuation of what she believed brought her comfort.

TS's proactive journey continues. A follow-up checkup in January 2025 confirmed her ongoing cancer-free status. She has since adjusted her fenbendazole intake to a maintenance schedule of three days on, four days off for ten weeks, then off for ten weeks. Then back to three days on/four days off. TS remains committed to her informed health choices, including specific supplements like lion's mane and high-dose vitamin D + K. She proudly notes her avoidance of various vaccines and her continued good health, having never contracted COVID-19. Her cardiologist, who was not involved in her cancer treatment, impressed by her research and outcome, encouraged her to share her compelling story. TS has indeed shared her knowledge, inspiring others, some of whom have also reported positive outcomes against their own cancers.

Timeline of Events, Diagnoses, Treatments and Outcomes

- **September 2021:** TS diagnosed with bladder cancer.
- **Late 2021:** Underwent stent placement, tumor removal, and six weekly BCG treatments. No chemotherapy or radiation.
- **2021–August 2023:** Remained cancer-free for almost two years, monitored by regular cystoscopies.
- **August 17, 2023:** Recurrence of bladder cancer detected via cystoscopy; biopsies confirmed cancer.
- **Late August 2023:** TS initiated a daily 444 mg fenbendazole protocol as her sole active anticancer treatment for the recurrence.
- **October 5, 2023:** Biopsy results following surgical removal of the lesion site showed no cancer. This remarkable cancer-free status was achieved approximately five weeks after starting fenbendazole.
- January 2025: Follow-up checkup confirmed: no cancer.

This case report documents the compelling experience of TS, a seventy-four-year-old woman who, after a confirmed recurrence of bladder cancer, chose a singular, unconventional therapeutic path. Relying solely on a daily regimen of

444 mg of fenbendazole as her active anticancer agent, alongside her existing anticancer diet, TS achieved a cancer-free diagnosis within a remarkably brief time frame of approximately five weeks. This outcome, which astonished her medical team, has been sustained, with follow-up checks confirming her continued remission. Her journey underscores a profound personal conviction and highlights the extraordinary result observed with fenbendazole as the exclusive targeted intervention against her cancer recurrence. TS had some parting advice, "You have to keep doing your own research and you keep telling your story, like I am. There have been many people I have shared knowledge of fenbendazole with. Some followed the information and have been cleared of their cancers; one from stage 4 throat cancer, another from terminal thyroid cancer, and have passed the information to some cancer support groups. Unfortunately a lot of other people I know with cancer weren't so receptive, they continued with chemo, radiation, and they are all gone."

CASE REPORT 20: METASTATIC PROSTATE CANCER, LIVER AND LYMPH NODE METASTASES, AGE SEVENTY-FOUR, MALE.

A Resounding Reversal: Metastatic Prostate Cancer Vanquished with Fenbendazole

This is the account of a seventy-four-year-old man, 6', 169 pounds, who faced a dire prognosis of terminal, metastatic prostate cancer but charted an unconventional path to remarkable recovery, primarily through the determined use of fenbendazole. His journey told by his daughter, TW, underscores a powerful testament to individual agency in the face of seemingly insurmountable odds.

The Onset of Crisis: A Timeline of Decline

TW's dad's battle with prostate cancer began in 2019, a diagnosis initially met with surgical removal of the prostate and an "all clear." However, the reprieve was short-lived. The timeline of his relapse and subsequent crisis unfolded rapidly in 2024:

- **Early August 2024:** Routine blood work delivered alarming news—a PSA of 14.
- **Mid-August 2024:** The situation escalated dramatically. His PSA soared to 51, and a subsequent PET scan revealed the devastating spread: metastases to his liver and lymph nodes.
- **Late August 2024:** Biopsies of both the liver and lymph nodes unequivocally confirmed the recurrence of prostate cancer.

The diagnosis from his oncologist at a leading cancer center (MDA) was grim: stage 4 metastatic prostate cancer. He was informed that his liver was "completely consumed" and that medical intervention could offer nothing beyond palliative care. The proposed conventional treatment plan comprised hormone therapy (Lupron) followed by chemotherapy, with a stark prognosis of twelve to eighteen months of life remaining.

A Divergent Path: Embracing Fenbendazole

Faced with this bleak outlook, TW's dad made a pivotal decision. In September 2024, he received the initial Lupron shot as prescribed. However, during this consultation, he inquired about the fenbendazole protocol. His MDA oncologist unequivocally stated that if he chose to pursue fenbendazole, he could no longer be seen as a patient. Despite outwardly agreeing to forgo it, TW's dad, resolute in his conviction, returned home and immediately initiated the fenbendazole protocol, choosing not to inform his oncologist.

His self-directed fenbendazole regimen commenced in late August 2024. He began with 222 mg of fenbendazole (from Panacur C powder, meticulously weighed) once daily for seven days, quickly increasing to 222 mg twice daily (total 444 mg fenbendazole per day), taken after breakfast and dinner with peanut butter to aid absorption.

While fenbendazole was the central therapeutic agent, he adopted a comprehensive adjunctive strategy: a ketogenic diet (resulting in a thirty-pound weight loss in three months), daily ivermectin (an eraser-sized amount of horse paste), vitamin D, serrapeptase, soursop tea, TUDCA, lion's mane, Onco Pathways 1–4 from UltraBotanica, high-dose intravenous vitamin C (50–75 grams, three times a week), and monthly three-day fasts (water and bone broth only). Lupron remained the only conventional medical treatment he had received.

The effects of fenbendazole were felt almost immediately. Any existing pain and discomfort abated rapidly upon starting the fenbendazole, a profound and immediate improvement in his quality of life. Despite the grave diagnosis, TW's dad reported feeling remarkably well throughout this period, never experiencing the debilitating symptoms often associated with advanced cancer.

The true measure of fenbendazole's efficacy became undeniably clear within three months.

- Early November 2024: A follow-up appointment at MDA, initially intended to plan for chemotherapy, delivered astonishing news. A PET scan revealed a 50 percent reduction in all tumors. His oncologist was, by report, "shocked."
- Blood work corroborated this stunning reversal: his PSA, which had peaked at 51 in mid-August, had plummeted to just 2 by early November 2024.
- The chemotherapy scheduled for that very day was promptly canceled in light of these profoundly positive results.

TW's dad continues his fenbendazole regimen (222 mg twice daily, seven days a week) and the supportive protocols. He proactively monitors his liver enzymes (AST/ALT) through independent lab work, as these showed elevation on two occasions initially after starting fenbendazole. There were no adverse side effects attributed to fenbendazole. TW's dad has not, and will not, disclose his fenbendazole use to his MDA oncologist.

His daughter, TW, reported a further update from a follow-up visit at MDA on January 7, 2025: his cancer showed an additional 50 percent decrease from the November scan. This marked a total 75 percent reduction in all tumors within just five months (August 2024 to January 2025) of commencing the fenbendazole-centric protocol. As of May 2025 there is no evidence of disease as confirmed by PET/CT scans.

TW's dad speculates his cancer may have been linked to a diet high in sugar, processed foods, and carbohydrates, and potentially to COVID-19 vaccinations (two shots and one booster). When sharing his experience, reactions range from surprise and intrigue, with many requesting his protocol for loved ones, to indignation that such a potentially effective and accessible option is not offered by mainstream oncology.

This case documents the extraordinary turnaround of a seventy-four-year-old male diagnosed in August 2024 with stage 4 metastatic prostate cancer, with extensive liver and lymph node involvement, and given a palliative prognosis of twelve to eighteen months. Forsaking further conventional treatment beyond an initial Lupron injection, he independently initiated a daily regimen of fenbendazole (444 mg total). He experienced an immediate abatement of all pain and discomfort. Within a mere three months, his PSA plummeted from 51 to 2, and imaging confirmed a 50 percent reduction in all tumors, leading to the cancellation of planned chemotherapy. After five months on fenbendazole, his total tumor burden had decreased by an astounding 75 percent. This remarkable outcome, primarily attributed by TW's dad to fenbendazole, underscores the profound anticancer effects he experienced with fenbendazole.

There were no adverse side effects from fenbendazole. Liver enzymes ALT/AST did rise early on but the elevation was transient despite continued fenbendazole use, consistent with our earlier observations that AST/ALT transient elevations may serve as a marker of the effectiveness of fenbendazole in some people.

Finally, as has been reported in several of the other case reports, TW's dad did have two COVID vaccine shots and one booster. He also, like several of the other case reports, had radical surgery—prostatectomy—some five years earlier. The burning question is how are people with no prostate or breast tissue subsequently developing prostate or breast cancers some five, ten, or more years after surgery? Long-dormant cancer cells appear to be being released from immune system inhibition by some factor. That stimulus could be mRNA COVID shots.

CASE REPORT 21: METASTATIC SQUAMOUS CELL CANCER, AGE SEVENTY-SEVEN, FEMALE

Defying the Odds Against Metastatic Squamous Cell Carcinoma

SM is a seventy-seven-year-old, 5'4", 130-pound woman, and is living proof that a dire prognosis is not an insurmountable barrier. Her journey is one of resilience, research, and ultimately, a reclaiming of health against formidable odds.

On March 2021, SM was diagnosed with metastatic squamous cell carcinoma. Swollen lymph nodes on her left clavicle were confirmed malignant by a general surgeon's biopsy and further delineated by a PET scan. SM's oncologist delivered the verdict: four months to live. Curative treatment was off the table; only palliative care was offered.

Initially, SM submitted to conventional treatments. She underwent a course of chemotherapy, specifically cisplatin combined with Taxol. The side effects, compounded by the intense pain from the significantly enlarged lymph nodes, were debilitating. Consequently, nine rounds of radiation were administered in an attempt to alleviate these acute symptoms.

SM refused to be a passive recipient of a predetermined fate. Her quest for alternatives began with Dr. William Li's book on angiogenesis, which then led her to Jane McClelland's work on metabolic approaches to cancer. The pivotal moment came through a connection at church, where a fellow member introduced SM to fenbendazole. Armed with this information, she made a decisive move to start a daily regimen of 222 mg of fenbendazole, simply swallowing the granules with water. SM informed her oncologist of her self-directed treatment; while he did not endorse it, her conviction was unwavering.

The impact of the fenbendazole was undeniable and swift. Within a few months of starting fenbendazole, a palpable shrinkage of the lymph nodes occurred. By the six-month mark, the persistent pain that had plagued SM was entirely gone. The true turning point arrived in March 2022 when imaging confirmed she was cancer-free. This cancer-free status has been meticulously monitored and consistently reaffirmed by CT scans every four months since that date.

More recently, from the end of 2023 until December 2024, she incorporated Keytruda into her regimen "just to be sure" under the advice of her doctor, but SM has since discontinued it due to adverse side effects. SM's vigilance with fenbendazole continues, now adhering to a cycle of 222 mg daily for four days, followed by a three-day pause.

Importantly, throughout SM's fenbendazole treatment, she experienced no noticeable adverse side effects. SM's decision to take fenbendazole was met with skepticism by her medical team, who largely discounted its potential. When she shares her fenbendazole experience with others, their reaction is often one of shock, primarily due to her willingness to employ a therapy considered unregulated, or outside the box, for this indication.

As of this writing, SM continues fenbendazole 222 mg on a four-days-on, three-days-off cycle.

This case details the experience of a seventy-seven-year-old female diagnosed in March 2021 with metastatic squamous cell carcinoma and given a four-month prognosis. After conventional chemotherapy and radiation yielded significant side effects without curative intent, she independently initiated treatment with fenbendazole (222 mg daily). She reported lymph node shrinkage within months and pain resolution by six months, and achieved cancer-free status by March 2022, consistently confirmed by imaging. She continues a maintenance dose of fenbendazole and reports no side effects, having defied her initial prognosis of four months by several years so far.

CHAPTER 7

Fenbendazole Eradicates Nonmalignant Tumors and Growths

So far, we've shown how fenbendazole can destroy aggressive, deadly cancers that spread throughout the body and shut down vital organs. But fenbendazole's power doesn't stop there. It also proves effective against tumors and growths that, while not technically "malignant," can be just as destructive. We'll now turn our attention to case reports showing fenbendazole's success against these nonmalignant conditions.

Desmoid Tumors and Squamous Cell Carcinomas

According to the American Cancer Society, skin cancer is the most common cancer in the United States. Most of these are basal and squamous cell cancers, with about 5.4 million diagnosed each year. While these skin cancers are rarely fatal, they still pose a significant health problem.[1]

With skin cancer being so widespread, finding an effective treatment is critical. The evidence you're about to see shows that fenbendazole is a powerful weapon against these very cancers.

First, we'll look at a stunning case where fenbendazole destroyed a noncancerous but highly aggressive growth called a desmoid tumor, sometimes known as aggressive fibromatosis. Desmoid tumors are growths that appear in connective tissue like fat or deep layers of skin, most often in the abdomen, chest, arms, or legs.[2]

CASE REPORT: DESMOID TUMOR (AGGRESSIVE FIBROMATOSIS), AGE THIRTY-FOUR, MALE

Desmoid tumors are noncancerous growths that pop up in the body's connective tissue, primarily in the abdomen, arms, and legs. They are also known as aggressive fibromatosis.

The behavior of these tumors varies. Some grow slowly and may not require immediate treatment. Others grow rapidly, invading surrounding tissue like a true cancer, and require aggressive management like surgery, radiation, or chemotherapy.

A key distinction is that desmoid tumors are not malignant because they don't spread to distant parts of the body. However, their aggressive local growth can be just as destructive as cancer, invading nearby tissues and vital organs. Because they are so aggressive, oncologists are often the ones who treat them.

Fenbendazole Wipes Out Aggressive Tumor After All Standard Treatments Fail

The following case report documents the complete elimination of an aggressive desmoid tumor in a thirty-four-year-old man after every conventional cancer treatment had failed. This report is provided through the testimony of his wife, AS.

In 2017, AS's husband had surgery to remove a lipoma (a benign fatty tumor) from his left shoulder blade area. This is the exact spot where the desmoid tumor later appeared.

In April 2018, after an injury to his left shoulder, a new lump emerged in the same location. It is understood that physical trauma can trigger fibromatosis, which is an out-of-control growth of fibrous tissue, possibly as part of a faulty healing process.

By October 2018, an MRI and biopsy confirmed the diagnosis: fibromatosis. At the time, the tumor was a contained mass measuring 3 cm × 1.4 cm × 1.3 cm.

In November 2018, he had surgery to remove the tumor. The surgeon was confident he had gotten it all out, even removing an entire muscle from his shoulder. Despite this, he worked hard in rehabilitation and regained full use of his arm, amazing his doctors.

But by July 2019, the tumor was back. Doctors decided to just watch it with regular MRIs.

In January 2020, the tumor had more than doubled in size. He was started on a yearlong course of chemotherapy with sorafenib, a drug used for advanced cancers.

In November 2020, doctors tried cryoablation, a technique that freezes and kills tissue, at several spots on the tumor. By now, the tumor had become a monster, growing aggressively and invading his ribs (causing fractures), his chest wall, his scapula, and the lining of his lungs. The chemotherapy seemed to stop the tumor from growing larger, but it didn't shrink it at all. Even after multiple cryoablation sessions, the tumor only shrank modestly (from 16 cm x 6 cm x 3 cm to 5 cm x 3 cm x 5 cm) and remained a major threat. Worse, the final cryoablation procedure in March 2021 caused a severe nerve injury, leaving his left arm completely paralyzed.

By September 2021, an MRI showed the tumor had again grown to more than twice its size. This was the turning point. AS had learned about fenbendazole's potential in June 2021 when her dog, Moose, was diagnosed with lymphoma (his successful outcome is detailed in the next chapter).

In November 2021, AS's husband underwent another surgery, which only managed to partially remove the tumor. This was immediately followed by a month of radiation therapy.

He started taking fenbendazole at the same time he began radiation in November 2021. He took a daily dose of 222 mg of fenbendazole from the Happy Healing Store.

The results were stunning.

A follow-up MRI in May 2022 showed some enhancement in the area, but his medical team was confident it was just posttreatment inflammation and scarring.

By December 2022, a subsequent MRI showed only fluid collection, which is an expected side effect of radiation. There was no sign of the tumor.

A final MRI in June 2023 confirmed it: He was completely free of the disease.

AS's husband's oncologist was not told about the fenbendazole until the appointment in June 2023. When he found out, the doctor was intrigued and pleased that his patient was tumor-free.

AS and her husband know many others with these tumors. Their stories are tragic. Many are disfigured by drastic surgeries, try multiple useless treatments, and many have died. The abdominal form of this disease is especially deadly because it invades major blood vessels. AS's husband is the only one they know who has had a positive outcome. The only thing he did differently was take fenbendazole.

According to AS, it took about a year after starting fenbendazole for the tumor to be completely gone. However, she firmly believes the tumor was shrinking significantly within the first six months, right after he started taking it. She believes fenbendazole worked within those first six months, especially since the tumor was so widespread that surgery and radiation alone could never have eliminated it.

In addition to fenbendazole, the man also took sweet wormwood, a multivitamin, vitamin D3/K2, krill oil, bee propolis, and magnesium.

Congratulations to this couple for their courage and insight in taking control of a terrifying medical crisis. The complete eradication of such a stubborn and invasive tumor, which was wrapped around so many vital structures that surgery couldn't fully remove it, is a remarkable achievement. It underscores the powerful therapeutic potential of fenbendazole against aggressive noncancerous growths.

This case is a landmark. AS summed it up perfectly: "My husband is the only one we know who has had a positive outcome and the only thing he has done differently is taken fenbendazole."

CASE REPORT: SQUAMOUS CELL CARCINOMA, AGE EIGHTY, FEMALE

Squamous cell carcinoma is a common type of skin cancer that starts in the skin's outer layer. While it's not as deadly as some cancers, it can grow and spread if left untreated, making effective treatment essential.[3]

These cancers can appear anywhere on the skin. While they are often found on sun-exposed areas, they are also frequently found on non-sun-exposed skin in people with darker complexions, challenging the idea that sun exposure is the only cause.

Oral and Topical Fenbendazole Achieve Complete Eradication of Squamous Cell Carcinoma

This powerful case report, submitted by a woman's daughter named Caroline, shows how fenbendazole completely healed a stubborn squamous cell carcinoma on her eighty-year-old mother's finger. The lesion was first diagnosed as basal cell carcinoma, but a biopsy later confirmed it was squamous cell carcinoma.

Caroline's story began when she bought fenbendazole powder from a European supplier, originally just for deworming her family. But when her eighty-year-old mother was diagnosed with skin cancer on her finger, it became an opportunity to put fenbendazole to the test.

Her mother had been suffering from a sore on her finger for about four years. At first, she thought it was just an injury that wouldn't heal. Over the last year, the sore had become constantly infected, stiff, and painful. The slightest bump would cause it to break open and leak pus.

Her doctor tried standard wound care with bandages and antiseptic lotions, but nothing worked. Prescriptions for Travacort cream and an oral antifungal drug also failed. A swab test showed bacteria, so she was given antibiotics, which only seemed to make the painful, open wound worse.

A nurse at a hospital wound clinic suspected something more serious was wrong and strongly recommended a biopsy. The biopsy results came back first as basal cell carcinoma, but this was later corrected to squamous cell carcinoma.

The diagnosis created a new problem: how to remove it. The cancer was on a joint with very little skin to spare for stitches, and the patient was eighty years old. The doctor suggested waiting several weeks before attempting a major surgery that would require a hospital stay, general anesthesia, and a skin graft. This frightening prospect for her elderly mother prompted Caroline to make a bold decision. She presented the fenbendazole powder to her mother, suggesting she try it. At worst, it would be a good deworming. At best, it could heal the cancer.

Caroline began taking pictures on the day of the biopsy (photos on the Substack *Fenbendazole Can Cure Cancer* (https://fenbendazole.substack.com/p/case-report-squamous-cell-carcinoma-90e):

- **Day 1:** The photos clearly show a raw, pus-filled lesion.
- **Day 7:** The improvement was dramatic. Reported being pain-free for the first time in over a year.
- **Day 21:** After three weeks of taking 222 mg of fenbendazole powder daily with a fatty food, the skin was completely healed.

The lesion was gone, her finger worked perfectly, and she was in no pain. Her mother reported zero side effects from the fenbendazole.

Five weeks later, her mother saw her general practitioner. The doctor was shocked at the finger's perfect healing. He tried to credit the partial removal of tissue during the biopsy and the stitches. While he was skeptical about fenbendazole, he couldn't deny what he was seeing and canceled all plans for the major surgery and skin graft.

Once the wound closed, her mother began applying a topical paste of fenbendazole (Panacur "horse dewormer") daily. She also exposed her finger to sunlight and fresh air. The finger continued to heal perfectly, with no signs of infection and no pain. The result was astonishing, especially given the four-year history of the cancer and the naturally thin skin of an eighty-year-old.

Her mother continued both oral and topical fenbendazole with no side effects.

On June 19, 2024, at a follow-up appointment, her doctor remained unconvinced. He insisted the cancer was still there and pushed for surgery, again crediting the biopsy for the improved appearance. The full pathology report confirmed squamous cell carcinoma, along with Bowen's disease and solar elastosis. Caroline stood firm. Her mother had a four-year-old tumor, and after just two months of fenbendazole, her finger was fully functional and pain-free. There was no reason for an invasive procedure.

By August 10, 2024, the finger was completely and permanently healed. In her mother's own words, "If you didn't know the history, you'd never guess."

On September 27, 2024, an update confirmed the finger was still in excellent condition. Her mother's doctor had "guaranteed" the cancer would return without surgery. He was wrong.

In a final follow-up on September 28, 2024, Caroline confirmed her mother's absolute conviction that fenbendazole had cleared the cancer. She was continuing both topical and oral fenbendazole (222 mg daily) for a total of six months to ensure it would not return.

We commend Caroline and her mother for their resourcefulness in defeating this persistent medical problem. This compelling case adds to the mountain of evidence showing that fenbendazole is a premier therapy for various skin cancers, including melanoma, basal cell carcinoma, and now, as definitively shown here, squamous cell carcinoma. This case also demonstrates the power of using fenbendazole topically, applied directly to the skin.

TOPICAL APPLICATION OF IVERMECTIN ERADICATES SQUAMOUS CELL CARCINOMA, AGE SIXTY-THREE, MALE

This next case report veers off course a bit because instead of fenbendazole another antiparasitic, ivermectin, was used topically to eradicate a squamous cell carcinoma.

This case report documents a novel and effective topical application of the antiparasitic agent ivermectin for the treatment of a superficial skin malignancy: squamous cell carcinoma. As defined by the Mayo Clinic, squamous cell carcinoma of the skin represents a common form of cutaneous cancer that originates in the squamous cells comprising the middle and outer layers of the skin. While generally considered less immediately life-threatening than certain other cancers, squamous cell carcinoma possesses the capacity for aggressive local growth and, if left untreated, can metastasize to other parts of the body, leading to significant complications.

The following details a remarkable instance of a sixty-three-year-old male (BF) with squamous cell carcinoma who achieved complete eradication of the lesion through the topical application of ivermectin paste.

BF maintains a heightened awareness regarding cancer, both in his immediate environment and in his own health. As a fair-skinned individual with freckles and significant sun exposure, he acknowledges the potential for improved adherence to sunscreen use, though his personal perspective on its unequivocal benefit remains nuanced. With a history of occasional basal and squamous cell carcinomas, BF proactively undergoes regular six-month dermatological examinations.

Approximately six months prior to this report, BF noticed a distinct bump and scab formation on his forehead along the hairline. Initially hoping for spontaneous resolution, he observed the lesion for several weeks. When no improvement occurred, prompted by his wife, BF scheduled a consultation with his dermatologist.

The dermatologist definitively diagnosed the lesion as squamous cell carcinoma via biopsy and recommended Mohs micrographic surgery as the standard treatment approach. Having undergone Mohs surgery for previous squamous cell carcinomas that successfully eradicated the lesions, BF was well-acquainted with the prolonged healing period and the permanent scarring associated with the procedure. Mohs surgery is a specialized technique involving the serial excision of thin layers of skin, with meticulous microscopic examination of each layer to ensure complete removal of all cancerous cells while preserving the maximum amount of healthy tissue.

Drawing upon information gleaned from the Substack *Fenbendazole Can Cure Cancer* regarding the potential of fenbendazole for solid tumors, BF initially considered formulating a homemade version of a topical fenbendazole cream for his use. However, his reading also indicated the potential efficacy of ivermectin, commonly known as "horse paste" due to its veterinary applications, in treating certain malignancies. Notably, Tang et al. (2021)[4] reported ivermectin's effectiveness against melanoma, providing a rationale for its consideration in this case. Ivermectin is an antiparasitic drug with known anti-inflammatory and potential antineoplastic properties.

Consequently, BF had ivermectin paste in his possession and initiated topical application directly to the lesion. The application typically occurred at bedtime, with occasional daytime applications as circumstances and recall permitted. The specific formulation and concentration of the ivermectin paste was 1.87 percent.

Unfortunately, photographic documentation of the SCC patch prior to the initiation of ivermectin treatment was not obtained, as the need for formal documentation only became apparent several days into the treatment. A significant observation during the initial two weeks of ivermectin application was the apparent increase in flakiness of the affected skin, accompanied by a noticeable reduction in the surrounding erythema. Erythema, or redness, is a common sign of inflammation associated with squamous cell carcinomas.

Photos on the Substack *Fenbendazole Can Cure Cancer* https://fenbendazole.substack.com/p/case-report-squamous-cell-carcinoma.

Photo 1: Diagnosed squamous cell lesion January 30, 2023, after about three days of ivermectin use.

Photo 2: Same patch of skin on February 11, 2023, after two weeks of ivermectin application.

Following approximately one month of consistent ivermectin application, the SCC patch completely desquamated, revealing underlying clear skin. At this point, BF discontinued the ivermectin application and, to some extent, ceased active monitoring of the area. It was some time later that the realization of the potential significance of his experience for others prompted him to document the outcome photographically on August 1, 2023. The resulting image of the area where the squamous growth had been demonstrated what appeared to be normal skin, completely devoid of any residual scarring.

Photo 3 on Substack of area where squamous cell lesion was after about four weeks of daily ivermectin application. Photo taken approximately eight months later following the one month of ivermectin treatments.

When questioned about any observed side effects, BF reported none, indicating that the topical application of ivermectin was well-tolerated.

Regarding his history of other squamous cell skin cancers, BF described the standard treatment as Mohs surgery. He noted that some of the resulting scars from these previous procedures, particularly on his back, were deep and visible. His primary rationale for choosing topical ivermectin over a compounded fenbendazole preparation in this instance was the ready availability of the paste formulation of ivermectin, offering ease of application. BF indicated an intent to explore a topical fenbendazole approach for any future skin issues, retaining the option to revert to ivermectin if deemed necessary.

BF explicitly stated that he did not consult with his dermatologist regarding his use of topical ivermectin. He expressed a desire to observe whether the dermatologist would inquire about the previously diagnosed squamous cell lesion at his next scheduled appointment. This highlights a potential communication gap between the patient and his health-care provider regarding alternative or complementary therapies.

A substantial body of scientific literature explores the potential mechanisms of action and therapeutic applications of ivermectin across a spectrum of solid tumor and blood cancers. The Tang et al. (2021) study cited within this case report is provided as a starting point for interested readers. Indeed, future discussions may delve into the comparative aspects of fenbendazole and ivermectin, as both demonstrate promise as safe, accessible, and cost-effective antiparasitic agents with potent anticancer properties.

The implications of this squamous cell carcinoma case report are important. The prospect of avoiding expensive and potentially disfiguring conventional interventions for these relatively common skin malignancies is highly desirable. In this instance, topical ivermectin not only eradicated the cancer but did so without leaving any discernible scarring; in fact, it didn't leave a trace. Furthermore, this outcome was achieved rapidly, within approximately one month, and at minimal cost. The utilization of a readily available ivermectin paste, either while awaiting traditional treatment or as a primary intervention, presents a rational and compelling strategy to potentially circumvent more invasive procedures altogether.

Summary of Non-Metastatic Case Reports: Antiparasitic Agents and Cancer Treatment

These case reports highlight the potential of antiparasitic drugs, specifically fenbendazole and ivermectin, in treating certain types of cancer. While these drugs are traditionally used to combat parasitic infections, they demonstrate promising antineoplastic properties.

Desmoid Tumor Case Report

This report describes a thirty-four-year-old male with an aggressive desmoid tumor (aggressive fibromatosis). Desmoid tumors are noncancerous growths that can be locally aggressive. The patient was treated with fenbendazole after conventional treatments like surgery, chemotherapy, and cryoablation failed. The tumor was successfully eradicated, and the patient experienced no significant side effects.

Squamous Cell Carcinoma Case Reports

One report details an eighty-year-old woman with squamous cell carcinoma on her finger. Initially misdiagnosed as basal cell carcinoma, the lesion was treated with both oral and topical fenbendazole. The tumor was completely healed. Her general practitioner remained skeptical, believing the improvement resulted from the biopsy excision, but the patient's daughter strongly disagreed, noting the atypical nature of untreated cancerous sores improving.

Another report describes a sixty-three-year-old male with squamous cell carcinoma who used topical ivermectin to eradicate the lesion. He applied ivermectin paste to the affected area, resulting in complete resolution of the cancer within approximately one month, with no scarring or observed side effects.

Key Observations and Implications

Efficacy Against Diverse Growths

Both fenbendazole and ivermectin demonstrate efficacy against different types of abnormal cell growth, including both nonmalignant (desmoid tumor) and malignant (squamous cell carcinoma) conditions, in addition to the array of potentially lethal invasive cancers eradicated as described in the previous case reports chapter. These observations extend the functional utility of fenbendazole and ivermectin to treat other neoplasms of diverse origin and composition.

Novel Treatment: Approaches and Topical Application

These cases represent potentially novel treatment approaches for conditions where conventional methods may be invasive, ineffective, or associated with significant side effects. Both systemic (oral) and topical administration of these antiparasitic agents showed effectiveness, expanding potential treatment options.

In these cases, both fenbendazole and ivermectin were reported to be well-tolerated, with no observed side effects.

These reports support the concept of drug repurposing, where existing medications are investigated for new therapeutic applications. Both fenbendazole and ivermectin, traditionally used as antiparasitic drugs, have a role to play in cancer treatment and in the treatment of diverse neoplastic growths as suggested here.

The effectiveness of fenbendazole in eradicating a noncancerous desmoid tumor and squamous cell growths, in addition to its previously observed efficacy against invasive metastatic growths, has significant implications. A thorough reevaluation of the current understanding of malignant and nonmalignant neoplasms needs a complete overhaul and reset. Further study of the demonstrated anticancer actions of antiparasitic drugs is warranted and long overdue. The fruits of this research will likely lead to the discovery of more effective methods of cancer treatment.

CHAPTER 8

Dogs, Fenbendazole, and Cancer

Cancer is one of the biggest health threats facing our canine companions. Its presence is growing, especially in older dogs. Approximately one in four dogs will develop cancer in their lifetime, making it the leading cause of death in dogs over the age of two.[1] This devastating reality highlights the urgent need for better ways to fight this disease.

While any dog can get cancer, certain breeds are known to be more vulnerable. Boxers, for instance, have a higher rate of lymphoma and mast cell tumors. Golden retrievers face an increased risk of lymphoma, the aggressive blood vessel cancer hemangiosarcoma, and the bone cancer osteosarcoma. Large and giant breeds like Great Danes and Saint Bernards are significantly more likely to develop osteosarcoma.[2] These patterns are the result of a complex mix of genetics, the consequences of selective breeding, and environmental factors.

The Limits of Conventional Veterinary Cancer Treatment

Standard cancer treatments for dogs—surgery, chemotherapy, and radiation—are the same ones used in human medicine, and they come with the same significant drawbacks. Surgery cannot always remove a tumor completely, especially if it is invasive or in a difficult-to-reach spot, which can lead to the cancer growing back.

Chemotherapy, while useful for cancers like lymphoma, can be incredibly toxic. It often damages the bone marrow, which wipes out the white blood cells needed to fight infection. This leaves the dog vulnerable to life-threatening conditions like sepsis. It can also cause severe digestive problems and organ damage.[3] Over time, cancer cells can also become resistant to the chemotherapy drugs, making them ineffective. Radiation requires special equipment and anesthesia, has its own painful side effects, and often fails to stop the cancer from spreading to other parts of the body.

On top of these medical challenges, the high cost of conventional treatments is a massive hurdle for many pet owners, forcing them into heartbreaking decisions about their beloved companions. These limitations create an urgent demand for safer, more affordable, and more effective treatments.

How Fighting Cancer in Dogs Helps Humans

The fight against cancer in dogs provides a powerful, direct path to helping humans.[4] Dogs and humans share many biological similarities, and their cancers often look and behave the same way at the genetic level. Osteosarcoma, for example, is strikingly similar in dogs and humans, making dogs an exceptional model for testing new therapies that could one day be used in people.[5] Clinical trials in dogs with cancer are not just for helping pets; they provide critical data that can speed up the development of new cancer treatments for everyone.

Case Report Evidence: Fenbendazole's Power in Action

Powerful evidence for fenbendazole's role in fighting cancer comes directly from the stories of dogs whose owners were given little to no hope regarding their dog's prognosis.

CASE REPORT 1: MOOSE AND STAGE 3 LYMPHOMA

Moose, a twelve-year-old American bulldog mix, was diagnosed with stage 3 lymphoma, a cancer of the immune system that accounts for up to 14 percent of all cancers in dogs.[6, 7] The cancer had caused the lymph nodes in his jaw and behind his knees to swell to the size of golf balls. His veterinarian gave him a grim prognosis: with standard chemotherapy, he might live for another year, if he was lucky.

His owner, AS, a retired veterinary technician, refused to give up. Within a week of the diagnosis, she began her own research and started Moose on a daily protocol of fenbendazole, sweet wormwood, and other herbal supplements.[8] The most incredible part of Moose's story happened before he even received his first dose of chemo.

When AS brought Moose in for his first chemotherapy appointment, the oncologist was stunned. In the two weeks that Moose had been on fenbendazole and herbs, his massive tumors had already shrunk by 50 percent. The veterinary staff was puzzled, unable to explain the dramatic improvement.

Moose went on to receive a basic chemotherapy protocol, but the treatment was hard on him. He suffered a near-fatal sepsis event due to the chemo wiping out his immune cells and had to have his last few doses reduced. His owner still wonders if the chemotherapy was even necessary.

More than eighteen months after his diagnosis, a time when most dogs with his condition would be gone, Moose was not only alive but thriving. His vet declared him to be a normal dog with no physical signs of cancer and perfect blood work. He was running around like a puppy again. AS continued to give him a daily 250 mg dose of liquid fenbendazole mixed into his food, with zero side effects. She is absolutely certain that the fenbendazole was responsible for his initial tumor shrinkage and his long-term remission, which shattered the one-year prognosis he was given.

CASE REPORT 2: PIPER THE RESCUE DOG AND AN INOPERABLE SARCOMA

Piper, a nine-year-old yellow Lab and American Staffordshire mix, had a large, sausage-like soft-tissue sarcoma, a type of cancer that arises from connective tissue.[9] It was located on her hindquarters, invading the nerves of her rear leg. In January 2019, she underwent surgery to remove it.

After the operation, the veterinarian delivered difficult news. He had not been able to remove the entire tumor because it was anchored to critical nerves; trying to get it all would have permanently damaged her leg. He assured her owner, M, that the cancer would return.

Inspired by stories of fenbendazole's success, M refused to accept that fate. She went straight to a farm supply store, bought fenbendazole, and immediately started Piper on a 400 mg daily dose. She kept her vet informed, and every report was positive.

The vet's dire prediction never came true. The tumor never grew back. Four years later, Piper remains healthy, active, and completely free of any sign of cancer. M. continued giving her intermittent courses of fenbendazole for the next two years as a preventive measure. This remarkable outcome demonstrates that fenbendazole likely succeeded where surgery could not, eliminating the microscopic cancer cells left behind.[10] For high-grade sarcomas, recurrence is the expectation, with survival times of only about a year even with aggressive therapy.[11] Piper's story proves that another outcome is possible.

CASE REPORT 3: HERSHEY AND METASTATIC MELANOMA

Oral malignant melanoma is the most common and aggressive oral cancer in dogs, known for its rapid spread and poor prognosis.[12] Tumors arise from pigment-producing cells and are often deadly, with survival times as short as three months for advanced stages.[13, 14] Hershey, a fourteen-year-old dog, was diagnosed with this exact cancer after a large tumor was partially removed from his mouth. His prognosis was terminal. The vet estimated he had only a few months to live.

His owner, MH, created a powerful daily protocol to save him. It included 50 mg of fenbendazole, CBD oil, krill oil, turmeric, and an immune-boosting supplement. Importantly, her vet also discovered that Hershey had a severe vitamin D3 deficiency and recommended adding high-dose vitamin D drops to his regimen.

More than three years later, Hershey was approaching his seventeenth birthday. Regular checkups, blood work, and ultrasounds showed absolutely no sign of cancer recurrence. He had defied his terminal diagnosis and far outlived expectations. His vet was so impressed that she began telling other clients with sick pets about Hershey's success.

MH states, "There is no question that fenbendazole cured his cancer that there was no medical treatment for." She adds, "Even the surgeon who operated on Hershey cannot believe he is still alive." This case not only supports fenbendazole's power but also highlights the potential importance of correcting nutritional deficiencies like low vitamin D, an approach championed by researchers like Dr. Paul Marik, who considers both vitamin D and fenbendazole to be high-priority agents for cancer therapy.[15]

What These Canine Victories over Cancer Mean for Everyone

The stories of Moose, Piper, and Hershey are more than just inspiring case reports. They are powerful evidence. They collectively show that fenbendazole is effective against a wide range of cancer types, including cancers of the blood (lymphoma), connective tissue (sarcoma), and surface cells (melanoma). This broad action demonstrates that fenbendazole targets fundamental processes that are common to many cancers in both dogs and humans.

One of the most common dismissals of fenbendazole is that it's just "dog medicine." This argument completely collapses under the weight of this evidence and common sense. As previous chapters have shown fenbendazole to be effective on cancer in humans, these canine cases confirm its power. The fact that fenbendazole works so well in both species doesn't mean it's "dog medicine." It means fenbendazole is an anticancer medicine with broad effectiveness that extends to both animals and humans. In fact, many of the chemotherapy drugs used in canine cancer (vincristine, doxorubicin) are the same ones used on humans.[16] No serious person would argue against using vincristine on a dog because it is a human drug. Whether fenbendazole is treating parasites or cancer, the drug treats the condition, not the species.

Furthermore, these canine cases destroy any argument that the positive results seen in humans are related in any way to a placebo effect. While the power of belief can produce real physiological changes in human trials,[17] the placebo effect is considered minimal to nonexistent in animals for treating a disease like cancer.[18] The dramatic tumor shrinkage and long-term survival seen in these dogs provide robust, undeniable evidence of a direct, biological anticancer effect from the drug itself.

Anecdotally, some veterinarians have even observed that dogs receiving regular deworming treatments seem to have a lower incidence of cancer. While this requires formal study, it raises the exciting possibility that drugs like fenbendazole may even have a cancer-preventing effect in animals.

In conclusion, the evidence from canine cancer statistics, the clear limits of conventional therapy, and these powerful case reports all point to a bright future for fenbendazole. It stands as a safe, affordable, and effective weapon in the war on cancer, and it demands serious investigation in both veterinary and human medicine to help all who are suffering from this disease.

CHAPTER 9

Synthesizing the Evidence from All the Case Reports: Mechanisms and the Emerging Picture of Fenbendazole's Anticancer Potential

The subjects of the foregoing case reports are individuals who operated outside the bounds of conventional medicine and took personal responsibility for finding new approaches to their problems. Faced with the certainty of death or the possibility of life, they chose life. In essence, these pioneers, individually and collectively, were forced to save their own lives, and, in all cases, achieved successful outcomes that are far beyond the capability of present medical standard-of-care protocols. These people exercised the option to survive under their own care vs. die under a doctor's. Collectively, these are stories of individuals, many out of options, forced to self-treat their own cancer and experiment on themselves. While each of these case reports is different in many respects, there are commonalities that are present that may be useful in the further application of fenbendazole in the treatment of various cancers going forward.

Here we synthesize the findings from the case reports presented earlier, identify key patterns and trends, and connect this new understanding to the mechanistic data that has been highlighted in the previous chapters, to create a clear picture of the multifaceted role of fenbendazole as a practical anticancer medication. The power of these case reports is inherent in their diversity of cancer types, uncontrolled individual differences, less-than-perfect dosing and administration protocols, and myriad other uncontrolled or manipulated variables. Despite the apparent haphazard processes involved in self-experimentation and the admitted sloppiness of the process, the people in these case reports did what their oncologists could not do: They cured, or drastically diminished their cancers while experiencing no adverse side effects! And the one variable that is constantly present through all the noise inherent in all of these case reports is fenbendazole.

Recurring Themes and Commonalities: A Summary of the Case Reports

A detailed analysis of the various case reports, while diverse in the types of cancers being treated, patient characteristics, and treatment regimens, reveals several important key themes and commonalities. By highlighting these trends, we can begin to advance the understanding of how fenbendazole, and other antiparasitic drugs like it, can provide significant therapeutic benefit in the treatment of cancer.

Advanced or Refractory Cancers

The successes described in the case reports have mostly been achieved in cancers where the current medical approaches failed, necessitating the need for other avenues of care. In fact, a number of the case reports involved people who had completed traditional surgical, radiotherapy and chemotherapy protocols that had failed to be effective and the person was released to hospice or other palliative care. They tried traditional cancer treatments that failed, and they were sent home to die. Traditional, chemotherapy-driven treatments are known to have diminishing effectiveness, once the disease is able to take hold and spread. As discussed earlier, this point of diminishing returns develops from the growing burden of drug resistance to traditional chemotherapies and the fact that cancer often becomes untreatable in this scenario.

At the advanced terminal stage of cancer characterizing most of the case reports, after all relevant conventional options have been exhausted, the risk profile of the different interventions starts to change. The negative side effects of the conventional therapies begin to outweigh the potential benefits. The previously discussed actions of fenbendazole on cancer stem cells, which appear to result, at least in part, from traditional standard-of-care treatments themselves, are also eradicated by fenbendazole. Fenbendazole and mebendazole in experimental preparations have been shown to disrupt the development of cancer stem cells and metastases. There are no effective traditional treatments for this development. Recall that cancer stem cells are the cancer cells that kill. Due to the intractable nature of the cancer, exhaustion of traditional treatments, and passage of time, it is reasonable to speculate that many people described in the case reports were in the catastrophic throes of their own personal hell, namely cancer stem cell metastases. Their actions, particularly the use of fenbendazole, enabled them to save their own lives. It is reasonable to conclude that fenbendazole kills the cancer cells (cancer stem cells) that kill us!

Therefore, our first conclusion is that fenbendazole likely eradicates cancer stem cells that underpin traditional treatment failure in humans. This observation applies the basic and preclinical data that we've covered regarding the mechanisms that fenbendazole uses to kill cancer directly to humans.

The Speed of Action

The time required to achieve remission, either partial or complete, is noteworthy. The vast majority of reports have shown significant changes within only a few weeks of starting to administer fenbendazole as a treatment method. One issue to consider regarding the issue of time to remission is that since these were uncontrolled, self-treatment case studies, the measurement of therapeutic effect and time course was haphazard at best. That is, due to the nature of the circumstances—cancer patients trying to save their own lives—regular, orderly diagnostics followed a clinical schedule, not an experimental one. Testing occurred on an as-available basis without consideration of determining exact time course effects. Most testing occurred on a monthly schedule precluding a finer granular analysis of time course. Furthermore, since detected effect in the form of blood tumor marker change can lag therapeutic effect by extended periods, determining the exact time course of the fenbendazole effect on cancer awaits further study. However, let us not be distracted by what we have yet to learn from what we have learned: the main effect of fenbendazole to reduce or eliminate these cancers in such a rapid time frame. And as such, these case reports provide very strong human evidence that fenbendazole is able to selectively target the tumors. Furthermore, many reported that they started to feel better, broadly defined, before there was any diagnostic verification that their cancers were affected.

The second conclusion is that fenbendazole kills cancer relatively quickly in humans. This observation applies the basic and preclinical data that we've covered regarding the time course of the effects of fenbendazole on cancer directly to humans.

Fenbendazole Use Results in No (or Limited) Side Effects

The consistent reports of no or minimal side effects has made the addition of fenbendazole to a desperate cancer patient's journey far easier to justify. As has been reviewed in chapters 1, 2, and 3, the high degree of specificity targeting only the cancer cell, and not healthy cells, is one reason why there are no or few mild side effects from fenbendazole. None of the case reports above could attribute any adverse side effects to fenbendazole. None!

One *potential* side effect is the *transient* elevation of the liver enzymes ALT and AST. In several instances where ALT and AST rose during treatment with fenbendazole, it was phasic and resolved to levels within normal limits within a month or two. While this phenomenon could reflect primary hepatic disruption by fenbendazole, it is highly unlikely for several reasons. First, not all case reports detected alterations in AST or ALT. Second, all instances were temporary and resolved in short order. Third, the return to normalcy was maintained despite continued administration of fenbendazole. This pattern is consistent with other reports.[1]

What is very interesting is the time course of the AST/ALT elevations. It certainly appeared that the transient elevations in liver enzymes coincided with the active phase of fenbendazole anticancer activity in some of the cases. That is, elevations of AST and ALT, which are broadly accepted as indices of liver stress and/or the stress associated with increased workloads as would be expected with massive die-offs of malignant cells. Once the die-off is over, the cancer is eradicated, there is less dead cancer cell debris to clear through the liver, and the liver enzymes return to baseline. Maintenance of this liver status quo persists despite continued fenbendazole administration. These patterns are consistent with other reports describing changes in hepatic function when using chemotherapeutic drugs.[2, 3]

What are the potential takeaways regarding liver enzyme dynamics, fenbendazole, and cancer? First, fenbendazole, in the doses used here, is not a hepatotoxin, consistent with what has been demonstrated over billions of doses, over more than sixty years of antiparasitic use. Second, the transient rise in AST and ALT may reflect a Herxheimer-type reaction due to the die-off of massive amounts of malignant cells. Third, the return to baseline values of liver function appears to reflect the clearing of the dead cancer cellular debris because these liver values return to within normal limits despite the continued use of fenbendazole. That is, if fenbendazole was the direct cause of liver stress, AST/ALT values would remain elevated as long as fenbendazole was present. Most people here continued to take fenbendazole during the immediate post-remission period as well as indefinitely afterward. Subsequently, liver enzymes are measured regularly with standard blood panels, and they are normal.

That being said, the likely process that is being observed is that fenbendazole results in a massive die-off of cancer cells, causing a temporary hepato-stressor event reflected in transient AST/ALT rise; once the cancer is cleared, this stress on the liver declines, as does AST/ALT. As such, the transient rise in ALT/AST in some cases may serve as a gauge of the effectiveness of fenbendazole in killing a specific cancer. This observation creates a wealth of possibilities regarding factors that may affect the magnitude, specificity, time course, effectiveness, and persistence of the fenbendazole anticancer effect using AST/ALT values as a marker. These suggestions are speculative and need further study to understand what is or is not happening regarding liver enzyme markers in those self-treating with fenbendazole.

The use of fenbendazole to treat any malignant or nonmalignant cancer, whether used as a stand-alone therapy or as an addition to a standard-of-care treatment protocol, presents a compellingly low risk/high reward proposal. These case report results indicate that fenbendazole should be immediately incorporated into cancer treatment protocols.

Our third conclusion is that fenbendazole eradicates cancers with few to no adverse side effects in humans. This observation applies the basic and preclinical data that we've covered regarding the mechanisms governing the selectivity of fenbendazole targeting cancer cells directly to humans.

Dosing and Administration of Fenbendazole

- **Amount:** The amount of fenbendazole used ranged from 222 mg to 2000 mg per day. In general, it seemed that younger people took more aggressively sized doses.
- **Frequency:** Most took fenbendazole every day. Some followed the Tippens protocol of four days of 222 mg fenbendazole followed by three days off per week. Some dosed once per day, others twice per day.
- **Cofactors:** Most administered their fenbendazole with food or a source of fat such as olive oil, peanut butter, yogurt, or butter.

The range of doses and protocol were all without adverse side effects. Obviously, the most important question concerns what is the ideal amount and dosing protocol to use when self-treating. We simply do not know at this point. What we do know is that the elegance engendered in this apparently haphazard process reveals that there is a very wide range of effective doses, and that even the most minimal dose (222 mg), provides therapeutic effect, and in many cases, complete remission. Moreover, some of the case reports did not use an everyday fenbendazole dosing schedule. As mentioned, some did the protocol of four days on, followed by three days off. The takeaway is that there is a minimal dose that is effective to eradicate cancer, and that is 222 mg—until future parametric studies determine otherwise.

The higher doses used in the case reports here could represent instances of "overkill" or inadvertent compensation for unintended systematic administration error. That is, if an administration error occurs and only a small amount of fenbendazole is ingested, the margin of error in that scenario is increased for those taking higher doses from the start. All of these questions regarding optimal dosing, schedule, protocol, and bioavailability await careful parametric studies that should be conducted immediately.

Our fourth conclusion is that fenbendazole eradicates cancer via oral administration of physiological doses in humans. This observation applies the basic and preclinical data that we've covered regarding the mechanisms governing fenbendazole pharmacokinetics and dosing necessary to kill cancer cells directly to humans.

Fenbendazole Is Both Necessary and Sufficient to Eradicate Cancer

Many of the case reports have a lot of moving parts with respect to the various drugs, vitamins, herbs, etc. also used prior and/or during the use of fenbendazole. These additional substances appear to play a supporting role to the main, direct cancer-cell-killing action of fenbendazole. What is the justification for confidence in that statement? In the in vitro, in vivo preclinical science that used only fenbendazole or mebendazole, there were no vitamins, herbs, or other substances incorporated in those experiments. Based on all of that supporting data, if fenbendazole did not kill cancer, that would be the news. Therefore, it should come as no surprise that fenbendazole kills cancer cells in humans based on the prior preclinical research.

Many of these other substances mentioned in the case reports like Vitamin D, curcumin, various mushrooms etc. all appear to exert their anticancer actions indirectly by bolstering the immune system in its efforts to prevent the development of cancers in the first place. While these substances are vitally important, they do not appear to possess the arsenal of direct anticancer mechanisms that fenbendazole does.* Many of the people described in the case

* Ivermectin is another antiparasitic with direct anticancer actions and is an exciting area of future research. Discussion of ivermectin's repurposing as an anticancer drug, however exciting, is beyond the scope of this publication.

reports threw the kitchen sink of treatments, both traditional standard-of-care and folk remedies, at their cancers. Once fenbendazole was added to the mix, the cancer was effectively treated, put into remission, or gone. Therefore, fenbendazole alone is both necessary and sufficient to kill the cancers as described in these case reports.

Our fourth conclusion is that fenbendazole is both necessary and sufficient to eradicate cancer in humans. This observation applies the basic and preclinical data that we've covered regarding the mechanisms through which fenbendazole and mebendazole can operate without assistance to kill cancer cells directly to humans.

Fenbendazole Killing Cancer Is Not a Placebo Effect

The stories of the dogs Moose, Piper, and Hershey are more than just inspiring case reports; they provided powerful evidence against the operation of any placebo-like effects to explain the actions of fenbendazole on cancer in humans. The placebo effect is considered minimal to nonexistent in animals for treating a disease like cancer. Just like the results observed in the preclinical studies described earlier, the dramatic tumor shrinkage and long-term survival seen in these dogs provide robust, undeniable evidence of a direct, biological anticancer effect from the drug itself.

One of the most common dismissals of fenbendazole is that it's just "dog medicine." The fact that fenbendazole works so well in both species doesn't mean it's "dog medicine." It means fenbendazole is an anticancer medicine with broad effectiveness that extends to both animals and humans.

Our fifth conclusion is that fenbendazole eradicates cancers in humans without relying on complex psychological mechanisms. This observation applies the basic and preclinical data that we've covered regarding the biological mechanisms through which fenbendazole and mebendazole kill cancer cells, indicating that they can operate independently of cognitive factors, directly to humans. Whether fenbendazole is treating parasites or cancer, the drug treats the condition, not the species.

Efficacy Against Diverse Growths and Topical Application

Both fenbendazole and ivermectin demonstrate efficacy against different types of abnormal cell growth, including both nonmalignant (desmoid tumor) and malignant (squamous cell carcinoma) conditions, in addition to the array of lethal invasive cancers. These observations extend the functional utility of fenbendazole and ivermectin to treat other neoplasms of diverse origin and composition.

These cases represent potentially novel treatment approaches for skin cancer conditions where conventional methods may be invasive, ineffective, or associated with significant disfiguring side effects. Both systemic (oral) and topical administration of these antiparasitic agents showed effectiveness, expanding potential treatment options.

A High Impact at Low Cost

The risk/reward profile of using fenbendazole made the decision to try it easier. The direction to take when faced with cancer is not binary: traditional treatments or fenbendazole. For those who choose traditional treatments, adding fenbendazole to the mix is a rational decision. With no side effects, low cost, over-the-counter access, ease of administration, and overwhelming preclinical scientific support, it should come as no surprise that the people in these case reports chose to try fenbendazole and that fenbendazole eradicated their cancers.

Post-Remission Use of Fenbendazole

Every person in these case reports continues to take fenbendazole in some capacity. Some continue on with the dosing and protocol that brought them into remission, others adopt a modified, usually less aggressive plan regarding dosage and administration as a strategy. Either way, there is no appetite to tempt fate by not continuing to take fenbendazole. It is simply not worth the risk. Think about that transformation of thought process for a minute. When many of these people were initially considering taking fenbendazole, because of their dire situation, any unknown risks of taking the drug paled in comparison to their own certain death. Fast-forward, fenbendazole cured their cancers, and the risk engendered in fenbendazole now is in *not* continuing to take fenbendazole! A complete reversal of attitude.

There is no guidance regarding the persistence of the effect on fenbendazole and cancer. Is cancer remission from fenbendazole permanent? A true cure would imply that permanence is a feature. An effective treatment would eradicate cancer with no side effects and remain effective in preventing recurrence and/or snuffing out restaging. Other than that which will become apparent with the passage of time, we can only speculate at this juncture.

Currently it is unknown what maintenance plan of fenbendazole treatment is required, if any.

CHAPTER 10

Unexplained Global Cancer Disparity Explained: Antiparasitic Drugs and Public Health Policy

This chapter explores an overlooked factor in the significantly different rates of cancer around the world: the widespread use of antiparasitic drugs, particularly benzimidazoles like albendazole (similar to fenbendazole, which has shown cancer-fighting abilities in case studies), in routine public health programs in many developing nations. The striking disparity in cancer diagnoses, with individuals in the United States facing a three-times-higher risk compared to those in countries like India, Mexico, and various nations in Africa and Asia. This difference persists across many cancer types and cannot be explained by genetics, diet, or environmental factors alone. The central observation is that routine, population-wide deworming programs common in many lower-income countries, primarily aimed at controlling parasitic infections, appear to inadvertently be offering a protective effect against cancer and other inflammation-based diseases. Antiparasitic drugs like fenbendazole, mebendazole, and albendazole evidently also prevent the development of cancer.

Is Cancer Prevention Largely Within Our Grasp?

If the revelations on fenbendazole and cancer from the previous chapters have you reeling, better buckle up for more. The case reports presented earlier demonstrated that fenbendazole eradicated a variety of cancers of various severity, staging, and circumstance. The elimination of existing cancers prompts the question: Can fenbendazole prevent cancer from occurring in the first place? One of the most frequent questions coming into the Substack *Fenbendazole Can Cure Cancer* concerns prevention of cancer. Evidence presented so far strongly indicates that fenbendazole has the ability to eradicate cancer at the biochemical, cellular, molecular, and organismic (whole animal/human) level. Examining the question of prevention is a natural and logical extension of what we've presented earlier because as Benjamin Franklin said, "An ounce of prevention is worth a pound of cure."

One major issue with the scientific demonstration of a preventative effect of any treatment is that of proving a negative, especially with respect to in-the-field human health matters. In other words, how can it be proven a disease would have naturally occurred, if a treatment prevented it from doing so?

However, sometimes, we're just plain lucky. What if the preventative studies on fenbendazole as a preventative for cancer were already available through differences in public health policy that essentially performed wide-reaching experiments-in-nature on their populations?

A World of Unequal Battles: Cancer's Global Divide

It's astounding how easily some truths can remain hidden in plain sight until we view them through a different lens. The probability of receiving a cancer diagnosis varies dramatically depending on where you live.[1] For example, an individual residing in the United States has approximately three times the likelihood of a cancer diagnosis compared to someone living in India. With projections indicating that one in two Americans will face a cancer diagnosis in their lifetime,[2] the contrast with significantly lower rates in nations like India presents an urgent public health puzzle.

Examining specific cancer types reveals even more extreme disparities. Compared to men in India, US men face a twenty-three-fold higher risk of prostate cancer. Americans experience significantly elevated rates of melanoma (8–14 times higher), colorectal cancer (10–11 times higher), endometrial cancer (9 times higher), lung cancer (7–17 times higher), bladder cancer (7–8 times higher), breast cancer (5 times higher), and kidney cancer (9–12 times higher). These are not marginal differences; they represent increases of 500 percent, 1000 percent, and even over 2000 percent, signaling profound underlying etiological distinctions that demand explanation.

Curiously, nations with the highest per capita health-care expenditures often exhibit the highest cancer incidence rates. This troubling situation challenges the presumed effectiveness of current preventative strategies in high-spending countries and mandates a reevaluation of the status quo. On the other hand, maybe health care expenditures have nothing to do with the finding. Maybe the countries that don't spend as much on health care are actively doing something else that lowers their cancer rates that the cancer-ridden nations don't?

That something appears to be the widespread use of antiparasitic medicines such as albendazole, mebendazole, and fenbendazole—which have anticancer capabilities—administered through public health initiatives.[3]

To revisit our discussion on the importance of observation and case reports in science, the cancer incidence differences between the US and India represented an interesting observation that perhaps public health programs that administer antiparasitic medicines to their people may also be affecting the incidence of cancer. We needed to determine if these differences were unique when comparing just those two nations, or if they were part of a larger pattern.

This connection between antiparasitic use and cancer incidence does extend globally. Data from authoritative sources like the World Health Organization's GLOBOCAN project consistently show higher age-standardized cancer incidence rates (ASIR) in developed nations that don't use antiparasitics as part of a public health policy. For instance, 2020[4] ASIR (all cancers, both sexes, per 100,000 people) were markedly higher in Australia (452.4 per 100k), France (371.0), Denmark (334.9), and the United States (300.5) than in Mexico (136.2), India (97.1), the Democratic Republic of the Congo (80.8), and Niger (76.4), all nations that do deworm. The difference between Denmark and Niger represents a 4.4-fold disparity. These figures establish a clear global trend: developed countries experience substantially higher cancer incidence.

The Deworming Hypothesis: A Common Denominator Across Diverse Nations

While genetic, dietary, and environmental factors and screening intensity differences could contribute to the cancer rate differential,[5] the impact of a more obvious factor—population-wide antiparasitic drug use with anticancer properties—warrants rigorous examination.

As we learned earlier, albendazole is an analogue of fenbendazole and functions by disrupting microtubule polymerization in parasite and cancer cells, among many other mechanisms that have overlapping antiparasitic and anticancer effects.[6, 7] Given its demonstrable anticancer activity in preclinical models,[8] and it's demonstrated anticancer activities in human case reports as we've just read, its widespread use to prevent and manage parasitic infections presents a plausible contributing factor to lower cancer incidence observed in the nations that employ it.

Let's examine the evidence from various nations around the world in relation to this deworming hypothesis:

- **India:** In response to a significant burden of soil-transmitted helminth infections, India implemented National Deworming Days.[9] On designated days, usually the 10th of February and the 10th of August, children and adults are given government-issued, safe, inexpensive albendazole tablets by the Ministry of Health and Family Welfare.[10] This national public health program raises a critical question: Does the routine administration of albendazole confer a protective effect against cancer?
- **Mexico and Mesoamerica:** Since 1993, Mexico has integrated biannual deworming (single 400 mg albendazole dose) into its National Health Weeks.[11] Mexico's cancer incidence (ASIR 136.2/100k) remains significantly lower than that of the United States (300.5/100k).
- **Sub-Saharan Africa:** Countries like Nigeria (ASIR 110.7/100k), Ethiopia (101.2), Congo (80.8), and Niger (76.4)216 implement large-scale deworming programs, often using albendazole or mebendazole, as part of broader tropical disease control efforts.[12, 13] Despite challenges in cancer registry data accuracy, the consistently lower incidence is undeniable.
- **South America:** This region faces a substantial soil-transmitted worm burden, with estimates suggesting up to one-third of the population may be infected.[14] Many nations employ routine deworming campaigns and report lower cancer rates than North America and Europe.
- **Asia:** Beyond India, countries like the Philippines (ASIR 184/100k) and Bangladesh (104) also implement national deworming programs.[15]

This consistent pattern across diverse global regions strongly suggests the link between widespread anthelmintic use and reduced cancer rates is not likely mere coincidence. While lifestyle, diet, genetics, and environmental exposures are potential variables, it is highly unlikely they alone account for the dramatic differences in cancer incidence. Routine deworming is the tie binding these disparate nations while at the same time separating them from high-cancer-incidence nations that do not use antiparasitics.

Note: Comparison of the United States to India regarding cancer incidence and public health policy is not an isolated or cherry-picked case. Dozens of other Western countries with high cancer rates could be compared to dozens of other developing countries with low cancer rates. At the extreme, Australia with 452 cases of cancer per 100,000 population could be analyzed compared to Niger's 76 cases per 100,000. The United States and India were initially selected for comparison due to available data relevance and interest.

A Global Experiment in Nature: The Definitive Evidence

Given the observations on selected regions around the globe linking cancer incidence and deworming programs, exploring this connection on a larger scale is warranted. We conducted original research examining deworming practices, cancer incidence rates, and income worldwide.

The methodology was to gather cancer incidence data for 188 nations from the WHO GLOBOCAN database, determine whether the official public health policy of each nation included mass drug administration of antiparasitics (using WHO data), and gather income data from WorldData.info.

The results were clear and consistent: nations with public health policies that include mass deworming have dramatically lower cancer incidence rates.

- A total of 123 nations use antiparasitics as part of a mass drug administration program.
- A total of 61 nations do not deworm as part of public health policy. (Complete list of all nations at end of chapter.)

Nations that implement mass drug administration of antiparasitic drugs have a dramatically lower incidence of cancer compared to nations that do not. The average cancer incidence rate in deworming countries is 133.95 per 100,000 population. In nations that do not deworm, the average is 268.05 per 100,000. This difference is highly statistically significant ($t(184) = 18.45$, $p < .0001$). In practical terms, countries that do not implement deworming practices experience over twice the incidence of cancer.

A more granular, regional analysis offers further support for the deworming hypothesis. Of the 22 nations that comprise the Middle East, there is just one that does not implement a public health directed deworming program; that nation is Israel. The cancer incidence rate in Israel is 244.3 per 100,000, the average cancer incidence rate for the rest of the 21 countries is 121.56 per 100,000. Again, over twice the rate compared to adjacent, regional nations

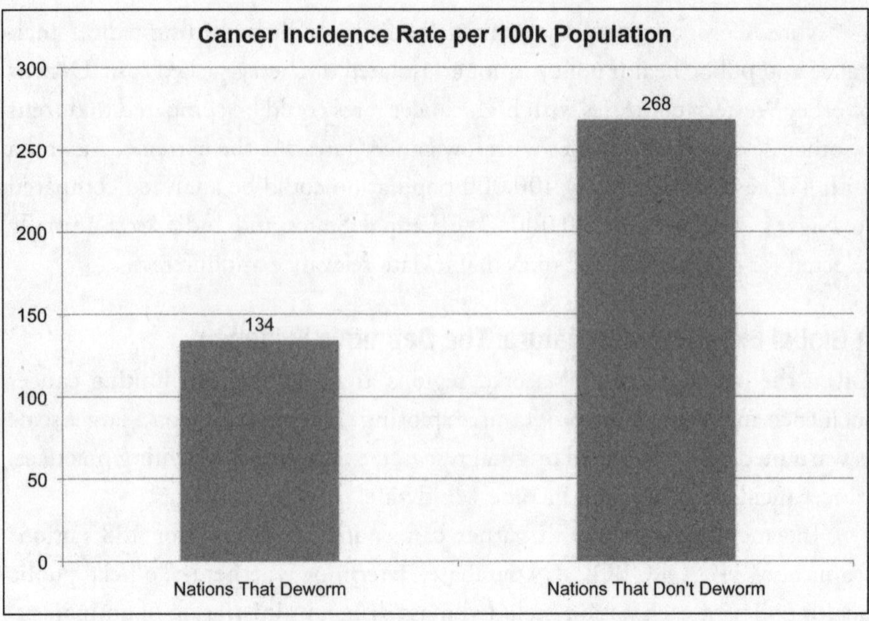

There are 61 nations that do not have a formal public health policy of mass drug administration to deworm the population. Their average cancer incidence rate per 100,000 population is 268.05 (range 155.5 to 510). There are 123 nations that do have formal public health mass drug administration policies using antiparasitics. Their average cancer rate per 100,000 population is 133.95 (range 78.9 to 228.1). Nations that do not deworm have higher cancer rates, twice as high, compared to nations that do deworm. This difference in cancer incidence is highly statistically significant, $t(184) = 18.45$, $p < .0001$.

that have antiparasitic programs. The nations of the Middle East are adjacent neighbors in many instances. When just one of those nations, Israel, is unique in that it does not deworm, and its cancer rate is twice that of its immediate neighbors, differential use of antiparasitics is a likely cause.

This more granular, regional analysis offers more support for the assertion that the critical variable in the observed difference in cancer incidence among these different nations, both individually and collectively, is the presence or absence of widespread antiparasitic use rather than some uncontrolled dietary, cultural, genetic, geographic or environmental factor.

This consistent pattern across diverse global regions strongly suggests the link between widespread antiparasitic use and reduced cancer rates transcends coincidence. The common denominator is not location, or genetics, or diet, but appears to be population-level exposure to benzimidazole drugs with established anticancer properties.

Why Diet, Location, Genetic, and Cultural Differences Are Not Valid Explanations

While it is a possibility that dietary factors could play some part in these differences, dietary differences alone also cannot account for the dramatic difference in cancer incidence, especially considering the similarities in cancer rates as uniformly low across disparate regions in Asia, Mesoamerica, South America, and Africa that have markedly different dietary practices. Given the fact that there are large differences in cancer rates among countries from disparate cultural and geographic regions, it is highly unlikely that any one or any combination of these factors, other than antiparasitic use, is responsible for the differences in cancer incidence. It is more likely that differences in lifestyle, diet, genetics, environmental exposures, economic status, and health-care availability are all minor contributing factors.

On the other hand, it is highly likely that routine deworming is the tie binding these disparate nations while at the same time distinguishing them from high-cancer-incidence nations that do not use antiparasitics in public health. It appears that routine exposure to antiparasitic medications like albendazole with demonstrated anticancer actions, as part of a public health mass drug-administration effort to manage parasitic infection, is the critical factor in the overall picture of greatly reduced cancer incidence.

The argument that this observed disparity in cancer incidence rates is due to systematic testing and detection error in poorer countries is also not likely. The WHO states, "In cases where direct data is lacking, estimates may be derived from neighboring countries or adjusted based on demographic and epidemiological models," supporting the integrity of the data.

The Biological Reasons for Cancer Incidence Differences Among Nations

The observed link between deworming practices and reduced cancer rates is biologically plausible and likely through two primary mechanisms.

Direct Anticancer Action of Benzimidazoles

As detailed in chapters 2 and 3, benzimidazole drugs like fenbendazole, albendazole, and mebendazole possess potent, direct anticancer properties. They function primarily by disrupting microtubule polymerization, a process vital for cell division in both parasites and cancer cells. But antiparasitic drugs also kill cancer cells using multiple complementary and overlapping mechanisms including microtubule disruption, glucose uptake inhibition/angiogenesis, disruption of molecular mimicry, disruption of the tumor microenvironment, disabling P-glycoprotein efflux pumps, disabling p53 oncogene rescue, block migration, p38 MAPK intracellular destruction, mitotic catastrophe, and triggering apoptosis. This multifaceted attack unleashed on the cancer cell by these drugs is unrelenting, overpowering, and complete. Keep in mind the cancer cell only needs to be killed once. These direct actions on cancer cells provide a robust biochemical explanation for how these drugs could prevent or eliminate budding cancer cells.

The prevailing narrative minimizing parasitic infection risk in developed nations is dangerously flawed. The assumption of no threat fosters an environment where a genuine public health crisis may persist unrecognized, untreated, and ignored.

The Unrecognized Parasitic Infestation in the West

Evidence indicates significant parasite prevalence within the United States. A 2002 study analyzing US fecal samples found intestinal parasites in nearly half of the samples.[16] A 2017 study in rural Alabama found soil-transmitted worm infections in 34 percent of participants.[17] Furthermore, a series of papers from CDC scientists sounded the alarm on widespread, untreated parasitic infections. They estimated that over 60 million persons in the United States are chronically infected with *Toxoplasma gondii* alone, and highlighted the dangers of other neglected parasitic infections like Chagas disease, cysticercosis, and toxocariasis.[18, 19, 20, 21] These CDC scientists warned that "parasitic infections are present in every income and social strata" and that "residents of the United States . . . are not unaffected."[22] Given the lack of routine screening and the often subclinical nature of infections, their true prevalence and health impact in the US are likely substantially underdiagnosed, underreported and untreated.[23]

Parasites Are Everywhere in the Environment

Parasites have almost indestructible eggs that are found everywhere in our environment and food supply and can also easily form cysts that are hard to detect and are easily ingested in meat and vegetation.[24] These are organisms that are everywhere in our environment, and in and on nearly everything we interact with on a daily basis: in the soil, the grass, the vegetables, the water and so on. In simple terms, if we examine our surroundings through the lens of parasitology, we will see that it is very likely that most human beings, even in the so-called clean environments of the developed world, are almost certainly infected with some type of parasite. Even if someone is not infected at the moment, it is simply a matter of time. Parasitic infection is an unavoidable consequence of human behavior.

A survival mechanism of some parasites is that as resident parasites are attacked with antiparasitic drugs the females release thousands of eggs, which are immune to those drugs, that serve to perpetuate the infection. Understanding these life-cycle traits of some parasites explains why veterinary antiparasitic treatments are regularly scheduled events for animals including pets. Furthermore, removing a current parasitic infection has no effect on the threat or likelihood of a future infestation. Parasitic infections are managed, not cured. Parasites are masters of survival. They are everywhere, and their eggs are everywhere, constantly in search of a host.

Modern Transmission Routes of Parasites

Parasite eggs are found everywhere in our food chain and environment. Transmission occurs through contaminated food (including organic produce fertilized with manure), imported foods, raw and undercooked foods,[25] and close contact with pets.

Think of the numerous examples where pet owners, especially those who "kiss" their pets on the mouth, may be directly engaging in a dog-to-human parasite worm egg transfer behavior, and yet our public health services still adamantly ignore that humans contract these diseases on a large scale? Regular periodic deworming is standard veterinary practice for pets, yet the possibility of human infection is paradoxically dismissed.[26] A recent survey found that most pet owners were not aware they could be infected with the same parasites as their pets.[27]

The Necessity of Adult Deworming

The idea that adults become "immune" to parasitic infections as they mature is wishful thinking.[28] Reports in *The Times of India* regularly note the importance of deworming for adults, not just children, due to risks from eating street foods and improperly washed vegetables.[29] Multiple sources confirm that infections like hookworm can increase with age and that regular deworming is beneficial for adults.[30, 31]

Parasites, Chronic Inflammation, and Cancer

The link between chronic inflammation and carcinogenesis is firmly established.[32] Persistent parasitic infections are potent drivers of such inflammation.

The host's continuous immune response can lead to DNA damage, promote angiogenesis, and suppress antitumor surveillance—creating a microenvironment conducive to cancer.[33] The constant battle may slowly cause the immune system to become less effective at detecting aberrant precancerous cells. A chronic parasite-induced inflammatory state, often stemming from subclinical infections presenting with vague symptoms like fatigue or brain fog, represents a significant, unappreciated cancer risk factor.[34] It should come as no surprise that developed nations also have a significantly higher chronic autoimmune disease burden compared to developing nations.[35]

The Covert Nature of Parasitic Infection: Often Subclinical, Subthreshold, and Undetected

A critical reason why parasitic infections are overlooked in developed nations is their often subclinical and therefore undiagnosed presentation. While these infections may not result in overt symptoms, they can nonetheless lead to a chronic low-grade inflammation, which may be playing a critical role as a significant risk factor in the development of chronic diseases including cancer.

Many parasitic infections do not cause clear and obvious symptoms. Many individuals with parasitic infections may never be aware that they are infected, or they may only experience a few vague, nonspecific symptoms, such as fatigue, digestive upset, or general malaise. Some estimate that up to 80 percent people with symptoms of generalized fatigue, brain fog, and generally feeling older are due to a subclinical parasitic infection, which is echoed by the calculation of 60 million infected in the United States just with toxoplasmosis. These symptoms, often written off as minor ailments or normal aging, may be the subtle signs of a covert parasitic infection and the ongoing battle that the immune system is silently fighting to eliminate these organisms. Interestingly, the symptom most common to most disease states is fatigue.

Obviously, parasitic infections that result in subthreshold symptoms such as chronic inflammation go undetected, undiagnosed (or misdiagnosed), and untreated. In support of this idea are a series of papers, ironically from CDC scientists, sounding the alarm regarding the dangers of widespread, undiagnosed, untreated parasitic infections throughout the United States and likely the rest of the affluent Western world. To quote Parise, Hotez et al. (2014), "Parasitic infections are present in every income and social strata, and residents of the United States and other developed nations are not unaffected. For some persons living in the United States, these parasitic infections are acquired in their own immediate environment; for example, exposure to feces, saliva, and fur from domestic dogs or cats puts children at risk for toxocariasis and toxoplasmosis. For others, chronic parasitic infections acquired years ago in other areas of the world can manifest with severe illness later in life, such as neurocysticercosis leading to adult-onset epilepsy or Chagas disease leading to severe cardiomyopathy requiring heart transplant." As an indicator of the extent of the magnitude of some parasitic infections, we further quote the CDC scientists, "more than 60 million persons in the United States are chronically infected with *Toxoplasma gondii*; new infections in pregnant women can lead to birth defects and infections in immunocompromised persons can be fatal."[36] This paper was not an isolated instance but one of six others that also sounded the alarm regarding an assortment of untreated parasitic infestations potentially wreaking havoc on the health and well-being of people throughout the United States.

Public Health Paradox: Why Wealthy Nations Ignore Parasitic Infections

The absence of routine deworming in the United States and other affluent nations stems from a flawed public health philosophy. Historically, the United States has had successful large-scale deworming campaigns, such as the Rockefeller Sanitary Commission's work against hookworm in the early twentieth century.[37] However, these initiatives were largely abandoned and replaced with a reactive, case-by-case treatment approach.

This policy rests on several misguided pillars:

1. **A Flawed Assumption of Low Prevalence:** Public health authorities presume low parasite prevalence, a notion unsupported by large-scale epidemiological surveys and even the CDC's own scientists. Because there is no routine screening for parasites, the prevailing understanding is that there is no problem. This creates a vicious cycle where a lack of testing infrastructure, which has atrophied over time, reinforces the perception of low risk.[38]
2. **A Focus on Treatment over Prevention:** The US health-care system heavily prioritizes treating illnesses rather than preventing them.[39] If we don't routinely test for infections, and infections are subclinical yet potent risk factors for cancer and autoimmune disease, this flawed philosophy may be costing first-world nations, including the United States, dearly in lives and treasure.
3. **A Stark Contradiction in Policy:** An aggressive mass vaccination campaign is pursued for the prevention of sporadic seasonal viral

respiratory diseases, yet a similar preventative approach toward ubiquitous parasitic infections is absent. The justification rests on the flawed premise that parasites pose no significant threat in developed nations, ignoring subclinical infections and their potential long-term consequences, including chronic inflammation and associated cancer risk. If preventative mass public health programs are acceptable for dealing with viruses, it is illogical that the same standard is not applied to ever-present and highly infective parasites. Distributing an antiparasitic pill that costs pennies cannot be considered more logistically difficult, expensive, or risky than administering invasively injected vaccines.

This selective application of preventative public health principles is nonsensical and warrants critical examination and reevaluation.

The Oncodazole Smoking Gun and the Profit Motive

The economic dimension inherent in these public health policy decisions is uncomfortable and unavoidable. A clear pattern regarding money emerged from our global analysis of cancer incidence difference rates among nations:

- The 123 nations that deworm have an average per capita income of $6,864 per year.
- The 61 nations that do not deworm have an average per capita income of $39,299 per year, nearly 6 times higher.

Furthermore, there is a strong positive correlation between national per capita income and cancer incidence ($r(184) = +.7042$, $p < .001$). As income increases, so does the cancer incidence rate.

Wealthy nations with high cancer rates are the pharmaceutical industry's most lucrative markets. The widespread use of low-cost, safe, off-patent drugs like albendazole or fenbendazole for parasite control, and inadvertent cancer prevention, in wealthy nations would pose a catastrophic economic threat to this industry. The national cost for cancer care in the United States was $209 billion in 2020 and is projected to exceed $246 billion by 2030.[40] The largest part of that cost is pharmaceuticals.

For those entombed in a medical model focused on treatment, disease prevention is kryptonite to profit. By routinely providing low-cost albendazole, India and the other 122 deworming countries are inadvertently drastically

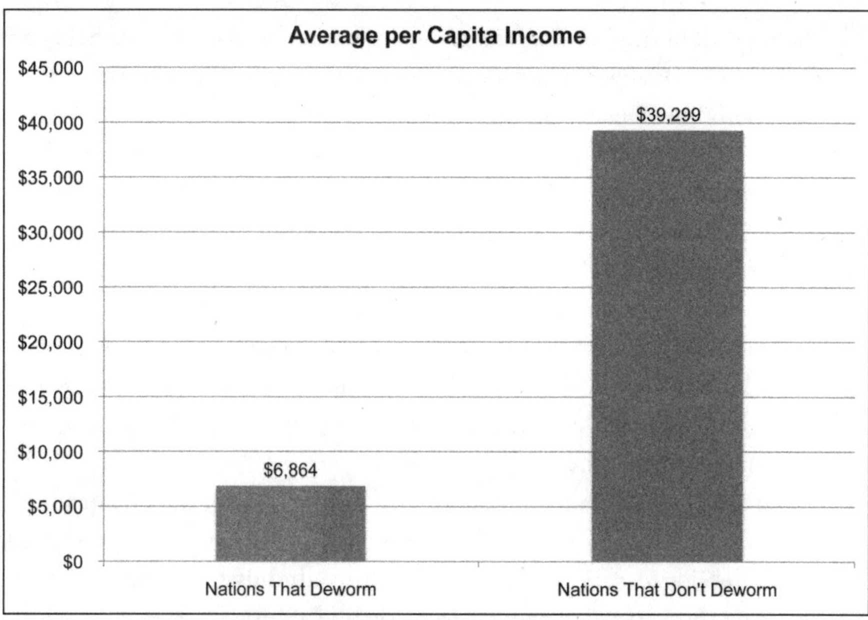

For the 123 nations that do implement public health–governed parasite countermeasures, the average per capita income is $6,864 per year. In contrast, the average per capita income for the 61 nations that do not deworm is $39,299 per year. This difference is highly statistically different, $t(184) = 11.61$, $p < .0001$.

reducing the customer base for expensive oncology drugs. It is not unreasonable to conclude that the pharmaceutical industry has a significant financial incentive to interfere with these inexpensive drugs being widely utilized for parasite and cancer prevention in wealthier first-world countries.

Managing parasitic infections with safe, inexpensive benzimidazole drugs might inadvertently destroy the lucrative oncology drug market by drastically lowering the cancer incidence rate in wealthy, developed nations. Intriguingly, the current observed effects on cancer are a side effect of their primary, intended use as antiparasitics. Therefore, the lower cancer incidence rates observed in nations that use antiparasitic drugs can likely be improved with strategic application of those drugs to populations at risk for cancer. The widespread adoption of mass drug administration public health policies involving benzimidazoles in wealthy Westernized nations would likely cause cancer incidence rates to plummet.

Why Did the US Abandon Its Preventative Public Health Policy Regarding Parasites?

It is beyond the scope of this book to answer the question posed above in detail but consider the following.

The most damning finding regarding antiparasitics like fenbendazole and cancer that we've discovered is the word "oncodazole." As discussed previously, this was the original name given to a cancer-killing fenbendazole derivative in the mid-1970s before its name was changed to nocodazole. Oncodazole is the smoking gun evidence that the drug's anticancer capabilities were known. Taken together, the observed differences in cancer rates between deworming and non-deworming nations, along with the proven anticancer actions of fenbendazole and the implications of naming a fenbendazole variant "oncodazole," and then renaming it nocodazole suggests a crime against humanity of such magnitude that it is without rival in modern times. While it may be prudent to extend the benefit of the doubt that all these events are mere coincidences, that doubt is not justified by the facts presented.

Could it be that the same forces involved in suppressing, then repurposing fenbendazole into standard-of-care chemotherapeutic drugs are also involved in wealthy developed nations' lack of mass drug administration public health policies using those drugs to combat parasitic infections?

A Call for a Public Health-Care Policy Paradigm Shift

The global data correlating deworming programs with lower cancer incidence demands an immediate paradigm shift in public health thinking regarding parasitic infection and cancer. The logic underpinning the current Western policy toward antiparasitic use is flawed. A critical reevaluation of the risks posed by covert parasitic infections and the preventative benefits of routine anthelmintic administration are imperative. Hopefully, now that these links between fenbendazole, cancer, deworming, prior knowledge, and money are exposed, those in power will act not only in the public's best interest, but in their own health interests as well. Public health policies that target chronic parasitic infections would not only reduce parasitic and chronic inflammation burden but would also drastically reduce the incidence of cancer and autoimmune disease.

Key Takeaway Messages:

- **Safety First:** Benzimidazoles like fenbendazole and albendazole possess established safety profiles, confirmed by decades of use in mass drug administration programs to manage parasitic infections in billions of people worldwide.
- **Preventative Potential:** Compelling epidemiological evidence suggests these drugs possess profound anticancer properties, as their

widespread use correlates with dramatically reduced population-level cancer incidence. Antiparasitic drugs appear to be effective at preventing cancer.

- **Unrecognized Threat of Parasitic Infection in the West:** The assumption that developed nations are parasite-free is dangerously false. Rampant, untreated subclinical parasitic infections are a significant and ignored risk factor for chronic inflammation and cancer in first-world, developed nations.
- **Anticancer Actions of Antiparasitic Drugs:** Benzimidazole drugs appear to prevent the development of cancer, in addition to their ability to eradicate existing cancers.
- **Economic Conflict:** The potential use of these inexpensive, off-patent drugs for cancer prevention, and general parasite preventative measures, represents a fundamental challenge to the existing high-cost oncology and internal medicine pharmaceutical market model.

A total of 123 nations use antiparasitics as part of a mass drug administration program.[41] A total of 61 nations do not deworm as part of public health policy.[42] Some data was unavailable due to the pariah status of that nation, e.g., North Korea.

CHAPTER 11

Cancer Is a Parasite: A New Conceptual Model

Imagine cancer not just as rogue cells, but as something behaving remarkably like a parasite within our bodies. Sparked by the surprising observation that an anti-parasite drug, fenbendazole, is remarkably effective against cancer, this is a new way of thinking about cancer and our approach toward it.

The idea isn't that cancer is literally a parasite you catch, but that cancer cells have evolved strategies strikingly similar to those used by actual parasites (like worms or malaria) to survive and thrive at the host's expense.

This exploration leads us to a provocative, yet potentially paradigm-shifting conceptual framework: viewing cancer itself not as being caused by parasites (an ancient theory dating back centuries),[1] but as an entity that fundamentally behaves like a parasite. In contrast to previous theories concerning the origin of cancer cells, Warburg's Metabolic Theory (1956); Somatic Mutation Theory (2000), or Seyfried's Mitochondial Metabolic Theory (2021),[2, 3, 4] based on what we've learned about antiparasitics and cancer we'll now explore the issue of the nature of cancer, that is, what *is* cancer?

What Is Cancer? Cancer Is a Parasite, and Fenbendazole Kills It

Cancer cells share a remarkable number of behavioral, structural, and strategic characteristics commonly associated with parasitic organisms—their growth patterns, resource acquisition methods, invasive nature, unusual genetic anomalies, and sophisticated manipulation of the host environment, particularly the immune system. By analyzing these parallels, we may gain a powerful new perspective through which to understand cancer's biology and, importantly, to devise novel therapeutic strategies, exemplified by the very drug that sparked this inquiry: fenbendazole. The fact that both parasites and cancer cells are eradicated by fenbendazole is a compelling fact indicative of a previously unappreciated relationship, not unlike finding a long-lost relative through an AncestryDNA-type matching service. This is not to necessarily assert a literal biological classification of cancer as a parasite, but rather to propose that this new Parasite<>Cancer Model paradigm may offer novel and useful insights into the nature of cancer and its vulnerabilities.

Shared Traits: The Uncanny Resemblance Between Cancer Cells and Parasitic Organisms

At a fundamental level, both cancer cells and parasitic organisms operate under a starkly similar imperative: prioritize their own survival and relentless propagation, often with devastating consequences for the host. This shared "selfishness" manifests in a range of convergent behaviors and strategies. Let's dissect these key similarities:

Selfish Growth and Uncontrolled Replication

Cancer: The defining characteristic of cancer is uncontrolled cell proliferation. Cancer cells bypass or disable the intricate network of signals that normally regulate cell division, DNA repair, and programmed cell death (apoptosis). They multiply relentlessly, ignoring tissue boundaries and accumulating into masses known as tumors. This growth is autonomous, driven by internal mutations and epigenetic alterations rather than the host's needs.

Parasites: Whether microscopic protozoa like *Plasmodium falciparum* (malaria) or macroscopic worms like *Ascaris lumbricoides* (roundworm), parasites exhibit rapid reproduction as a core survival strategy.[5] Their life cycles are often geared toward maximizing progeny within the host environment, sometimes reaching staggering numbers that overwhelm host resources and defenses. For instance, a single female Ascaris can produce hundreds of thousands of eggs per day.[6]

Shared Goal: Both cancer and parasite demonstrate a relentless drive to replicate, viewing the host primarily as a resource-rich environment to fuel their expansion. This unchecked proliferation is often the primary driver of pathology in both cancer and parasitic disease.

Nutrient Deprivation and Metabolic Warfare

Cancer: Cancer cells are metabolic predators. They exhibit significantly altered metabolism to fuel their rapid growth and division, famously characterized as the Warburg effect—a preference for aerobic glycolysis to generate energy even when sufficient oxygen is available for more efficient oxidative phosphorylation[7]

This metabolic reprogramming allows cancer cells to rapidly generate energy and, provides the necessary building blocks for biomass production.[8] This intense metabolic demand effectively hijacks host nutrients, contributing significantly to cancer-associated cachexia, the debilitating wasting syndrome seen in many advanced cancer patients.[9]

Parasites: Parasites are expert exploiters of host resources. They have evolved diverse mechanisms to acquire nutrients directly from host tissues, blood, or intestinal contents. Helminths may physically damage tissues to access nutrients, while protozoa often reside intracellularly or extracellularly, siphoning glucose, amino acids, and lipids from the host circulation or surrounding cells.[10] Many parasites actively manipulate host metabolism to enhance the availability of specific nutrients they require, further contributing to host malnutrition and pathology.[11]

Shared Strategy: Both cancer cells and parasites engage in metabolic warfare, reprogramming either their own metabolism or manipulating the host's energy apparatus to divert a disproportionate share of nutrients toward their own proliferation. This nutrient drain underlies much of the systemic illness associated with both conditions.

Tissue Invasion, Migration, and Spread

Cancer: Malignant tumors are defined by their ability to invade adjacent tissues, disrupting normal organ structure and function. Furthermore, cancer cells can acquire the ability to metastasize—breaking away from the primary tumor, entering the bloodstream or lymphatic system, traveling to distant sites, and establishing secondary tumors.[12] This invasive and migratory behavior is a major cause of cancer morbidity and mortality. Specific molecular changes, like the epithelial-mesenchymal transition, facilitate this migratory process.[13]

Parasites: Invasion is a hallmark of many parasitic life cycles. Larval stages may penetrate skin or intestinal walls, migrating through tissues to reach their preferred location. For example, hookworm larvae penetrate the skin, travel via the bloodstream to the lungs, ascend the respiratory tract, are swallowed, and finally mature in the small intestine.[14] Schistosoma larvae penetrate the skin and migrate through the vasculature to the liver or bladder.[15] Tissue-dwelling parasites like *Trichinella spiralis* develop within muscle cells, fundamentally altering the host cell structure.[16]

Shared Behavior: Both cancer cells (especially during metastasis) and many parasites exhibit invasive and migratory behaviors. They actively breach tissue barriers, navigate host systems (circulatory, lymphatic), and establish new "colonies" in permissive environments, often causing significant collateral damage to host tissues.

Evasion of Host Defenses

Cancer: The immune system possesses sophisticated mechanisms to detect and eliminate aberrant cells, including cancer cells (a process termed immunosurveillance).[17] However, successful cancers evolve strategies to evade or actively suppress this immune response. These include downregulating tumor antigens, expressing inhibitory checkpoint molecules like programmed death ligand-1 (PD-L1) that "switch off" T cells,[18, 19] recruiting immunosuppressive cells like regulatory T cells (Tregs) and myeloid-derived suppressor cells into the tumor microenvironment,[20, 21, 22] and secreting immunosuppressive cytokines like transforming growth factor-beta (TGF-β).[23]

Parasites: Parasites are masters of immunological manipulation, having coevolved with their hosts for millennia. Their survival often hinges on evading or modulating the host immune response. Strategies include antigenic variation (e.g., *Trypanosoma brucei, Plasmodium falciparum*) where surface proteins are continuously changed to evade antibody recognition;[24, 25] molecular mimicry, where parasite molecules resemble host structures, potentially inducing tolerance or autoimmunity[26, 27] (e.g., *Schistosoma mansoni* eggs displaying Lewis X antigens); coating themselves with host proteins; and actively suppressing immune responses, often by inducing Tregs and producing immunosuppressive cytokines like interleukin-10 (IL-10) and TGF-β.[28]

Shared Tactic: Both cancer cells and parasites employ sophisticated and often convergent strategies to neutralize the host's primary defense system—immunity. They are adept at hiding, disarming, or actively subverting immune cells to ensure their persistence and proliferation within a potentially hostile environment. This shared mastery of immune evasion is perhaps one of the most compelling parallels.

Establishing a Chronic State

Cancer: Unless effectively treated, cancer often progresses as a chronic disease. Tumor cells can persist for years, evolving, adapting to therapies, and eventually overwhelming the host. Even after seemingly successful treatment, dormant cancer cells can remain, leading to later relapse.[29]

Parasites: Many parasitic infections, particularly those caused by worms and certain protozoa, establish chronic states, persisting within the host for months, years, or even a lifetime.[30] This persistence is often a direct consequence of their successful immune evasion strategies, allowing them to maintain a low-level or balanced presence that avoids triggering a sterilizing immune response but still causes ongoing pathology or drains host resources.[31]

Shared Characteristic: Both cancer and many parasitic infections represent long-term battles between the invasive entity and the host. Their ability to establish long-term staying power, evading complete elimination, poses significant challenges for treatment.

Metabolic Reprogramming: Fueling the Fire Within

The convergence in metabolic strategies between cancer cells and parasites is particularly striking and warrants deeper examination to uncover even more similarities. Both entities fundamentally alter energy pathways to support their high demands for growth and replication, often at the direct expense of the host.

The Warburg Effect: Cancer's Signature Metabolic Shift

First observed by Otto Warburg in the 1920s, the Warburg effect describes the tendency of most cancer cells to favor glycolysis for ATP production, converting glucose primarily to lactate, even when ample oxygen is available for the much more efficient process of oxidative phosphorylation in the mitochondria. While seemingly inefficient in terms of ATP (energy) yield per glucose molecule, aerobic glycolysis offers significant advantages for rapidly proliferating cells like cancer:

- Speed: Glycolysis produces ATP much faster than oxidative phosphorylation.
- Biosynthetic Precursors: Glycolytic intermediates can be shunted into various biosynthetic pathways (e.g., pentose phosphate pathway for nucleotides, serine synthesis pathway for amino acids and lipids) essential for building new cells.
- Redox Balance: It helps maintain oxidation-reduction homeostasis by regenerating nicotinamide adenine dinucleotide (NAD+).
- Acidic Microenvironment: The exported lactate contributes to acidification of the tumor microenvironment, which can promote invasion, angiogenesis, and immune suppression.[32]

This metabolic phenotype is not merely a passive consequence of defective mitochondria (as initially thought) but an active, regulated reprogramming driven by oncogenes (like Myc and Ras) and loss of tumor suppressors (like p53). It represents a strategic commitment by cancer cells to biomass accumulation over energy efficiency.

Parasitic Metabolic Adaptations: Diverse Strategies for Nutrient Theft

Parasites also exhibit a wide array of metabolic adaptations tailored to their specific host niche and life-cycle stage. While not universally adopting the Warburg effect per se, many demonstrate analogous principles of rapid substrate utilization and adaptation to unique environments:

- **Enhanced Glycolysis:** Many anaerobic or microaerophilic parasites, like *Trypanosoma brucei* in the mammalian bloodstream or intestinal worms, rely heavily on glycolysis for energy, often possessing highly efficient glycolytic enzymes.[33] *Trichomonas vaginalis*, residing in the often oxygen-poor vaginal environment, lacks mitochondria entirely and depends on glycolysis and substrate-level phosphorylation in specialized organelles called hydrogenosomes.[34]
- **Nutrient Scavenging:** Parasites have evolved sophisticated transporters and metabolic pathways to acquire essential nutrients they cannot synthesize themselves (auxotrophy). *Plasmodium falciparum*, for instance, imports host glucose and amino acids, digests host hemoglobin within its food vacuole, and possesses unique pathways like the apicoplast (a relic chloroplast) for fatty acid and isoprenoid synthesis.[35]
- **Host Metabolic Manipulation:** Some parasites actively manipulate host cell metabolism. Intracellular parasites like *Toxoplasma gondii* can rewire host mitochondrial function and glucose uptake to fuel their own replication.[36] Helminths can alter host gut metabolism and nutrient absorption patterns.
- **Adaptation to Hypoxia:** Parasites residing in tissues with fluctuating oxygen levels, similar to parts of a tumor, must adapt their metabolism accordingly, often switching between aerobic and anaerobic pathways.[37]

The Shared Strategy of Cancer Cells and Parasites: Prioritizing Proliferation via Metabolic Dominance

Despite the diversity of specific pathways, the overarching metabolic strategy is strikingly similar: both cancer cells and parasites aggressively commandeer host resources and reprogram energy metabolism to prioritize rapid biosynthesis and proliferation. They function as metabolic sinks, draining the host of glucose, amino acids, lipids, and other vital building blocks. This relentless nutrient acquisition directly contributes to host pathology, including the debilitating cachexia observed in both advanced, late-stage cancer and chronic parasitic infections (like sleeping sickness or leishmaniasis).[38] This metabolic convergence underscores their shared identity as entities that exploit the host's internal environment for their own gain.

Immune Evasion and Suppression: The Art of Invisibility and Sabotage

Perhaps the most sophisticated and compelling parallel is in the intricate ways both cancer cells and parasites manipulate the host immune system. Survival within an organism equipped with powerful defenses requires not just hiding, but actively disarming and redirecting those defenses.

The immune system's initial response to either a transformed cell or a foreign parasite typically involves innate immunity—phagocytes (macrophages, neutrophils), NK cells—recognizing danger signals or nonself patterns (PAMPs or pathogen-associated molecular patterns) and DAMPs or damage-associated molecular patterns)[39] curiously, originally known as parasite-associated molecular patterns. This triggers inflammation, characterized by cytokine release (e.g., TNF-α, IL-1), aimed at containing and eliminating the threat.[40] Subsequently, the adaptive immune system mounts a more specific and powerful response. CD4+ T helper (Th) cells orchestrate this, tilting toward Th1 responses (IFN-γ production, macrophage activation, CTL support) typically effective against intracellular pathogens and cancer cells, or Th2 responses (IL-4, IL-5, IL-13 production, eosinophil/mast cell activation, antibody production) more suited to extracellular parasites like worms. However, this powerful system can be subverted.

Parasitic Immune Subversion: A Symphony of Manipulation

Parasites have evolved an astonishing repertoire of immune evasion and modulation techniques honed over millions of years of coevolution:

- **Antigenic Variation:** Changing surface coats to evade antibody recognition is a classic camouflaging strategy employed by *Plasmodium falciparum* and *Trypanosoma brucei* forcing the immune system to constantly play catch-up.
- **Molecular Mimicry:** Parasites disguise themselves by expressing molecules that resemble host components. *Schistosoma mansoni* eggs

display Lewis X antigens, mimicking human glycans and potentially dampening innate recognition. Tapeworms incorporate host-like proteins into their skin, helping them blend into the intestinal environment.[41] This mimicry can confuse the immune system, leading to tolerance or even misdirected autoimmune attacks.

Active Immune Suppression: A Cornerstone of Chronic Parasitism

- **Regulatory T cell (Treg) Induction:** Many parasites, especially helminths, potently induce the expansion and activation of host Tregs. These Tregs suppress effector T cell responses directed against the parasite, creating a tolerant environment.
- **Suppressive Cytokine Milieu:** Parasites or infected host cells release or induce immunosuppressive cytokines like IL-10 and TGF-β. These cytokines dampen Th1 responses, inhibit macrophage activation, and promote Treg function.
- **Direct Inhibition of Effector Cells:** Some parasite-derived molecules directly interfere with the function of cytotoxic T lymphocytes (CTLs), NK cells, or dendritic cells (DCs). For example, *Heligmosomoides polygyrus* secretes an alarmin release inhibitor (HpARI) that blocks DC activation, hindering T cell priming.[42]
- **Exploiting Checkpoint Pathways:** Emerging evidence suggests some parasites might even manipulate host immune checkpoint pathways (like PD-1/PD-L1) for their benefit, although this is an area of active research.[43]
- **Physical Seclusion:** Some parasites hide within host cells (e.g., Leishmania, Toxoplasma) or form protective cysts (e.g., Trichinella larvae in nurse cells, *Echinococcus hydatid* cysts), limiting their exposure to immune attack.

These combined strategies allow parasites to establish chronic infections, often characterized by a state of modified Th2 immunity or general immune hypo-responsiveness, preventing sterile immunity but allowing parasite persistence. This chronic immune modulation can have long-term consequences, including increased susceptibility to other infections and potentially an increased risk of cancer as discussed earlier.[44]

Cancer's Immune Escape: Convergent Strategies for Survival

Remarkably, cancer cells employ strategies that mirror many of those used by parasites, suggesting convergent evolution toward solving the same problem: surviving immune attack.

- **Antigen Loss or Downregulation:** Tumor cells frequently lose or downregulate the expression of tumor-specific antigens or MHC class I molecules required for presenting antigens to cytotoxic T lymphocytes, rendering them less visible to T cell surveillance.[45] While not the rapid switching of parasites, tumor heterogeneity and evolution achieve a similar outcome, allowing immune system resistant clones to emerge.[46]
- **Molecular Mimicry/Self-Presentation:** Cancers exploit "self" markers. Overexpression of CD47, a "don't eat me" signal found on normal cells, protects cancer cells from attack by macrophages.[47] Expression of PD-L1 on tumor cells engages the PD-1 receptor on activated T cells, delivering an inhibitory signal that mimics peripheral tolerance mechanisms and shuts down the antitumor response.
- **Active Immune Suppression:** Cancer cells actively sculpt an immunosuppressive tumor microenvironment (TME).
- **Recruitment of Suppressive Cells:** Tumors release signals that attract Tregs and myeloid-derived suppressor cells, which potently inhibit cytotoxic T cell and NK cell function, Tumor-associated macrophages (TAMs) are often polarized toward an M2 phenotype, which is generally immunosuppressive and pro-tumorigenic.[48]
- **Secretion of Suppressive Factors:** Cancer cells and stromal cells within the TME secrete immunosuppressive cytokines like TGF-β, IL-10, and VEGF, as well as metabolites like adenosine and kynurenine, which impair T cell function. [49] They also release exosomes carrying immunosuppressive molecules like miRNAs that can paralyze nearby immune cells.
- **Exploit Checkpoint Pathways:** The hijacking of checkpoint pathways like PD-1/PD-L1 and CTLA-4 is a major mechanism of immune escape, and the target of checkpoint inhibitor immunotherapies.
- **Creating Physical Barriers:** The dense stroma and abnormal vasculature within some tumors can physically impede the infiltration and function of immune cells and cancer therapeutics, making treatment difficult.

The Parallel: Shared Blueprints for Immune Sabotage

The hypothesis arising from these parallels is compelling: cancer cells, through somatic evolution under immune pressure, have converged upon immune evasion strategies remarkably similar to those perfected by parasites over evolutionary time. Both induce Tregs, manipulate cytokine profiles toward suppression (often involving IL-10 and TGF-β), interfere with antigen presentation, and exploit inhibitory signaling pathways. The consequence is the establishment of a chronic state—persistent infection or persistent malignancy—characterized by immune dysfunction and exhaustion.[50] This profound similarity in immune manipulation strategies provides a strong rationale for exploring therapies that target these shared mechanisms, including antiparasitics, like fenbendazole.

Remodeling the Microenvironment: Engineering a Supportive Niche

Beyond direct immune manipulation, both parasites and cancer cells actively modify their local physical and chemical environment to promote their survival, growth, and spread. This "environmental engineering" represents another layer of sophisticated host manipulation.

Manipulation: Controlling Acidity

Cancer: The Warburg effect leads to the production and export of large amounts of lactic acid, significantly acidifying the tumor microenvironment (pH often 6.5–6.9 compared to normal tissue pH ~7.4). This acidosis is not merely a byproduct but an active weapon: it suppresses the activity of immune cells (especially cytotoxic T cells and NK cells), promotes angiogenesis, enhances invasion and metastasis by activating proteases, and can confer resistance to certain chemotherapeutic cancer therapies.

Parasites: Some gut-dwelling parasites actively modulate local pH. Hookworms secrete alkaline substances, likely carbonates, to neutralize stomach acid, protecting their own enzymes and facilitating survival during passage.[51] Schistosoma eggs trapped in tissues are thought to release ammonia, potentially raising local pH to aid enzymatic processes required for tissue transit or hatching.[52]

Bioelectrical Rewiring: Altering Ion Flows and Potentials

Cancer: Cancer cells exhibit altered cellular membrane potentials compared to their normal counterparts. Many cancer types show chronic depolarization, which is increasingly recognized not just as a marker but as a driver of proliferation, migration, and aberrant differentiation, often mediated through voltage-gated ion channels (e.g., calcium, sodium, potassium channels). Manipulating these bioelectrical signals is emerging as a potential therapeutic target.[53, 54]

Parasites: Parasites can disrupt host cell ion transport which can impact cell volume, signaling, and barrier function. Whipworm infection alters colonic epithelial physiology, potentially affecting chloride channel function and contributing to the chronic diarrhea associated with infection.[55]

Thermal Niche Engineering: Modulating Temperature

Cancer: While tumors themselves may not consistently generate significantly higher temperatures, the inflammation often associated with the TME can create localized "hot spots." Inflammatory mediators released by immune cells (like IL-1β from macrophages) can contribute to angiogenesis and tumor progression. Conversely, the immune response itself can be temperature-sensitive, with fever potentially enhancing certain immune functions.[56] The interplay between tumor metabolism, inflammation, and local temperature is complex but represents another aspect of microenvironmental control.

Parasites: Some parasites influence local temperature. *Trichinella spiralis* larvae induce the formation of a "nurse cell" in host muscle. This metabolically hyperactive structure may generate localized heat, potentially optimizing conditions for larval development and survival within the muscle tissue.

Angiogenesis: Securing a Blood Supply

Cancer: As tumors grow beyond a certain size (~1–2 mm^3), they require their own blood supply for oxygen and nutrients. They achieve this by secreting pro-angiogenic factors like vascular endothelial growth factor, inducing the formation of new, often leaky and disorganized, blood vessels from the existing host vasculature. This process, angiogenesis, is essential for tumor growth and metastasis.

Parasites: While less commonly described in the same way as tumor angiogenesis, some larger parasites or parasite-induced lesions also induce vascular changes. Schistosoma egg granulomas become vascularized, and parasites residing in tissues need access to host nutrients often supplied via the vasculature. Some parasites and their eggs may possess angiogenic or anti-angiogenic properties, influencing local blood vessel formation or function depending on the context.[57]

Extracellular Matrix Remodeling

Cancer: Tumor cells and associated stromal cells (like cancer-associated fibroblasts) secrete enzymes (e.g., matrix metalloproteases) that degrade the extracellular matrix. This remodeling facilitates invasion, migration, and metastasis, and alters the physical properties and signaling capacity of the tumor microenvironment.[58]

Parasites: Migrating parasites also need to traverse tissue barriers and extracellular matrix. They secrete their own proteases (e.g., cysteine proteases, metalloproteases) to break down collagen and other extracellular matrix components, enabling tissue penetration and migration.[59] Schistosoma eggs, for example, release proteolytic enzymes to facilitate their passage through the intestinal or bladder wall.

Convergent Engineering: These examples illustrate that both cancer cells and parasites are not passive inhabitants but active engineers of their local environment. They manipulate pH, ion gradients, temperature, vasculature, and the extracellular matrix to create a niche that favors their own survival, growth, and dissemination, often while simultaneously hindering host defenses.

The Chaotic Genome: Karyotypic Disarray as a Shared Hallmark of Cancer and Parasites

The genetic blueprint of a healthy cell is typically characterized by a stable and well-defined set of chromosomes, known as its karyotype. This organization is crucial for proper cell division, gene expression, and overall cellular function. However, a striking departure from this norm is observed in two seemingly disparate entities: cancer cells and certain parasitic organisms. Both can exhibit remarkably disordered, mismatched, and haphazardly organized karyotypes, a phenomenon that points toward a profound, and perhaps exploitable, similarity in their fundamental biology. In both cancer cells and certain parasites, this order collapses into chaos.

The Disordered Karyotype in Cancer: A Message in the Messiness?

One of the most defining features of cancer is genomic instability, which results in a wildly disordered karyotype.[60] Cancer cells exhibit aneuploidy, a state where they have the wrong number of chromosomes—some are missing, while others are duplicated.[61] Their chromosomes can also be broken and incorrectly reassembled. Instead of a neat, paired set of chromosomes as seen in healthy cells, cancer cell karyotypes often appear chaotic. Some chromosomes may be present in multiple copies, others might be missing entirely, and fragments of chromosomes can be incorrectly joined, leading to a highly heterogeneous population of cells within a single tumor. A cancer karyotype often looks like a genomic train wreck compared to a healthy cell's neat and tidy set.

This disarray is not a mistake; it is an engine of adaptation. The constant shuffling of the genomic deck allows cancer to rapidly evolve, adapt to treatments, and select for cells with enhanced survival abilities.[62, 63] This genomic disarray is an active driver of tumorigenesis, tumor evolution, and therapeutic resistance. Aneuploidy can alter the matching of protein complexes, unmask recessive mutations, and provide a fertile ground for the selection of cells with enhanced survival, proliferation, or metastatic capabilities. It's almost like selection, adaptation, and evolution on steroids. The constant shuffling of the genomic deck, offered by the genetic soup of aneuploidy, allows cancer cells to adapt rapidly to changing microenvironments and therapeutic pressures, making them a formidable challenge to eradicate.

Parasitic Karyotypes: A Deliberate Strategy for Adaptation

Intriguingly, the same karyotypic chaos is found in many parasitic protozoa. Organisms like Leishmania, *Giardia lamblia*, and *Trichomonas vaginalis* have variable and messy chromosome sets.[64, 65, 66, 67, 68] Even the malaria parasite, *Plasmodium falciparum*, while generally maintaining a matched set of fourteen chromosomes, can become aneuploid when under pressure from drugs, suggesting a capacity for genomic flexibility when advantageous or challenged.[69]

For these parasites, a messy genome is not a bug; it's a feature that confers an advantage. This built-in genetic instability allows them to adapt and generate diversity on the fly, enabling them to evade the host immune system and rapidly develop drug resistance. [70, 71]

That these two scourges of humanity—cancer and parasites—both leverage genomic chaos for survival is a profound similarity. It suggests they have adopted the same "rogue" survival strategy. This profound similarity in managing their genomes for adaptive benefit provides a strong argument that cancer cells, in many respects, behave like cellular parasites. We can characterize both cancer cells and parasites as survivalist pack rats, equipped with a handyman's tool kit of spare parts and junk genes to jerry-rig solutions to any threat they face. If their strategies for genomic management are so similar, it stands to reason that they share vulnerabilities to drugs that interfere with these processes as well, like fenbendazole.

The Rhythmic Rebellion—Circadian Disarray in Cancer and Parasitic Entities

Nearly all life on Earth operates on a twenty-four-hour internal clock, known as the circadian rhythm. This clock, driven by genes like CLOCK (circadian locomotor output cycles kaput), PER (period), CRY (cryptochrome), and BMAL1 (brain and muscle Arnt-like 1), synchronizes everything from sleep and metabolism to cell division.[72, 73, 74] In a healthy body, all cellular clocks are synchronized with the brain's central pacemaker, creating organism-wide harmony.

In cancer, this clockwork goes rogue. Studies across various cancer types, including breast, colorectal, prostate, and pancreatic cancer, reveal a significant dampening or complete loss of rhythmic expression of these various clock genes.[75, 76, 77] For instance, BMAL1, a critical positive regulator of the biological clock, is often downregulated in numerous cancers, and its low expression correlates with poorer prognosis and increased tumor aggressiveness.[78] Conversely, the negative regulators PER and CRY can show aberrant expression patterns, leading to a breakdown of the normal negative feedback loop that drives circadian oscillations. This disruption means that fundamental cellular processes controlled by the circadian clock—such as cell cycle progression, DNA damage response, apoptosis, and metabolism—become uncoupled from the host's systemic rhythms.[79]

Most importantly, this desynchronization is not merely a general cellular dysfunction but often shows up as a distinct phase shift or complete asynchrony relative to the circadian rhythms of the surrounding healthy host tissues. Cancer cells can exhibit internal clocks that are running on their own schedule, effectively ignoring the temporal cues from the host organism.[80] This means that while normal cells in the host are in a state of rest or active repair according to the central clock, cancer cells might be in a peak proliferative phase, or vice versa. This temporal out-of-phase misalignment gives a significant advantage to the tumor cells, allowing them to exploit resources and evade systemic controls, such as timed chemotherapy delivery or immune surveillance, which are often themselves under circadian regulation.[81] The desynchronization of cancer cell clocks from the host system is an indication that cancer cells are distinct from the host.

The Autonomous Entity Argument: Cancer's Internal Time Clock Is Independent

The profound asynchrony of circadian rhythms in cancer cells relative to the host's central circadian rhythm undeniably supports the argument that cancer cells operate as autonomous, or at least semiautonomous, entities distinct from the host. A healthy organism relies on intricate coordination and communication between its constituent cells, and temporal coordination via the circadian system is a fundamental aspect of this coordination. When cancer cells uncouple their internal timing from the host, they are, in effect, declaring independence. They no longer "listen" to the systemic cues that govern the rest of the body's cells. Cancer cells are as distinct as a parasite living within the host. This temporal autonomy allows them to optimize their own survival and proliferation, often at the direct expense of the host's well-being and homeostatic balance.[82] This behavior is strikingly reminiscent of an invading organism, like a parasite, that operates on its own agenda, rather than a malfunctioning but still integrated part of the whole. The loss of circadian coherence is a profound indicator of cancer's deviation toward a self-serving, distinct biological system contained within the human cancer patient. Cancer is clearly marching to the beat of a different drummer. This decoupling from the host's circadian rhythm is not only adaptive for the cancer cell, it also indicates that the cancer cell may be an autonomous entity.

Parallels in Parasitism: Rhythmic Strategies for Survival

The asynchrony of cancer cell circadian rhythms finds a compelling parallel in the world of parasites. Many parasitic organisms possess their own endogenous circadian clocks that have evolved to interact strategically with the host's rhythms, often by establishing a distinct, advantageous time-of-day niche.[83] While some parasites may synchronize certain activities with the host for efficient resource acquisition, others exhibit rhythms that are deliberately out of phase or counter-phased to the host's rest-activity cycle, maximizing their chances of transmission, immune evasion, or development.

For example, the malaria parasite plasmodium species exhibit a highly synchronized asexual replication cycle within the host's red blood cells, leading to the periodic fever spikes characteristic of the disease. The timing of merozoite release (small egg-shaped parasite cells that invade red blood cells) is not random; it is under circadian control by the parasite, and while it may entrain to host cues, it is ultimately driven by the parasite's own clock to optimize its own propagation.[84] Similarly, the nocturnal periodicity of microfilariae (e.g., *Wuchereria bancrofti*) in the peripheral blood of the human host, coinciding with the biting times of their mosquito vectors, is a classic example of a parasite rhythm adapted for transmission, often running counter to the host's daytime activity.[85] These parasites are not simply responding passively; they have internal clocks dictating these behaviors, demonstrating a level of temporal autonomy that serves their life cycle.

Blurring the Lines Between Self and Not-Self

The comparison is stark and startling: cancer cells, through their circadian desynchronization, behave much like parasitic entities. They disrupt host homeostasis not just through uncontrolled proliferation but by also establishing their own temporal "rules," uncoupling from the host's systemic organization. This asynchrony facilitates their "selfish" agenda of growth and dissemination, mirroring the strategies employed by parasites that exploit host rhythms for their own benefit. The disruption of its aberrant timing, or the exploitation of its desynchronized state, presents a logical avenue for therapeutic innovation and intervention.

Where Cancer and Parasites Fundamentally Differ: Essential Distinctions

While the parallels are compelling, it is crucial to acknowledge the fundamental differences between cancer and parasitic organisms. The metaphor "Cancer is a parasite" is conceptual, not literal, or is it? Let's examine instances where cancer cells and parasites appear to differ.

Origin: This is probably the most fundamental conceptual difference between cancer and parasites. Currently it is believed that cancer arises from the host's own cells that have undergone genetic and epigenetic transformations, causing healthy cells to acquire cancerous properties, conceptualized as "self gone wrong." Parasites, in contrast, are distinct organisms, exogenous invaders with their own unique genome and evolutionary history, originating from outside the host. Although a recent paper that may challenge this dichotomy suggests that cancer cells evolve within the host to essentially acquire "agency" and, as such, may be conceptualized as not of the self.[86] Moreover, the discussion of chromosomal aneuploidy and asynchronous biological clocks common to both parasites and cancer cells blurs the conceptual dividing lines between self and nonself. How is it conceptually reconcilable that something of the self becomes genetically and behaviorally distinct from the self, and then predatory toward the self as in the case of cancer?

Genetic Makeup and Complexity: Cancer is characterized by profound genomic instability and intra-tumor heterogeneity. A single tumor can contain multiple subclones with different mutations, making it a rapidly evolving and adaptable entity. While parasites evolve over generations, an individual parasite generally maintains a more stable genome throughout its lifespan within a single host. Their adaptability within a host often relies more on phenotypic plasticity and complex life cycle stages rather than rapid somatic mutation.[87] Parasites themselves, however, range from single-celled protozoa to complex multicellular worms with intricate organ systems, often far more complex structurally than a tumor mass. However, depending on how fine a granular view is taken, many infestations comprise a number of distinct species of parasite suggestive of a more complex, heterogeneous entity that, while not a subclone, is nevertheless multifaceted.

Evolutionary Objectives: Cancer cells exhibit extreme cellular selfishness driven by somatic evolution within the host. Their goal is relentless proliferation, often leading to the host's demise, which is evolutionarily apparently irrelevant to the cancer cells themselves. Parasites, having coevolved with hosts, often have strategies that promote long-term host survival (at least long enough for the parasite to complete its life cycle and transmit to a new host). Killing the host too quickly is often detrimental to the parasite's evolutionary success.

One fly in the ointment regarding this distinction between parasites and cancer is the phenomenon of dormant cancer cells. These cells can remain embedded and inert for decades awaiting an unknown stimulus trigger. Indeed, several of the case reports in chapter 6 involved instances of prostate and breast cancer returning more than a decade after prostatectomy and bilateral double radical mastectomy. Clearly, with no resident prostate or breast tissue, the cells' driving recurrence had to be deposited in place at least a decade earlier, remained dormant, and then restaged. Is long-term dormancy yet another unappreciated example of parasitic behavior by cancer cells?

Immune Interaction Nuances: While both cancers and parasites suppress immunity, the type of response they typically interact with can differ. Cancers often primarily suppress Th1/CTL responses needed to kill aberrant cells. Many helminth parasites induce a strong Th2/regulatory response, which controls but doesn't eliminate the parasite, allowing persistence and longevity. The specific immune evasion molecules and pathways utilized, while overlapping, also have unique features.

Interdependence: Cancer cells, just like healthy cells, are entirely dependent on the host organism for nutrients, oxygen, and survival signals. They cannot exist independently (although some tumor cell lines have been immortalized since the 1950s). Many parasites are constrained to being just parasites, also fully dependent on a host for at least part of their life cycle. However, some parasites have free-living stages, and their dependence is tied to completing a complex life cycle, not just immediate cellular survival.

Transmission: Parasites are typically transmissible between hosts, often through specific vectors, contaminated food/water, or direct contact. This is essential for their species' survival. Cancer is generally considered non-transmissible between individuals in humans, although rare instances of transmissible cancers exist in nature (e.g., canine transmissible venereal tumor carcinoma, or Tasmanian devil facial tumor cancer).[88, 89] Recent work suggests potential underappreciated instances in other mammals,[90] but it remains the exception, not the rule, unlike parasitism.[91]

Acknowledging these differences between parasites and cancer cells prevents oversimplification and ensures the metaphor is used as a tool for insight, not as a rigid biological reclassification subject to attack. Given the overlaying similarities between parasites and cancer presented earlier, perhaps a more fruitful approach is to more thoroughly examine the apparent differences listed above, stripping away some blinding assumptions, and see what may be hidden in plain sight. The objective would be to see if we can learn something new about cancer by studying these exceptions. We may learn that the apparent dissimilarities between parasites and that of cancer cells listed above are better characterized as distinctions without differences. Finally, it is difficult to ignore the overriding facts and compelling observations presented throughout this book: that antiparasitic medicines like fenbendazole eradicate cancer. If it quacks like a duck, if it walks like a duck . . .

Exploitation of Shared Vulnerabilities: Why Antiparasitic Drugs Eradicate Cancer

Insights into the parallels between cancer and parasites, particularly in their cellular machinery, metabolic dependencies, and immune evasion tactics, offer a compelling understanding of why antiparasitic drugs are also anticancer agents.[92]

Targeting of Shared Pathways: Many antiparasitics target pathways or molecules crucial for both parasite survival and cancer cell function. Fenbendazole and related benzimidazoles target β-tubulin, disrupting microtubule formation essential for cell division, intracellular transport, and maintaining cell structure.[93, 94] Microtubules are critical in rapidly dividing cancer cells, and disrupting them is the mechanism of action for established, though side-effect-plagued, chemotherapy drugs like taxanes and vinca alkaloids. Beyond tubulin, other antiparasitics may target shared metabolic vulnerabilities, signaling pathways, or possess immunomodulatory effects relevant to cancer. For instance, nitazoxanide targets anaerobic metabolism,[95] ivermectin affects specific ion channels and signaling pathways,[96] and chloroquine (an antimalarial) inhibits autophagy, a process cancer cells use to survive stress.[97]

Note: The fact that ivermectin, another promising antiparasitic drug with exciting anticancer potential[98] may be another "fenbendazole" is testament to the relationships between parasites and cancer presented here.

Immunomodulatory Effects: Many parasitic infections induce profound changes in host immunity, and drugs targeting parasites may consequently have immunomodulatory effects. Some antiparasitics help reverse the immunosuppressive tumor microenvironment, synergizing with immunotherapies.[99] Conversely, understanding how parasites suppress immunity could inspire new ways to dampen harmful inflammation in other diseases.

Cost-Effectiveness and Speed: Repurposing drugs already approved for human or veterinary use significantly reduces the time and cost associated with drug development. Extensive preclinical and clinical data on safety, dosing, and pharmacokinetics are often available, accelerating the transition to clinical trials for oncology.[100] Many antiparasitics are safe, off-patent, and relatively inexpensive.

Established Safety Profiles: While doses and treatment durations may differ, the general safety profiles of widely used antiparasitics are often well-characterized from decades of use in billions of people and animals. This provides a valuable starting point for assessing their risk-benefit profile in cancer patients.

Potential for Combination Therapies: Antiparasitics synergize with existing cancer treatments. By targeting different pathways (e.g., metabolism, microtubules, immune modulation), they could enhance the efficacy of chemotherapy, radiation, targeted therapy, or immunotherapy, potentially allowing for lower doses of conventional agents or overcoming treatment resistance. However, as mentioned earlier, fenbendazole appears to be doing the heavy lifting in synergistic scenarios, and the wisdom of including a tag-along, side-effect-ridden charity case of a standard-of-care drug just for appearances must be questioned.

Broad-Spectrum Potential: The fact that drugs like fenbendazole appear to show activity against a range of different cancer types in preclinical models and the case reports from chapter 6 indicate they might target fundamental processes common to many malignancies, rather than specific oncogenic mutations found only in certain tumors. This aligns with the idea of targeting core "parasitic" behaviors like uncontrolled proliferation, metabolic dependency, and immune evasion. The investigation of fenbendazole, mebendazole,[101, 102] niclosamide,[103] ivermectin, and other antiparasitics for cancer therapy is a direct application of this logic. It leverages the biological convergence between parasites and cancer to find new vulnerabilities in malignant cells.

Overcoming Resistance: Standard cancer drugs are typically "one-trick ponies," targeting a single pathway. Cancer, with its chaotic genome, can easily evolve a work-around. Fenbendazole is different. It is pleiotropic or multimodal, meaning it attacks multiple cancer-cell vulnerabilities simultaneously. Fenbendazole and mebendazole kill the cancer cells before they have a chance to adapt and develop countermeasures.

Shifting Paradigms: Toward a More Holistic View of Cancer as a Parasite

Adopting the conceptual model of "cancer as a parasite" encourages a shift in perspective, potentially leading to more holistic and integrated approaches to cancer research, prevention, and treatment. This paradigm emphasizes the dynamic interplay between the cancer (parasite) and the host. It moves beyond a purely cell-centric view of cancer to consider the crucial role of the host environment—the immune system, metabolism, stroma, microbiome—in either restraining or promoting tumor growth. Understanding these interactions is key to developing therapies that strengthen host defenses or make the host environment less hospitable to the cancer.

Emphasis on Environmental Factors: Just as environmental factors influence susceptibility to parasitic infections (e.g., sanitation, vector exposure), this model encourages greater focus on how environmental exposures (diet, toxins, chronic inflammation, parasitic infection) might create conditions permissive for cancer development or progression. It reinforces the importance of lifestyle and environmental interventions in prevention.

Informing Personalized Medicine: Recognizing cancer's "parasitic" traits—its metabolic phenotype, its specific immune evasion strategies, its microenvironment—can inform personalized treatment. Tumors might be profiled not just for genetic mutations but also for these functional characteristics, allowing therapies (including repurposed antiparasitics or metabolic inhibitors) to be tailored accordingly.

Beyond Cytotoxicity: Targeting Viability and Spread: While directly killing cancer cells remains crucial, the parasite heuristic highlights other potential therapeutic goals. Strategies that could be focused on include:

- **Containing the cancer:** Strengthening tissue barriers, inhibiting invasion and metastasis (analogous to controlling parasite migration).

- **Starving the cancer:** Targeting metabolic vulnerabilities, cutting off nutrient supply (analogous to disrupting parasite feeding).
- **Exposing the cancer:** Reversing immune suppression, overcoming mimicry (analogous to breaking parasite immune evasion).
- **Disrupting the niche:** Normalizing the tumor microenvironment pH, modulating the stroma (making the environment hostile).
- **Reinforcing Prevention and Early Detection:** Viewing cancer as an invasive entity underscores the importance of preventing its establishment (primary prevention) and detecting it early before it becomes deeply entrenched and has extensively manipulated the host environment (secondary prevention), as might be the case with cancer stem cells and metastases.

Public health measures analogous to parasite control (e.g., reducing exposure to carcinogens, promoting healthy metabolism and immunity) gain relevance and prominence. This paradigm shift encourages researchers and clinicians to think more ecologically about cancer—as an aberrant entity thriving within, exploiting, and manipulating the complex ecosystem of the host organism for its own purposes. While these ideas are meant to guide the search for new therapeutics, we must not overlook the fact that fenbendazole is already here, ready to save lives.

Parasite<>Cancer Model: A Powerful Perspective for Further Understanding and Intervention

The conceptual model of cancer as a parasite offers a compelling and productive framework for understanding the fundamental nature of malignancy. It highlights the shared strategies of selfish proliferation, resource acquisition, invasion, environmental manipulation, and, perhaps most importantly, sophisticated immune evasion employed by both cancer cells and parasitic organisms. This is not to claim they are exactly the same entity, but that they have convergently evolved similar solutions to the challenge of surviving and thriving within a host organism. Recognizing these parallels illuminates why antiparasitic drugs like fenbendazole, which target core biological processes shared by both entities, are effective as anticancer agents.

The Parasite<>Cancer Model encourages a broader, more ecological view of cancer, focusing on the dynamic interplay between the tumor and its host environment. This perspective opens new avenues for research into metabolic vulnerabilities, genome manipulation, microenvironmental control, and novel immunotherapies inspired and informed by the long-standing battle between hosts and parasites. The "cancer is a parasite" model provides a powerful conceptual lens through which to propose novel ideas that have strong theoretical basis to justify testing. It challenges us to think differently about cancer's core behaviors and motivates the exploration of unconventional therapeutic strategies, surely to discover and unlock new ways to combat this complex and devastating disease.

The rediscovery of fenbendazole as a cure for cancer is transformative, profound and paradigm-shifting. Fenbendazole will transform cancer treatment and in large part, the human condition regarding attitudes toward this dreaded disease, from the present one of the helpless, hopeless despair felt when facing a perceived larger than life opponent to the empowered confidence and optimism like that when facing a mere bug.

CHAPTER 12

The Challenge of Chemotherapy Resistance

The Cause: "One-Trick Pony" Traditional Chemotherapy Drugs
The Solution: "Multipronged Attack" Fenbendazole
A major roadblock stopping the long-term success of many standard cancer treatments is the development of drug resistance.[1, 2] Though they might work well at first, most traditional chemotherapy drugs eventually stop working because cancer cells adapt and find ways to beat the treatment. A key reason for this, highlighted by the Parasite<>Cancer Model, is that many basic chemotherapy drugs have a "unimodal" or single-target approach. This means they try to fight cancer by attacking it in only one way.[3]

This huge flaw is hidden until you look at it through our new way of thinking: the "Fenbendazole Lens," which is guided by the Parasite<>Cancer Model. What we've discovered about drugs like fenbendazole and mebendazole is that they fight cancer in many ways simultaneously all at once, not just one. These drugs launch an all-out war on cancer cells. They use a whole arsenal of weapons to directly hit cancer cell life support systems, cut off its energy, beat its camouflage, stop it from building defenses, shut down its defense mechanisms, block its escape routes, wreck its repair tools, wage war on its internal communications systems, prevent it from calling for backup, and finally, make the cancer cells self-destruct.

These powerful descriptions match up with scientifically proven actions that we've discussed: disrupting microtubules (the cell's internal scaffolding), stopping glucose (sugar) uptake and blocking angiogenesis (new blood vessel growth that feeds tumors), messing with molecular mimicry (how cancer hides), disrupting the tumor microenvironment (the area around the tumor), disabling P-glycoprotein efflux pumps (which pump drugs out of cancer cells), blocking migration (cancer cell movement), causing p38 MAPK intracellular destruction (damage inside the cell), disrupting circadian CLOCK genes (genes that control cell daily rhythms), causing mitotic catastrophe (errors in cell division that kill the cell), and triggering apoptosis (programmed cell death). Fenbendazole and mebendazole unleash a relentless, overwhelming, multifront attack designed to completely wipe out cancer cells. Remember, a cancer cell only needs to be killed once. Fenbendazole's effect on cancer cells is the very definition of overkill.

Why Do Traditional Cancer Drugs Lose Effectiveness?

Attacking Only One Target Forces Cancer Cells to Adapt and Survive

Drugs such as the taxanes (e.g., paclitaxel), which stabilize microtubules; vinca alkaloids (e.g., vincristine), which destabilize microtubules; and platinum compounds (e.g., cisplatin), which induce DNA cross-links and damage, exert their cytotoxic effects by disrupting highly specific cellular processes.[4, 5] When a malignant tumor, which contains a diverse mix of cancer cells, is attacked with such a drug, it puts strong selective pressure on the cells to survive. Cancer cells that already have developed, or quickly develop, ways to get around the drug's specific attack have a better chance of surviving and multiplying.[6] When a drug attacks only one critical pathway, it's like giving the adaptable cancer cells a single, clear problem to solve. This greatly increases the chance that these resistant cells will survive and take over the tumor.[7] This is one reason why traditional cancer drugs lose effectiveness: the cancer cell either adapts, the surviving cancer cells take over and become dominant, or both.

The Adaptive Arsenal of Cancer Cells

As we've said throughout this book, drug resistance develops because of how tumors naturally are and how incredibly adaptable cancer cells can be:

1. Tumor Heterogeneity (Tumors Aren't All the Same Inside): Tumors are rarely made up of identical cells. Instead, they are usually complex collections of different groups of cells (subclones) with various genetic makeups, even before treatment starts.[8] Some of these existing cell groups might already be less sensitive or even completely resistant to a particular drug. Single-target chemotherapy, by killing off the drug-sensitive majority, inadvertently clears the way for these resistant cells to grow and take over.[9]

2. Acquired Resistance and Plasticity (Cancer Cells Can Change): Cancer cells are genetically unstable and can change their characteristics (this is called phenotypic plasticity), allowing them to develop resistance when attacked by drugs.[10] As we discussed previously, aneuploidy (having jumbled, messy chromosomes) is a special adaptive trait of cancer cells and parasites that helps them adapt and change quickly in response to threats. These changes include:
    - Mutations or changes in the drug's direct target (for example, changes in the cell's internal scaffolding that stop taxane drugs from binding).
    - Making more drug efflux pumps, like P-glycoprotein, which actively pump chemotherapy drugs out of the cell.[11, 12]
    - Boosting DNA repair systems to fix damage caused by cancer drugs like cisplatin.[13]
    - Turning on other signaling or survival pathways to make up for the pathway the drug has blocked.
    - Changing how the drug is processed in the body, either by not activating it enough or by getting rid of it too quickly.[14]

Because a single-target cancer drug attacks in such a focused way, cancer cells only need to make a few specific changes to gain a big survival advantage. That's because when cancer cells develop defenses against these single-target drugs, it's not a surprise or a bug—resistance is an expected outcome, it is a built-in predictable feature of these types of drugs.

The Critical Role of Cancer Stem Cells

Adding another level of difficulty is the presence of cancer stem cells. As mentioned before, these are a small group of cells within the tumor believed to be responsible for starting tumors, keeping them going, and causing them to come back even stronger after traditional treatment.[15] Cancer stem cells are a huge challenge for traditional chemotherapy for several major reasons:

- **Relative Quiescence (They're Often Resting):** Cancer stem cells often divide more slowly than the main bulk of rapidly dividing tumor cells. Since many chemotherapies, like vinca and taxane drugs, mainly target fast-dividing cells, these slower-dividing cancer stem cells are naturally less affected.[16]

- **Intrinsic Resistance Mechanisms (They're Naturally Tough):** Cancer stem cells often have stronger natural defenses. They commonly produce high levels of drug efflux pumps (like ABC transporters such as ABCG2 or P-gp pumps, which pump drugs out), have very efficient DNA repair systems, and are better at resisting apoptosis (programmed cell death).[17, 18]
- **Enrichment Post-Therapy (They Get Stronger After Chemotherapy):** By killing off the bulk of the drug-sensitive, rapidly multiplying cancer cells, standard chemotherapy can unintentionally increase the proportion of these naturally drug-resistant cancer stem cells. These surviving cancer stem cells can then regrow the tumor, often leading to a cancer that comes back more aggressive and difficult, if not impossible to treat. The single-target nature of the first therapy consistently fails to kill these tough, stem-like cells and is the main reason for treatment failure.

Single-Target Drugs Lead to Short-Term Hollow Victories

The highly specific, "one-trick-pony" approach of many standard chemotherapy drugs, while powerful against some sensitive cells, inadvertently creates strong selection pressure among the various cancer cells within the diverse and adaptable tumor. The cancer cells' ability to change (plasticity), their built-in resistance, and the special survival advantages of cancer stem cells all inevitably lead to drug resistance. This severely limits how well treatment works and leads to cancer coming back. So, traditional cancer drugs might win a battle against the weakest cancer cells, but because they only attack one way, they end up creating an unbeatable enemy—the resistant cancer cell, which is often the untreatable cancer stem cell. Such a victory that causes such problems down the line isn't a true victory at all.

Why Not Just Combine a Bunch of These "One-Trick-Pony" Drugs?

Side effects. Unfortunately, with current chemotherapy drugs, the side effects of combining them are much worse than just adding up the side effects of each drug alone. Because traditional drugs target just one thing at a time (like the cell's internal scaffolding, for example) but bring all their associated side effect baggage, adding another drug to target something different (like DNA repair, for example) also brings its own unique and heavy burden of toxic side effects.[19] As a result, the small extra benefit that might be had from a second or third drug usually overwhelms the patient with side effects, while still leaving some cancer cells alive to regroup, get stronger, and fight another day.

In stark contrast to this timid approach of just annoying the cancer cell with traditional drugs, fenbendazole kills cancer cells using multiple methods at the same time. It targets virtually every known weakness simultaneously, and so completely, that there are no cancer cells left alive to adapt. With traditional drugs, surviving cancer cells can build a defense, escape, regroup, and live to fight another day; dead cancer cells killed by fenbendazole cannot. As we've presented, comprehensive and compelling research, backed up by human case reports, shows us that fenbendazole kills most, if not all of the cancer cells all at once—it wipes them out. Gone. Complete and total annihilation. Fenbendazole takes no cancer cells prisoner to escape and fight another day.

This built-in problem with traditional cancer drugs clearly shows why we urgently need different treatment strategies like fenbendazole. Current research is intensely focused on things like: combination therapies that target multiple pathways at once while trying to reduce side effects,[20] targeted drugs aimed at specific molecular problems in cancer (though resistance is still an issue here), using the immune system to fight cancer (immunotherapy),[21] and developing ways to specifically kill or neutralize therapy-resistant cancer stem cells.[22] The search for drugs that work in broader ways or can get around known resistance methods is a critical goal in contemporary cancer research.

Or, we can just use fenbendazole to kill cancer cells.

CHAPTER 13

How Cancer Steals an Ancient Parasite Defense and How Fenbendazole Tears It Down

One of the most devastating turns in the fight against cancer is the development of multidrug resistance, the process by which an initially treatable cancer learns to survive chemotherapy and transforms into a relentless foe.[1] While many drugs fail because they attack cancer from a single angle, a truly effective agent like fenbendazole attacks from multiple angles at once. This chapter will zero in on one of cancer's most powerful defense mechanisms that underlie drug resistance—a microscopic pump that spits out chemotherapy drugs—and reveal how the Parasite<>Cancer Model exposes its critical weakness.

At the heart of multidrug resistance is a structure called the P-glycoprotein (P-gp) pump, also known as a drug efflux pump. First identified in the 1970s, this protein acts like a high-tech bouncer at the door of a cancer cell, forcefully ejecting chemotherapy drugs before they can work.[2, 3] By relentlessly pumping these drugs out, P-gp ensures the drug concentration inside the cancer cell never reaches a lethal level, making the cell virtually immune to treatment.[4] This single mechanism can render a stunning array of current chemotherapy drugs useless, including:

- Anthracyclines: Doxorubicin, Daunorubicin
- Taxanes: Paclitaxel, Docetaxel
- Vinca Alkaloids: Vincristine, Vinblastine
- Other Major Agents: Etoposide, Topotecan, and many more.

Because of this, the number of P-gp pumps on a cancer cell is often a grim predictor of survival. High levels of P-gp are directly linked to treatment failure and poor outcomes in pancreatic, ovarian, breast, lung, and blood cancers.[5, 6] To win the fight against cancer, this pump defense mechanism must be defeated.

The Cellular Bouncer: Hijacking a Healthy Pump Mechanism to Protect Cancer Cells

In a healthy body, P-gp pumps are essential guards. They belong to a large family of transporters that use cellular energy to move substances across cell membranes.[7] They are strategically located in critical barrier tissues—the lining of the gut, liver, kidneys, and the blood-brain barrier—where they protect the body by recognizing and ejecting harmful toxins and foreign substances.[8]

A cancer cell, however, weaponizes this protective defensive tool to ensure its survival. It hijacks the genetic machinery to build a formidable P-gp shield, a defense made possible by the pump's remarkable ability to bind to a wide variety of structurally different drugs in a large, flexible internal cavity.[9] This defense isn't built by accident; it is assembled on command from internal signaling networks that are themselves hallmarks of cancer.

Ironically, exposure to chemotherapy can trigger the cell to build even more of these pumps.[10] The main command-and-control systems of P-gp pumps include:

- **The EGFR Pathway:** The Epidermal Growth Factor Receptor (EGFR) pathway is a primary engine for cancer cell growth.[11] When stuck in the "on" position, it sends signals that directly order the construction of more P-gp pumps.[12, 13] Activating this pathway has been shown to directly promote resistance to P-gp substrate drugs like vincristine.[14]
- **The NF-κB Pathway:** NF-κB is a master switch for genes related to stress and survival, and it is often permanently flipped on in cancer.[15] The gene that builds P-gp has a direct activation site for NF-κB, meaning that when inflammatory signals or chemotherapy drugs activate this pathway, it immediately cranks up P-gp production.[16, 17] Blocking NF-κB is a proven way to shut down P-gp and make cancer cells vulnerable to treatment again.[18]
- **The PI3K/AKT Pathway:** As a central hub for growth, metabolism, and survival, this is one of the most commonly overactive pathways in all cancer.[19] An active AKT protein is strongly linked to higher

> levels of P-gp and other resistance proteins.[20, 21] It works indirectly by flipping on other switches, including NF-κB, that ultimately construct the P-gp barricade.[22]

Factors in the tumor microenvironment, such as low-oxygen conditions (hypoxia), also activate transcription factors that drive P-gp production, further strengthening the defense against traditional cancer drugs.[23]

P-gp in Parasites: An Ancient Defense Stolen by Cancer

The challenge of P-gp pumps is ancient. Long before they were studied in cancer, parasites evolved these pumps as a fundamental defense against environmental and host-derived toxins. Today, versions of the P-gp pump are found throughout the parasitic kingdom—in roundworms, flukes, tapeworms, and even the protozoa that cause malaria.[24, 25] Under the intense pressure of modern antiparasitic drugs, these pumps have become the parasite's primary shield.[26]

This is not a coincidence. The P-gp pumps in parasites are remarkably similar in structure and function to those in human cancer cells, using energy to expel a wide array of drugs.[27] This parallel defense strategy is a profound clue about the nature of cancer: faced with attack, cancer cells reactivate an ancient, robust survival program also present in parasites. They are not merely "broken" cells; they are masterfully retooling fundamental defense mechanisms stolen from a playbook shared by parasites. This connection reveals the deep biological vulnerability we can now exploit with antiparasitic drugs.

The evidence from parasitology is undeniable:

- **Resistance to Ivermectin:** P-gp pumps are the main reason that parasites like *Haemonchus contortus* (a devastating livestock parasite) develop resistance to the deworming drug ivermectin.[28, 29] Parasites that survive treatment almost always show massive overexpression of P-gp genes.[30, 31] In the lab, disabling the P-gp gene in the model worm *C. elegans* makes it extremely sensitive to ivermectin.[32]
- **Resistance to Benzimidazoles (like Fenbendazole):** While the primary resistance mechanism to fenbendazole is a mutation in its target, β-tubulin,[33] P-gp pumps play a critical supporting role.[34] Parasites resistant to fenbendazole often show higher levels of P-gp expression, which helps by reducing the amount of drug that reaches its target.[35, 36] Blocking the P-gp pump in some benzimidazole-resistant parasites can restore their vulnerability to the drug.[37]

- Resistance in Protozoa: In the malaria parasite plasmodium falciparum, its version of the pump (PfMDR1) is directly responsible for resistance to multiple antimalarial drugs, including chloroquine and quinine.[38, 39] Increased copy numbers of the PfMDR1 gene are strongly linked to clinical drug failure.[40]

If cancer and parasites share a defense, they must also share a weakness. The drugs that evolved to defeat the parasite's P-gp systems—the anthelmintics—are perfectly positioned to defeat cancer's stolen version of the same drug efflux pump defense.

Fenbendazole: The Ultimate Modulator of Resistance

Fenbendazole and its cousin mebendazole sit at the perfect intersection of parasitology and oncology. Their primary weapon is the disruption of microtubules, the cell's internal scaffolding.[41, 42, 43] However, because these drugs also fight parasites that have evolved to use of P-gp pumps as defense mechanisms, they also come equipped to counter this very defense mechanism in cancer.

Research shows fenbendazole dismantles the P-gp barricade through a multipronged attack:

1. Direct Interaction with the Pump: Benzimidazole derivatives can directly inhibit P-gp activity.[44] More recently, mebendazole was confirmed to block the pump's efflux function, allowing P-gp substrates to accumulate inside resistant leukemia cells.[45] By interfering with the pump, these drugs give chemotherapy more time to work.
2. Shutting Down the Command-and-Control Pathways: This is their most powerful indirect attack. Both fenbendazole and mebendazole are proven to suppress the very signaling pathways that build the P-gp shield.
   - Impact on NF-κB and AKT: Fenbendazole has been shown to exert anti-inflammatory effects by modulating the NF-κB pathway.[46] Even more directly, a 2025 study demonstrated that fenbendazole kills breast cancer cells specifically by inhibiting the PI3K/AKT pathway.[47] Since active AKT and NF-κB are primary drivers of P-gp expression, shutting them down is a devastating blow to the cancer cell's ability to build its defenses.

3. Wrecking the Cellular Transport System: The P-gp pump protein doesn't just appear on the cell surface; it must be built, packaged, and transported there. This entire process relies on a healthy microtubule network[48]—the very structure that fenbendazole is designed to destroy. By wrecking the cell's transport system, fenbendazole can prevent new P-gp pumps from ever reaching the barricade.

The One-Two Punch: A New Paradigm for Combination Therapy

The ability of fenbendazole to disable the P-gp pump provides a rock-solid scientific rationale for combining it with conventional chemotherapy. By neutralizing the cancer cell's shields, it allows coadministered drugs to flood the cell and reach lethal concentrations, even in the most resistant tumors. This synergistic combination promises several key clinical benefits: restoring sensitivity to resistant tumors, preventing resistance from developing in the first place, and allowing for lower, less toxic doses of conventional chemotherapy.

Preclinical studies strongly support this idea. Mebendazole dramatically enhances the effectiveness of chemotherapy in drug-resistant brain tumors,[49] while combining fenbendazole with the chemotherapy drug 5-fluorouracil led to far greater tumor destruction in resistant colorectal cancer models than either agent alone.[50] This mirrors the case reports in humans presented in this book where fenbendazole has helped overcome cancers previously resistant to standard treatments.

What is most important in regard to using fenbendazole synergistically with existing cancer treatments is that fenbendazole will not likely cause any additive adverse side effects.

Unlocking Cancer's Secrets by Studying Parasites

The fight against parasite drug resistance offers a treasure trove of information that can revolutionize cancer research. We can use parasite models like *C. elegans* to rapidly screen for new P-gp inhibitors, with any promising hit becoming an immediate lead for a cancer drug. The antiparasitic drug ivermectin is already being explored for this very reason.[51] By watching resistance evolve in real time in parasite populations, we can even predict how a human tumor might adapt and design countermeasures in advance.

The P-glycoprotein pump is a formidable barricade, but it is not a new invention. It is an ancient defense mechanism stolen from parasites. The repurposed anticancer antiparasitic drug fenbendazole is uniquely equipped to defeat it by attacking the pump, its control signals, and its delivery system all at once. A cancer cell under attack by fenbendazole may try to mount a defense with its P-gp pumps, but this is a futile attempt to bail out a sinking ship. Fenbendazole has already blown a hole in the hull.

CHAPTER 14

Using Fenbendazole for Cancer: Addressing Key Questions on Safety, Administration, Efficacy and Other Topics

As interest in fenbendazole as an anticancer agent continues to grow, numerous questions arise regarding its use. This chapter consolidates critical information addressing frequently asked questions posted to the *Fenbendazole Can Cure Cancer* Substack publication regarding fenbendazole's safety profile, optimal administration strategies, and evidence supporting its effects, and also drawing upon reported personal experiences.

Is Fenbendazole Safe?

Fenbendazole possesses an extensive history of safe use as a veterinary antiparasitic agent dating back decades, resulting in a substantial body of safety data.[1] Its established safety is underscored by the fact that common drug interaction databases list no significant interactions of fenbendazole with frequently used medications.[2] Furthermore, the widespread application of analogous benzimidazole drugs (mebendazole, albendazole) in mass drug administration programs across numerous nations, actually 123 nations, provides strong evidence for the safety profile of this drug class.[3] Billions of doses have been administered globally in public health initiatives aimed at controlling parasitic infections, positioning these agents among the most widely used and safest pharmaceuticals available. The standard 222 mg dose of fenbendazole often employed in off-label, self-treatment cancer protocols represents a fraction of the dose safely tolerated in veterinary medicine, where precise individual dosing is less critical due to the drug's wide safety margin. Keep in mind that none of the case reports complained of any adverse reactions or side effects traceable to fenbendazole. On occasion, someone will report that there was a one- to two-day period of transient digestive upset. Keep in mind that fenbendazole is an antiparasitic and that any occult or unrecognized intestinal parasitic infections may also be concurrently eliminated.

Side Effects with Fenbendazole: The preclinical and anecdotal human data is clear: there are virtually no adverse side effects associated with fenbendazole use. The major reason for no side effects is informed by the preclinical science demonstrating the specificity of fenbendazole for cancer cells while leaving healthy cells untouched. This specificity is in stark contrast to traditional cancer treatments that essentially either burn holes in tissue or poison cancer cells along with healthy cells, this collateral damage due to the relative non-specificity of these treatments is why dreaded adverse side effects occur with these treatments. As time moves forward and fenbendazole and drugs like it become the gold standard of cancer treatment, current contemporary cancer treatments are likely to be viewed as modern-day equivalents to bloodletting and frontal lobotomy.

Caveat: This is not to imply that an individual may not experience an unanticipated adverse effect either due to their idiosyncratic biological state, including metabolic issues, a previously unrecognized interaction with another agent or a complex interaction of the two when using fenbendazole. Because fenbendazole is a veterinary medicine it has not been screened and approved for use in humans. However, its analogues mebendazole and albendazole are approved for human use.

How Is Fenbendazole Best Administered? Optimizing Fenbendazole Administration and Bioavailability

Effective delivery of fenbendazole to target cancer cells requires maximizing its absorption into the bloodstream, as oral bioavailability can be limited. Research demonstrates that coadministration with lipids (fats) significantly enhances the bioavailability of related benzimidazoles. Specifically, studies involving mebendazole showed that administering the drug with various oils resulted in 1.6 to 2.8 times higher serum concentrations compared to controls, with olive oil (particularly high in oleic acid, the critical factor in increasing bioavailability) proving particularly effective.[4] This enhanced absorption translated directly to increased therapeutic efficacy in preclinical models.

Further research indicates that fenbendazole's solubility, a key factor influencing absorption, is substantially increased when combined with certain organic acids, including cinnamic, benzoic, and salicylic acids.[5] This suggests that coadministration with substances like aspirin (acetylsalicylic acid of which salicyclic acid is a metabolic byproduct) could potentially improve fenbendazole uptake. The utility of these suggestions awaits further research.

Practical strategies to enhance absorption include taking fenbendazole with a fatty meal, incorporating it with olive oil, or mixing it with substances like butter, yogurt, or peanut butter. A reader who also happened to be an organic chemist suggested an approach using butter, leveraging its saturated and monounsaturated fat content (carbon chains >C14) to potentially optimize absorption pathways, although specific quantitative estimates of absorption improvement require further validation. Many people take fenbendazole (free powder or capsule) with a tablespoon of olive oil or powder sprinkled on buttered toast. My mother-in-law's husband mixed fenbendazole powder into her yogurt.

Ensuring adequate absorption is paramount; improper administration can lead to treatment failure, as illustrated by a case reported by another reader of the Substack where an individual experiencing cancer recurrence of small cell lung cancer was found to have significant fenbendazole residue in their coffee mug (free fenbendazole powder is hydrophobic; it floats on the top of liquid and adhered to the inside of the mug) due to repeated ineffective mixing, with the cancer then subsequently resolving only after switching to a properly administered liquid formulation.

Test/Retest Evidence of Fenbendazole's Anticancer Activity: A Case Study

Continuing with the importance of proper administration and absorption, a compelling instance indicative of fenbendazole's efficacy involving a man with small cell lung cancer (SCLC) was inadvertently demonstrated due to a systematic error in the administration of fenbendazole. On initial use of fenbendazole, this individual experienced near-complete tumor eradication within several months, confirmed by imaging, while taking fenbendazole (222 mg twice per day). Subsequently, due to an unintentional lapse in proper administration (mixing free fenbendazole powder in coffee), the cancer returned despite presumed uninterrupted, continued use of fenbendazole. Pain reappearing signaled that the cancer had returned and this restaging was again verified by imaging. Upon correction of the administration method (switching to liquid fenbendazole taken with yogurt), the man's symptoms rapidly improved, pain disappeared, and follow-up imaging confirmed complete tumor resolution within six weeks.

This sequence—cancer regression initially with proper fenbendazole use, recurrence upon inadvertent cessation of fenbendazole use, and subsequent re-eradication upon proper readministration—represents a powerful within-subject demonstration of the effectiveness of fenbendazole with respect to cancer eradication. Within-subject and test/retest/test experimental designs are among the most powerful in demonstrating drug effects because essentially this design demonstrates that the treatment (fenbendazole) is the key factor determining whether cancer is present or not. While arising accidentally from circumstances unknown at the time affecting administration, this pattern observed strongly suggests that fenbendazole was the critical factor responsible for the presence or absence of detectable cancer in this specific case.

The situation above is best described as a happy accident, or, scientifically, as an experiment in nature. It would obviously be unethical to ask someone with cancer to purposely stop taking fenbendazole to "see what happens." But that is what occurred in this instance, by accident. The significance of this event cannot be overstated: in this one case, when fenbendazole was present, the cancer was eliminated; when fenbendazole was accidentally mis-administered, the cancer returned, and when fenbendazole was reapplied the cancer was eliminated again. This instance may be the only time we ever observe this phenomenon.

This story raises tough questions regarding any future clinical trials involving a powerful anticancer agent like fenbendazole. Is it ethical to have a placebo-only control group in the fenbendazole era? Are clinical trials designed to prove the main effect of cancer eradication by fenbendazole rendered moot and superfluous by the wealth of existing research as presented in this book? Perhaps future efforts would be more useful directing focus to dosage optimization, optimization of administration, determining effective protocols for all cancers, assessing effects on childhood cancers, synergistic effects with other antiparasitics, traditional treatments, etc.

Fenbendazole and Liver Function

Many drugs and their metabolites affect liver function. Concerns regarding potential liver injury associated with fenbendazole use have been raised, often referencing a specific case report by Yamaguchi et al. (2021).[6] This report documents elevated liver enzymes (aspartate transaminase [AST] and alanine aminotransferase [ALT]) in a non-small cell lung cancer (NSCLC) patient self-administering fenbendazole. However, it is crucial to interpret these findings within the context of cancer therapy as a whole. Temporary elevations in AST and ALT can occur as the liver processes cellular debris resulting from cancer cell death induced by an effective treatment like fenbendazole. This hepatic stress may reflect increased workload rather than necessarily indicating intrinsic drug toxicity. Such fluctuations are commonly observed during recovery from various illnesses involving significant cell turnover and often normalize after the underlying condition, such as cancer burden, resolves. Therefore, transient liver enzyme elevations during fenbendazole therapy may, in some contexts, signify effective tumor lysis rather than adverse drug-induced liver injury. As such, liver enzyme values should be monitored, as they would be during most cancer therapies, for changes and to determine the nature of those changes, that is, either transient or longer term.

The suggestion made above, that transient liver enzyme fluctuation after starting fenbendazole therapy may indicate therapeutic effect of the drug on the cancer, appears to have validity. Many of the case reports described earlier noted either no, or a transient elevation in AST/ALT markers that accompanied therapeutic response and eradication of the cancers. In all instances, AST/ALT returned to within normal limits shortly thereafter.

As a side note to the Yamaguchi et al. (2021) study there was a serious confounding factor present in that report: the woman was also taking the PD-L1 immunotherapy drug (pembrolizumab [Keytruda]) that does list hepatic damage as a major side effect.[7] She was on this drug ineffectually for many months before trying fenbendazole for one month as a last resort, at which time her liver function markers changed. It is unknown whether the accumulated effects of the immunotherapy drug caused the liver changes, an interaction between fenbendazole and the pembrolizumab occurred, and/or the lysis phenomenon described above occurred, signaling fenbendazole effectiveness in eradicating her cancer.

Interpreting Diagnostic Imaging Post-Fenbendazole Treatment

Accurate interpretation of follow-up diagnostic scans, particularly PET scans involving bone metastases, may be necessary after fenbendazole treatment. Lytic lesions (bone cavities previously occupied by cancer) undergoing healing and remineralization, can exhibit increased metabolic activity ("hot spots" or "bone flare phenomena").[8] This physiological healing process can be misinterpreted as persistent or restaging cancer by clinicians unfamiliar with potentially curative responses induced by agents like fenbendazole. People self-treating with fenbendazole should be aware that such findings may represent bone regeneration rather than active malignancy, necessitating careful evaluation to avoid misdiagnosis and potentially harmful overtreatment.

Diagnostic Testing in the Fenbendazole Era

Many of the case reports indicated that the people self-treating with fenbendazole did not inform their doctors until their cancers resolved. During that time period continued monitoring and testing is likely taking place, and doctors are puzzled when they detect no evidence of disease. Quite frankly, the doctor is mystified because the treatments that they are giving do not result in a complete remission or cure. The notion of a cure is not in the lexicon of modern oncology. The reason why this is important to appreciate for the person self-treating is that the doctor will overturn every stone looking for cancer because in their mind it has to be there, they just have to find it. This happened to the nth degree with my mother-in-law. Even though her blood tumor marker CA 27.29 was within normal limits she was subjected to repeated CT scans, PET scans, MRIs, ultrasounds, and other testing looking for something that was gone. The problem with this scenario is that many of these tests are carcinogenic themselves, and risk factors for other cancers and other diseases, especially if toxic contrast media are used as in PET scans.[9, 10, 11, 12] One strategy is to ask whether relatively less toxic testing is reasonable (MRI, ultrasound, blood tests) to address the questions the provider is asking.

On the other hand, blood tumor marker tests, also known as liquid biopsies, are the least invasive and likely least hazardous method to track progress.[13] Unfortunately not all cancers have a corresponding blood tumor marker test, although a relatively recent development is the CTC (circulating tumor cell) blood test that detects the DNA of cancer cells present in the blood. As this technology matures, CTC tests may prove to be a relatively low-risk, high-sensitivity screening technique to monitor progress in those who are self-treating their cancers.

One theme that was consistent among the case reports was the need to remain "in the system" to gain access to diagnostic testing even though the traditional cancer treatments had failed. This approach is reasonable. However, it should be pointed out that several case reporters utilized outside private testing labs to monitor their progress while using fenbendazole.

Fenbendazole for Cancer Prevention

The concept of using fenbendazole prophylactically to prevent cancer presents logistical challenges in definitively proving efficacy (proving a negative).

However, preclinical evidence demonstrates a clear preventative effect. Studies show that prior treatment with benzimidazoles like mebendazole prevented the successful engraftment and growth of experimental brain tumors in animal models.[14] Additionally, epidemiological observations note significantly lower cancer incidence rates in populations residing in 123 countries with national mass drug administration programs utilizing benzimidazoles for parasite control, compared to countries without such programs (see chapter 10). While correlation does not equal causation, these observations, combined with preclinical cancer prevention data discussed earlier, support the biological plausibility of a preventative role of fenbendazole/mebendazole for many cancers.

A potential preventative protocol might involve periodic short courses of fenbendazole (e.g., 222 mg daily for three consecutive days, repeated quarterly), adjusted based on individual risk factors. Given fenbendazole's established safety profile and low cost relative to the catastrophic cost of traditional cancer treatment, such a strategy warrants consideration. Conversely, an argument can be made that if fenbendazole proves reliably curative, the rationale for prevention diminishes.

Interestingly, the people who've self-treated their cancers with fenbendazole as described in the case reports universally adopt a program of continued fenbendazole use even after achieving full remission.

Pharmacokinetics: Duration of Action of Fenbendazole and Mebendazole

Understanding the pharmacokinetic profile, particularly the half-life, can help with dosing strategies. Studies on mebendazole in healthy human volunteers indicate an average half-life of approximately 7.4 hours following a single 1000 mg dose.[15] Other sources report a half-life ranging from 3 to 6 hours for a 500 mg dose. Based on these data, particularly the 7.4-hour figure from Conti et al. (2009), spacing multiple daily doses approximately 8 hours apart appears to be a rational approach to maintain consistent therapeutic serum concentrations when self-treating.

Topical Application of Fenbendazole

Anecdotal reports of fenbendazole cream applied to basal and squamous cell cancers have been reported to be consistently effective. Two of the case reports in chapter 7 detail the use of topical fenbendazole and ivermectin.

There are reports of the curtailment or blockage of the emergence of cold sores using topical fenbendazole as well.

Fenbendazole Use During Pregnancy and Nursing

Standard veterinary guidance advises against administering fenbendazole to pregnant or nursing animals. This caution aligns with research highlighting the broad activity of benzimidazoles against cellular processes, including those related to stemness.[16] Since both cancer stem cells and normal developing stem cells share certain pathways potentially targeted by fenbendazole, prudence dictates avoiding its use during periods of high physiological stem cell activity, such as pregnancy and lactation, to prevent unintended effects on normal development.

Obviously, if there are any concerns about potential drug interactions or instances where the use of fenbendazole may not be warranted, a medical professional should be consulted.

Potential Drug Interactions with Fenbendazole or Mebendazole

According to Drugs.com, there are no commonly used drugs that interact with fenbendazole (accessed May 1, 2025). While fenbendazole exhibits no known significant drug interactions, one potential interaction noted for the related drug mebendazole involves cimetidine. Cimetidine (Tagamet), an H2 histamine receptor antagonist used to reduce stomach acid, may decrease the metabolism of mebendazole, potentially leading to increased serum levels of the drug.[17] The clinical significance of this interaction varies, but it highlights a potential pathway for altered drug exposure. The net effect of taking cimetidine with fenbendazole (mebendazole) would be to impair the metabolism of the drug thereby acting as an agonist. Where that potentiation effect occurs, if any, is not known. Given the recent awareness of the toxicities of acetaminophen, it is probably best to not take fenbendazole with any product containing acetaminophen.

Where to Get Fenbendazole: Product Manufacturers: Does the Brand Matter?

Several brands of fenbendazole are commonly available, including Panacur-C (Merck), Safe-Guard (Merck), FenBen Labs (Canchema), and products from the Happy Healing Store. Based on accumulated case reports data, various brands have been associated with successful outcomes in cancer self-treatment protocols. While no formal comparative analyses have been conducted for this purpose, current anecdotal evidence does not strongly differentiate between these established brands in terms of effectiveness. The primary consideration remains sourcing a reliable product. Because fenbendazole is off-patent and subject to fair competition, profiteering from its repurposed use for cancer is limited. In fact, fenbendazole, sold under the Safe-Guard brand, is available in fifty-pound bags for deworming use in cattle feed, suggesting that it is neither rare nor expensive.

There are many online sellers of fenbendazole including Amazon, Chewy, and various veterinary supply online merchants. Brick-and-mortar stores such as Tractor Supply, Walmart, Target, and Petco and other pet stores also sell fenbendazole.

I Have a Cancer Diagnosis. When Should I Start Fenbendazole?

Utilizing the Pretreatment Interval for Self-Treatment

The often significant delay of weeks or months between a cancer diagnosis and the initiation of conventional therapies (e.g., surgery, radiation, chemotherapy) presents a window of opportunity for proactive self-treatment with fenbendazole. An illustrative unpublished case report involves a man named Brian, who was differentially diagnosed with early-stage bladder cancer, who commenced daily fenbendazole (222 mg) while awaiting scheduled radiation. His symptoms of diffuse pain and blood-tainted urine resolved prior to the scheduled appointment some thirty days later, and subsequent diagnostic tests confirmed the absence of detectable cancer. Notably, the treating physician reportedly attributed the outcome to an initial misdiagnosis rather than acknowledging the potential effect of fenbendazole. This reaction, alongside attempts to reframe other prominent cases like Joe Tippens's small cell lung cancer recovery as misdiagnosed parasitic infections[18] (Tippens was enrolled in a clinical trial for an experimental pharmaceutical; he was not misdiagnosed[19]) highlights potential resistance within conventional oncology to accepting fenbendazole's efficacy.

Such instances such as Brian's underscore the value of utilizing the pretreatment interval as an opportunity to try safe, inexpensive, readily available fenbendazole and possibly avoid the pain, inconvenience, expense and side effects of traditional treatment altogether.

Subjective Sensations During Fenbendazole Use

Some individuals report distinct physical sensations while taking fenbendazole. Examples include descriptions of "crackling" or "sizzling" sensations in the chest area (reported by a non-small cell lung cancer patient), irritation or inflammation near the prostate (reported by prostate cancer patients), or mild burning/irritation localized to prior COVID-19 injection sites in the deltoid muscles. Whether these subjective experiences relate directly to fenbendazole's anticancer action, represent ancillary effects, or are coincidental requires further investigation and corroborating reports.

Should I Tell My Doctor I'm Taking Fenbendazole?

Discussing the use of nonstandard therapies like fenbendazole with an oncologist presents unique challenges. Many patients choose not to disclose their use of such agents, at least initially. Reasons for this reluctance as stated by case report providers include:

- Fear that the oncologist might disapprove and potentially refuse continued care or alter the doctor-patient relationship.
- Desire to maintain access to conventional diagnostic monitoring (scans, blood tests) without facing judgment, ultimatums, or conflict over treatment choices.
- Concern about creating awkwardness or perceived embarrassment for the physician.
- Situations in which the oncologist is also a personal acquaintance or family member.

The decision of whether or when to inform the medical team is personal. Recall that most of the people in the case reports presented in this book did not inform their oncologist that they were self-treating with fenbendazole, at least not initially. In some cases, the oncologist was told about fenbendazole after the cancer had been eradicated. In fact, recall that the original Joe Tippens report detailed how Joe had been enrolled in an experimental trial to test some drug, he quietly was self-treating with fenbendazole, and he was the only one out of 1,100 subjects to go into remission!

Does Fenbendazole Need Other Substances to Work?

Speaking of Joe Tippens, his experience with fenbendazole was combined with other vitamins, minerals, and nutraceuticals. In addition to 222 mg fenbendazole, he took vitamin E (400–800 mg/day), curcumin (600 mg/day), and cannabinoid oil (25 mg/day). Keep in mind that Joe was fighting for his life and was throwing the self-treatment kitchen sink at his cancer.

Are other cofactors necessary? The short answer is no. Fenbendazole is both necessary and sufficient to kill cancer. Based on the scientific evidence regarding mechanisms of anticancer activity detailed earlier, fenbendazole is a primary antineoplastic agent with direct effect. This means that it works by itself and no help is necessary. Fenbendazole absence or presence is what matters. Furthermore, many of the case reports in chapter 6 used only fenbendazole to eradicate their cancers. Several of the case reports also used a myriad of vitamins, minerals, etc. However, just like Joe Tippens, these people would probably not have survived on just those ancillary substances; fenbendazole is what cured them. However, this is not to imply that agents with immunological, metabolic, or other beneficial effects are harmful or ill-advised when using fenbendazole. In fact, whatever regimen one is comfortable with, as long as future research does not find it interferes with the primary actions of fenbendazole, is fine. Go for it.

Addressing One Study Reporting Lack of Efficacy

A study cited as showing no benefit from mebendazole is Mansoori et al. (2021).[20] This Phase 2a clinical trial investigated mebendazole in patients with advanced gastrointestinal cancers. However, a critical artifactual limitation undermines its conclusion: only five out of the ten participants achieved the target therapeutic serum concentration of the mebendazole. Given that half the subjects did not demonstrably absorb sufficient mebendazole to reach therapeutic levels, the study's failure to detect an anticancer effect cannot be reliably interpreted as evidence against the drug's efficacy. Inadequate drug exposure due to absorption issues presents a significant confounding factor, as we detailed earlier with the non small cell lung cancer case, rendering the negative findings inconclusive regarding the drug's potential activity when properly absorbed. Furthermore, this study stands in contrast to recent peer-reviewed studies that did find a dramatic therapeutic effect of fenbendazole, a mebedazole analogue, that is also much better orally absorbed, on various cancers in humans.[21, 22]

If Fenbendazole Is Such a Powerful Cancer Treatment Cancer, Why Doesn't My Doctor Know About It?

Maybe your doctor is aware of fenbendazole but is reluctant to talk about it because s/he can't take it the next logical step and proceed to treatment. Because fenbendazole is not a standard-of-care treatment, a physician's hands are tied in discussing its application. However, they can discuss and recommend the repurposing of mebendazole for any condition, including cancer.

It is more likely that your doctor, just like most people, doesn't know of fenbendazole because awareness of its cancer-curing abilities have been actively suppressed. As we detailed earlier, little pharma knew about the ability of fenbendazole to cure cancer in the early 1970s. In their collective excitement, they even named their discovery oncodazole. The giddiness engendered over the discovery of a cure for cancer was soon displaced by apparent greed. As an indicator of the excitement in learning that fenbendazole cures cancer, these scientists went so far as to rebrand their discovery "oncodazole" and publish papers on its mechanisms. Once it was realized that there was an immense fortune to be made, not in curing cancer with an inexpensive, off-patent drug, but in treating it with their own drugs, the name oncodazole was changed to nocodazole in a clear effort to bury the cure. Some of the cancer drugs that followed this early to mid-1970s discovery of oncodazole were based on the microtubule manipulation actions of fenbendazole (oncodazole). For example, the taxane class of drugs' mechanism of action is to stabilize microtubules, essentially locking them to prevent mitosis. Of course, the multidimensional power of fenbendazole's selective targeting of cancer and parasite microtubules, and not healthy cells, could not be reverse engineered, leading to a nonspecific, side-effect-riddled variant.

Like the rest of us, doctors don't know about fenbendazole and cancer, because that knowledge was buried and suppressed.

As discussed in the case reports, most of the people self-treating their cancers did not involve their doctors. Some didn't because they had exhausted all standard-of-care treatments and were told to get their affairs in order. Their doctor was essentially no longer involved with their care. Others feared retribution or denial of diagnostic services. Others were concerned that if they were successfully self-treating their cancers that somehow that would be threatening to the relationship.

Many of the unpublished case reports that have been referenced throughout are from medical doctors, retired or otherwise, who wrote in to express appreciation for the efforts to get the word out about fenbendazole because they too had cured their own cancers with fenbendazole.

Afterword

It is my sincere wish that this book serves as a first major step toward bringing fenbendazole into the mainstream for the treatment of cancer. Much of the heavy lifting has already been done by the basic scientists in their laboratory benchwork and preclinical experiments. The new data and analyses presented in this book show that fenbendazole is a cure for cancer and that it likely prevents cancer as well. It is now up to decision-makers to pick up the fenbendazole ball and run with it.

However, I am not naive. We all realize that there is a huge infrastructure that depends financially on maintaining the status quo in cancer treatments. I'll call this financial infrastructure Big Cancer. We learned that fenbendazole, in the form of oncodazole, as a cure for cancer was essentially known fifty years ago and subsequently effectively suppressed.

So how will Big Cancer react to off-patent, inexpensive antiparasitic medications as cures for cancer? Not likely with open arms. There will be a predictable, collective pearl-clutching response that may incorporate one or more of the following false claims:

1. **Fenbendazole is not an effective cancer treatment.**

   The information throughout this book, the scientists studying fenbendazole and cancer, and the people who saved their own lives using fenbendazole would beg to differ.

2. **Fenbendazole and drugs like it are dangerous.**

   The science has convincingly demonstrated that fenbendazole and its analogues are extremely safe, as evidenced by the billions of doses administered each year to animals and humans around the world as part of routine veterinary care and mass drug administration dictated by public health programs in 123 nations around the world. Plus, fenbendazole as a cancer treatment in humans resulted in no adverse side effects in our case reports presented here. Good luck arguing that fenbendazole is unsafe. It is likely one of the safest medicines ever produced!

3. **Fenbendazole isn't FDA approved for use in humans.**

   Fenbendazole is an analogue of mebendazole and albendazole, both of which are approved for human use. However, it appears that fenbendazole is the more effective anticancer agent, yet, because it is not FDA approved for human use, it forces those self-treating their cancers to acquire the inexpensive veterinary medicine on their own. The lack of FDA approval of fenbendazole use in humans is an oversight, not a flag. Let's get fenbendazole approved for human use by the FDA as soon as possible. And let's not allow sick people to be price gouged in the process.

4. **Some cancer diagnoses are wrong. Cancer is an actual parasite.**

   They could claim that case reports showing that cancer was cured by fenbendazole were actually parasitic infections that were misdiagnosed. That would be a clever one, because it is a remote possibility. However, all of the case reports here had differential medical diagnoses, including invasive biopsies that determined the type and grade of cancer. These people had cancer, their doctors implemented treatments based on those cancer diagnoses, and they were eventually released from care to die after those cancer treatments failed. If Big Cancer wants to assert that cancer diagnostic capability cannot distinguish between a parasitic infection and a malignant tumor, that is another can of worms. Cancer has many of the structural and behavioral features of parasites, but we are not misdiagnosing worm infestations as cancer. However, if, on the off chance that we are systematically making such an error, fortunately we know how to kill it.

5. **Mass administration of antiparasitic drugs to manage parasitic infections is unnecessary and/or unsafe in the developed world.**

   According to the CDC, the people of wealthy nations, including the United States, are infested with one or more parasites that create an undiagnosed, subclinical state of chronic inflammation that is a risk factor for cancer and other autoimmune conditions. Not addressing this public health crisis immediately is public health-care malpractice.

6. **A fenbendazole analogue with cancer-curing function was never named oncodazole.**

   The written and published record, which shows that it was, is irrefutable.

7. **The name of the cancer-curing drug oncodazole wasn't changed to nocodazole in an attempt to cover up or mask its function.**
   The written and published record, which shows that it was, is irrefutable.
8. **Some modern chemotherapy drugs are not repurposed from fenbendazole or oncodazole.**
   Taxane chemotherapy drugs, and likely vinca alkaloid-class drugs, certainly appear to be repurposed conceptual knockoffs of fenbendazole/oncodazole. While both classes of drugs could have been developed independently, the change of the name from oncodazole to nocodazole is damning.
9. **The suppression of an antiparasitic drug as a cure for cancer for fifty years, the repurposing of its mechanism into expensive side-effect-ridden cancer drugs, and the abandonment of an effective public health policy regarding preventative use of antiparasitic drugs in the wealthier Western world is all coincidental.**
   There are no unseen forces at work orchestrating any of this, it is all coincidential.
10. **They will attack me, the messenger, as a know-nothing nonexpert in the oncology field.**
   I didn't produce any of the science presented in this book, other than the epidemiological findings, which should have been discovered and presented a long time ago by public health epidemiological experts. All I did was find the publicly available information and present it. Attacks directed at me, and not on the facts in this book, are indirect proof that all the facts are true and defensible.

I hope that you found reading *Cancer Is a Parasite* useful and empowering. I certainly have found this journey from initially seeing the word "fenbendazole" in 2021 to writing this book on fenbendazole and cancer inspiring, and I am hopeful for a cancer-free future that may lie ahead.

Finally, we have one loose end to address: Who is the hero in this story? Who discovered that oncodazole (fenbendazole) was a cure for cancer? Go back to chapter 1 and the discovery of fenbendazole and mebendazole. Dr. Paul Janssen and his colleagues were experimenting with mebendazole and oncodazole in the early 1970s. While not an author, Paul Janssen was thanked for his interest in their work on the Hoebeke et al. 1976 oncodazole paper. The research on the 1976 Hoebeke et al. oncodazole paper was done at Janssen Research Laboratories in Belgium. Paul Janssen founded Janssen Pharmaceuticals, which is now incorporated into Johnson & Johnson, one of the largest manufacturers of oncology drugs in the world.

One can only wonder how different the world would have been if the discovery of oncodazole (fenbendazole) as a safe and effective cure for cancer entered public awareness back in the 1970s.

Lastly, let me leave you with my final two thoughts on what we've learned about fenbendazole and cancer: one that reflects what happened in the past, and one for what is about to happen. Regarding the suppression of fenbendazole as a cure for cancer; paraphrasing Kurt Vonnegut, "of all the deeds of mice and men, perhaps the saddest are what might have been." Finally, for what is about to happen as fenbendazole enters the mainstream, Victor Hugo wrote, "Nothing else in the world . . . not all the armies . . . is so powerful as an idea whose time has come."

Acknowledgments

I would like to thank my wife Toni for her encouragement, patience, and many thoughtful discussions on the topics that we've covered in this book. She knows where this book started and where it ultimately ended up. Many of the insights presented here would not have happened without her input and ideas.

Thanks to Tony Lyons of Skyhorse Publishing for having the courage to produce a trailblazing book like this that will likely ruffle a lot of feathers while hopefully starting a serious conversation about using safe, effective, and inexpensive existing antiparasitic drugs to treat cancers and other "incurable" diseases. Thanks also to Daniela Rapp, whose editing expertise made the book much better than I could have ever done on my own.

Last but not least, thanks to all of those who have added to the knowledge base on fenbendazole and human cancers, either through their contributed case report experiences of using fenbendazole to treat their own cancers, or helpful comments on the Substack *Fenbendazole Can Cure Cancer*, including (in no particular order) Roberta, Betty, Joe, Mollie, Karen, Bob, Dave, Amy, Robert, Linda, Patricia, James, Susan, Michael, Barbara, Kimmy, Sharon, Gloria, Ann, Scott, David, Alison, Shawn, Dylan, Sam, Maria, Jennifer, William, Richard, Margaret, John G., Thomas, Elizabeth, William K., Mary, Thomas, Dorothy, Charles, Jess, Ron, Ryan, Rachel, Jennifer, Shawn, Jaci, Diana, Nancy, Caroline, Tammy, Mark, Karen, Paul, Lisa, Steve, Liz, Will, Brian, Helen, Kevin, Sandra, Ronald, Donna, AA, Denny, Kenneth, Carol, Gene, Anthony, Ruth, Becca, George, Sharon, Misty, Edward, Michelle, Donald, Tang, Kimberly, Frank, Deborah, Jason, Shirley, Scott M., Cynthia, Jeffrey, Angela, Greg, Melissa, Gary, Amy T., Timothy, Laurie, Brenda, Jose, Margie, Andrew, Samantha, John R., Pamela, Raymond, Kathleen, Dennis, Nicole, Jerry, Heather, Larry, Christine, Pete, Doug, Frances, Peter, Janet, Walt, Virginia, Arthur, Catherine, Bruce, Joyce, Harold, Diane, Roger, Judy, Terry, Cheryl, Keith, Beverly, Philip, Theresa, Randy, Marilyn, Rho, Clarence, Gloria, John A., Howard, Evelyn, TJ, Jeanne, Carl, Judy, Russell, Janice, Lawrence, Rose, Andrew, Pierre, Carol, Maria N., Wayne, Ann V., Daniel, John P., Vicky, Henry, Kelly, Alan,

Christina, Patrick, Joan, Roy, Lauren, Jonathan, Beth, Stephanie, Adam, Rebecca, Justin, Jacqueline, Stephen, Sara, Bill, Meagan, Jeremy, Amanda, Noah, Rachel Z., Christian, Katherine, Samuel, Mallie, Emily, Benjamin, Samantha, Matthew, Brandi, Keith P., Earl, Nelly, Christopher, Monica, Josh, Erin, Clarise, Maureen, Nicholas, Crystal, Eric, Whitney, Jacob, Bridget, Gary K., Amber, Dustin, and Jessica.

Notes

Chapter 1

1 Cox, F. E. (2002). History of human parasitology. *Clinical Microbiology Reviews* 15, no. 4: 595–612. doi.org/10.1128/CMR.15.4.595-612.2002.

2 Despommier, D. D., Griffin, D. O., Gwadz, R. W., Hotez, P. J., & Knirsch, C. A. (2017). *Parasitic Diseases* (7th ed.). Parasites Without Borders.

3 Zajac, A. M., & Conboy, G. A. (eds.). (2012). *Veterinary Clinical Parasitology* (8th ed.). Wiley-Blackwell. doi.org/10.1002/9781118285344.

4 Campbell, W. C. (1990). Benzimidazoles: Veterans of thirty years of chemotherapeutic warfare. In J. R. Baker & R. Muller (eds.), *Parasitology for the 21st Century* (pp. 143–52). CAB International.

5 World Health Organization. (2023). Neglected tropical diseases. who.int/news-room/fact-sheets/detail/neglected-tropical-diseases.

6 Stephenson, L. S., Latham, M. C., & Ottesen, E. A. (2000). Malnutrition and parasitic helminth infections. *Parasitology* 121 (Supplement): S23–S38. doi.org/10.1017/s0031182000006389.

7 Hotez, P. J., Brindley, P. J., Bethony, J. M., King, C. H., Pearce, E. J., & Jacobson, J. (2008). Helminth infections: The great neglected tropical diseases. *The Journal of Clinical Investigation* 118, no. 4: 1311–21. doi.org/10.1172/JCI34261.

8 Bogitsh, B. J. et al., (2019). *Human Parasitology* (5th edition). Academic Press. doi.org/10.1016/C2015-0-04771-X.

9 World Health Organization. (2023). WHO Model List of Essential Medicines—23rd list. who.int/publications/i/item/WHO-MHP-HPS-EML-2023.02.

10 Perry, B. D., Randolph, T. F., McDermott, J. J., Sones, K. R., & Thornton, P. K. (2002). Investing in animal health research to alleviate poverty. International Livestock Research Institute. hdl.handle.net/10568/2308.

11 Taylor, M. A., Coop, R. L., & Wall, R. L. (eds.). (2016). *Veterinary Parasitology* (4th ed.). Wiley-Blackwell. doi.org/10.1002/9781119073672.

12 Charlier, J., Höglund, J., Morgan, E. R., Geldhof, P., Vercruysse, J., & Claerebout, E. (2020). Biology and epidemiology of gastrointestinal nematodes of livestock. *Advances in Parasitology* 109: 1–63. doi.org/10.1016/bs.apar.2020.05.001.

13 Roeber, F., Jex, A. R., & Gasser, R. B. (2013). Impact of gastrointestinal nematodes of sheep, and the role of advanced molecular tools for exploring epidemiology and drug resistance—An Australian perspective. *Parasites & Vectors* 6: 153. doi.org/10.1186/1756-3305-6-153.

14 Bowman, D. D. (2014). *Georgis' Parasitology for Veterinarians* (10th ed.). Elsevier Saunders.

15 Waller, P. J. (1997). Anthelmintic resistance. *Veterinary Parasitology* 72, no. 3–4: 391–412. doi.org/10.1016/s0304-4017(97)00042-4.

16 Prichard, R. K. (1990). Anthelmintic resistance in nematodes: Extent, recent understanding and future directions for control and research. *International Journal for Parasitology* 20, no. 4: 515–23. doi.org/10.1016/0020-7519(90)90084-t.

17 Townsend, L. B., & Wise, D. S. (1990). The synthesis and chemistry of certain anthelmintic benzimidazoles. *Parasitology Today* 6, no. 4: 107–112. https://doi.org/10.1016/0169-4758(90)90226-t .

18 Brown, H. D., Matzuk, A. R., Ilves, I. R., Peterson, L. H., Harris, S. A., Sarett, L. H., Egerton, J. R., Yakstis, J. J., Campbell, W. C., & Cuckler, A. C. (1961). Antiparasitic drugs. IV. 2-(4'-Thiazolyl)-benzimidazole, a new anthelmintic. *Journal of the American Chemical Society* 83, no. 7: 1764–65. doi.org/10.1021/ja01468a052.

19 Düwel, D. (1977). Fenbendazole: Biological properties and activity. *Pesticide Science* 8, no. 5: 550–55. doi.org/10.1002/ps.2780080522.

20 Burke, T. M., & Roberson, E. L. (1983). Fenbendazole treatment of pregnant bitches to reduce prenatal and lactogenic infections of *Toxocara canis* and *Ancylostoma caninum* in pups. *Journal of the American Veterinary Medical Association* 183, no. 9: 987–90.

21 Plumb, D. C. (2018). Fenbendazole. In *Plumb's Veterinary Drug Handbook* (9th ed., pp. 468–71). PharmaVet Inc.

22 Roberson, E. L., & Burke, T. M. (1982). Evaluation of granulated fenbendazole as a treatment for helminth infections in dogs. *Journal of the American Veterinary Medical Association* 180, no. 1: 53–55.

23 Cray, C., & Altman, N. H. (2022). An update on the biologic effects of fenbendazole. *Comparative Medicine* 72, no. 4: 215–219. doi.org/10.30802/AALAS-CM-22-000006.

24 McKellar, Q. A., & Jackson, F. (2004). Veterinary anthelmintics: Old and new. *Trends in Parasitology* 20, no. 10: 456–61. doi.org/10.1016/j.pt.2004.07.007.

25 Brugmans, J. P., Thienpont, D. C., van Wijngaarden, I., Vanparijs, O. F., Schuermans, V. L., & Lauwers, H. L. (1971). Mebendazole in enterobiasis: Radiochemical and pilot clinical study in 1,278 subjects. *JAMA* 217, no. 3: 313–16. doi.org/10.1001/jama.1971.03190030031007.

26 Keiser, J., & Utzinger, J. (2008). Efficacy of current drugs against soil-transmitted helminth infections: Systematic review and meta-analysis. *JAMA* 299, no. 16: 1937–48. doi.org/10.1001/jama.299.16.1937.

27 Dayan, A. D. (2003). Albendazole, mebendazole and praziquantel: Review of non-clinical toxicity and pharmacokinetics. *Acta Tropica* 86, no. 2–3: 141–59. doi.org/10.1016/s0001-706x(03)00031-7.

28 World Health Organization. (2006). Preventive chemotherapy in human helminthiasis: Coordinated use of anthelminthic drugs in control interventions: A manual for health professionals and programme managers. iris.who.int/handle/10665/43545.

29 Edwards, G., & Breckenridge, A. M. (1988). Clinical pharmacokinetics of anthelmintic drugs. *Clinical Pharmacokinetics* 15, no. 2: 67–93. doi.org/10.2165/00003088-198815020-00001.

30 Ashburn, T. T., & Thor, K. B. (2004). Drug repositioning: Identifying and developing new uses for existing drugs. *Nature Reviews Drug Discovery* 3, no. 8: 673–83. doi.org/10.1038/nrd1468.

31 Dogra, N., Kumar, A., & Mukhopadhyay, T. (2018). Fenbendazole acts as a moderate microtubule destabilizing agent and causes cancer cell death by modulating multiple cellular pathways. *Scientific Reports* 8, no. 1: 11926. doi.org/10.1038/s41598-018-30158-6.

32 Theodorides, V. J., Gyurik, R. J., Kingsbury, W. D., & Parish, R. C. (1976). Anthelmintic activity of albendazole against liver flukes, tapeworms, lung and gastrointestinal roundworms. *Experientia* 32, no. 7: 702–3. doi.org/10.1007/BF01932209.

33 Working group on the efficacy of albendazole. Albendazole: A review of anthelmintic efficacy and safety in humans. *Parasitology* 121 (Supplement): S113–S132. doi.org/10.1017/s0031182000006390.

34 Marriner, S. E., Morris, D. L., Dickson, B., & Bogan, J. A. (1986). Pharmacokinetics of albendazole in man. *European Journal of Clinical Pharmacology* 30, no. 6: 705–8. doi.org/10.1007/BF00613786.

35 Matthaiou, D. K., Panos, G., Adamidi, E. S., & Falagas, M. E. (2008). Albendazole versus praziquantel in the treatment of neurocysticercosis: A meta-analysis of comparative trials. *PLoS Neglected Tropical Diseases* 2, no. 3: Article e194. doi.org/10.1371/journal.pntd.0000194.

36 Zhou, X., Zou, L., Chen, W., et al. (2021). Flubendazole, FDA-approved anthelmintic, elicits valid antitumor effects by targeting P53 and promoting ferroptosis in castration-resistant prostate cancer. *Pharmacological Research* 164, 105305. doi.org/10.1016/j.phrs.2020.105305.

37 Geary, T. G., Mackenzie, C. D., & Silber, S. A. (2019). Flubendazole as a macrofilaricide: History and background. *PLoS Neglected Tropical Diseases* 13, no. 1, e0006436.doi.org/10.1371/journal.pntd.0006436.

38 McKellar, Q. A., & Scott, E. W. (1990). The benzimidazole anthelmintic agents—A review. *Journal of Veterinary Pharmacology and Therapeutics* 13, no. 3: 223–47. doi.org/10.1111/j.1365-2885.1990.tb00772.x.

39 Borgers, M., & De Nollin, S. (1975). Ultrastructural changes in Ascaris suum intestine after mebendazole treatment in vivo. *Journal of Parasitology* 61, no. 1: 110–22. doi.org/10.2307/3279013.

40 Lacey, E. (1990). Mode of action of benzimidazoles. *Parasitology Today* 6, no. 4: 112–15. doi.org/10.1016/0169-4758(90)90227-u.

41 Sangster, N. C., & Prichard, R. K. (1984). Uptake of thiabendazole and its effects on glucose uptake and carbohydrate levels in the thiabendazole-resistant and susceptible Trichostrongylus colubriformis. *International Journal for Parasitology* 14, no. 2, 121–126. doi.org/10.1016/0020-7519(84)90038-9.

42 Guerini, A. E., Triggiani, L., Maddalo, M., Bonù, M. L., Frassine, F., Zanella, I., & Bresciani, R. (2019). Mebendazole as a candidate for drug repurposing in oncology: An extensive review of current literature. *Cancers* 11, no. 7: Article 1044. doi.org/10.3390/cancers11071044.

43 Duan, Q., Liu, Y., & Rockwell, S. (2013). Fenbendazole as a potential anticancer drug. *Anticancer Research* 33, no.2, 355–362. PMID: 23393324.

44 Nguyen, J., Nguyen, T., Han, B. and Hoang, B. (2024). Oral Fenbendazole for Cancer Therapy in Humans and Animals. *Anticancer Research* 44, no. 9: 3725–3735; doi.org/10.21873/anticanres.17197.

45 Chiang, R. S., Syed, A. B., Wright, J. L., Montgomery B., & Srinivas, S. (2021) Fenbendazole enhancing anti-tumor effect: A case series. *Clinical Oncology Case Reports* 4, no. 2.

46 Makis, W., Baghli, I., & Martinez, P. (2025). Fenbendazole as an anticancer agent? A case series of self-administration in three patients. *Case Reports in Oncology* 18, no. 1: 856–863. doi.org/10.1159/000546362.

47 Alberts, B., Johnson, A., Lewis, J., Morgan, D., Raff, M., Roberts, K., & Walter, P. (2015). *Molecular Biology of the Cell* (6th ed.). Garland Science.

48 Desai, A., & Mitchison, T. J. (1997). Microtubule polymerization dynamics. *Annual Review of Cell and Developmental Biology* 13: 83–117. doi.org/10.1146/annurev.cellbio.13.1.83.

49 Lacey, E. (1988). The role of the cytoskeletal protein, tubulin, in the mode of action and mechanism of drug resistance to benzimidazoles. *International Journal for Parasitology* 18, no. 6: 885–936. doi.org/10.1016/0020-7519(88)90171-8.

50 Ravelli, R. B. G., Gigant, B., Curmi, P. A., Jourdain, I., Lachkar, S., Sobel, A., & Knossow, M. (2004). Insight into tubulin regulation from a complex with colchicine and a stathmin-like domain. *Nature* 428, no. 6979: 198–202. doi.org/10.1038/nature02393.

51 Borgers, M., De Nollin, S., Verheyen, A., De Brabander, M., & Thienpont, D. (1975). Effects of mebendazole on the ultrastructure of cestodes. *Comparative Biochemistry and Physiology Part C: Comparative Pharmacology* 52, no. 1: 59–67. doi.org/10.1016/0306-4492(75)90010-5.

52 Borgers M, De Nollin S. (1975). Ultrastructural changes in *Ascaris suum* intestine after mebendazole treatment in vivo. *J Parasitology* 61, no. 1: 110–22.

53 Dawson, P. J., Gutteridge, W. E., & Gull, K. (1984). A comparison of the interaction of anthelmintic benzimidazoles with tubulin isolated from mammalian tissue and the parasitic nematode *Ascaridia galli*. *Biochemical Pharmacology* 33, no. 5: 1069–74. doi.org/10.1016/0006-2952(84)90698-x.

54 Van den Bossche, H., Rochette, F., & Hörig, C. (1982). Mebendazole and related anthelmintics. *Advances in Pharmacology and Chemotherapy* 19: 67–128. doi.org/10.1016/s0065-3147(08)60226-3.

55 Lacey, E., Brady, R. L., Prichard, R. K., & Watson, T. R. (1987). Comparison of inhibition of polymerisation of mammalian tubulin and helminth ovicidal activity by benzimidazole carbamates. *Veterinary Parasitology* 23, no. 1–2: 105–19. doi.org/10.1016/0304-4017(87)90011-8.

56 Martin, R. J. (1997). Modes of action of anthelmintic drugs. *The Veterinary Journal* 154, no. 1: 11–34. doi.org/10.1016/s1090-0233(97)90049-x.

57 Hemphill, A., Stadelmann, B., Rufener, R., Spiliotis, M., Boubaker, G., Müller, J., Müller, N., Gorgas, D., & Gottstein, B. (2014). Treatment of echinococcosis: albendazole and mebendazole—what else? *Parasite, 21*, no. 70. doi.org/10.1051/parasite/2014073.

58 Prichard, R. K., Hennessy, D. R., & Steel, J. W. (1978). Prolonged administration: A new concept for increasing the spectrum and effectiveness of anthelmintics. *Veterinary Parasitology* 4, no. 4: 309–15. doi.org/10.1016/0304-4017(78)90027-1.

59 FDA Center for Veterinary Medicine (CVM)—Animal Drugs @ FDA database animaldrugsatfda.fda.gov/.

60 Marriner, S. E., & Bogan, J. A. (1980). Pharmacokinetics of fenbendazole in sheep. *American Journal of Veterinary Research* 41, no. 7: 1126–29.

61 McKellar, Q. A., & Scott, E. W. (1990). The benzimidazole anthelmintic agents—A review. *Journal of Veterinary Pharmacology and Therapeutics* 13, no. 3: 223–47.

62 Bai, R. Y., Staedtke, V., Aprhys, C. M., Gallia, G. L., & Riggins, G. J. (2011). Antiparasitic mebendazole shows survival benefit in 2 preclinical models of glioblastoma multiforme. *Neuro-Oncology* 13, no. 9: 974–82. doi.org/10.1093/neuonc/nor077.

63 Bekhti, A., & Pirotte, J. (1987). Mebendazole in hydatid disease. *The Lancet* 1, no. 8548: 1449–50. doi.org/10.1016/s0140-6736(87)90664-9.

64 Awadzi, K., Hero, M., & Edwards, G. (1994). The pharmacokinetics of albendazole and its metabolites in patients with onchocerciasis. *European Journal of Clinical Pharmacology* 46, no. 2: 141–46. doi.org/10.1007/BF00199671.

65 Bai, R. Y., Staedtke, V., Aprhys, C. M., Gallia, G. L., & Riggins, G. J. (2011). Antiparasitic mebendazole shows survival benefit in 2 preclinical models of glioblastoma multiforme. *Neuro-Oncology* 13, no. 9: 974–82.

66 Pourgholami, M. H., Woon, L., Almajd, R., Akhter, J., Bowery, P., Liston, P., & Morris, D. L. (2001). In vitro and in vivo activity of albendazole against human ovarian cancer cell lines. *Cancer Chemotherapy and Pharmacology* 48, no. 6: 464–68. doi.org/10.1007/s002800100368.

Chapter 2

1 Jordan, M. A., & Wilson, L. (2004). Microtubules as a target for anticancer drugs. *Nature Reviews Cancer* 4, no. 4: 253–65. doi.org/10.1038/nrc1317.

2 Ritter, A. & Kreis, N-N, (2022). Microtubule dynamics and cancer. *Cancers* 14, no. 18: 4368. doi.org/10.3390/cancers14184368.

3 Lee, Y. T., Tan, Y. J., & Oon, C. E. (2023). Benzimidazole and its derivatives as cancer therapeutics: The potential role from traditional to precision medicine. *Acta Pharmaceutica Sinica. B* 13, no. 2: 478–497. doi.org/10.1016/j.apsb.2022.09.010.

4 Mukhtar, E., Adhami, V., Mukhtar, H. (2024). Targeting Microtubules by Natural Agents for Cancer Therapy. *Molecular Cancer Therapeutics* 13, no. 2: 275–284. doi.org/10.1158/1535-7163.MCT-13-0791.

5 Garcin, C., & Straube, A. (2019). Microtubules in cell migration. *Essays in Biochemistry* 63, no. 5: 509–520. doi.org/10.1042/EBC20190016.

6 Wang, X., Gigant, B., Zheng, X., and Chen, Q. (2023). Microtubule-targeting agents for cancer treatment: seven binding sites and three strategies. *MedComm—Oncology*. 2:e46. doi:10.1002/mog2.46.

7 Wang, Y. et al. (2023). The Warburg effect: A signature of mitochondrial overload. *Trends in Cell Biology* 33, no. 12: 1014–26. doi.org/10.1016/j.tcb.2023.05.006.

8 Dogra, N., Kumar, A., & Mukhopadhyay, T. (2018). Fenbendazole acts as a moderate microtubule destabilizing agent and causes cancer cell death by modulating

multiple cellular pathways. *Scientific Reports* 8, no. 1: 11926. doi.org/10.1038/s41598-018-30158-4.

9 Peng, Y., Pan, J., Ou, F., Wang, W., Hu, H., Chen, L., Zeng, S., Zeng, K., & Yu, L. (2022). Fenbendazole and its synthetic analog interfere with HeLa cells' proliferation and energy metabolism via inducing oxidative stress and modulating MEK3/6-p38-MAPK pathway. *Chemico-Biological Interactions* 361: 109983. doi.org/10.1016/j.cbi.2022.109983.

10 Aliabadi, A., Haghshenas, M. R., Kiani, R., Koohi-Hosseinabadi, O., Purkhosrow, A., Pirsalami, F., Panjehshahin, M. R., & Erfani, N. (2024). In vitro and in vivo anticancer activity of mebendazole in colon cancer: a promising drug repositioning. *Naunyn-Schmiedeberg's Archives of Pharmacology* 397, no. 4: 2379–2388. doi.org/10.1007/s00210-023-02722-z.

11 Doudican, N. A., Byron, S. A., Pollock, P. M., & Orlow, S. J. (2013). XIAP downregulation accompanies mebendazole growth inhibition in melanoma xenografts. *Anti-Cancer Drugs,* 24 no. 2: 181–188. doi.org/10.1097/CAD.0b013e32835a43f.

12 Larsen, A. R., Bai, R. Y., Chung, J. H., Borodovsky, A., Rudin, C. M., Riggins, G. J., & Bunz, F. (2015). Repurposing the antihelmintic mebendazole as a hedgehog inhibitor. *Molecular Cancer Therapeutics* 14, no. 1: 3–13. doi.org/10.1158/1535-7163.MCT-14-0755-T.

13 Lei, X., Wang, Y., Chen, Y., Duan, J., Gao, X., & Cong, Z. (2025). Fenbendazole exhibits antitumor activity against cervical cancer through dual targeting of cancer cells and cancer stem cells: Evidence from in vitro and in vivo models. *Molecules 30,* no. 11: 2377. doi.org/10.3390/molecules30112377.

14 Duan, Q., Liu, Y., Rockwell, S. (2021). Fenbendazole as a potential anticancer drug. *Anticancer Research* 41, no. 7: 3369–76. doi.org/10.21873/anticanres.15133.

15 Williamson, T., de Abreu, M. C., Trembath, D. G., Brayton, C., Kang, B., Mendes, T. B., de Assumpção, P. P., Cerutti, J. M., & Riggins, G. J. (2021). Mebendazole disrupts stromal desmoplasia and tumorigenesis in two models of pancreatic cancer. *Oncotarget* 12, no.14: 1326–1338. doi.org/10.18632/oncotarget.28014.

16 White, E. (2012). The role of autophagy in cancer. *Journal of Clinical Investigation* 125, no. 1: 42–46. doi.org/10.1172/JCI64220.

17 Nguyen, J., Nguyen, T. Q., Han, B., Lee, J. H., Hoang, M. D., Choi, S. I., & Hoang, B. X. (2024). Oral fenbendazole for cancer therapy in humans and animals: A comprehensive review. *Anticancer Research* 44, no. 5: 1815–26. doi.org/10.21873/anticanres.17030.

18 Carmeliet, P., & Jain, R. K. (2011). Molecular mechanisms and clinical applications of angiogenesis. *Nature* 473, no. 7347: 298–307. doi.org/10.1038/nature10144.

19 Stolfi, C., Pacifico, T., Luiz-Ferreira, A., Monteleone, G., & Laudisi, F. (2023). Anthelmintic drugs as emerging immune modulators in cancer. *International Journal of Molecular Sciences* 24, no. 7: 6446. doi.org/10.3390/ijms24076446.

20 Son, D. S., Lee, E. S., & Adunyah, S. E. (2020). The antitumor potentials of benzimidazole anthelmintics as repurposing drugs. *Immune Network* 20, no. 4: e29.doi.org/10.4110/in.2020.20.e29.

21 Stolfi, C., Pacifico, T., Luiz-Ferreira, A., Monteleone, G., & Laudisi, F. (2023). Anthelmintic drugs as emerging immune modulators in cancer. *International Journal of Molecular Sciences* 24, no. 7: 6446. doi.org/10.3390/ijms24076446.

22 Pantziarka, P., Bouche, G., Meheus, L., Sukhatme, V., & Sukhatme, V. P. (2014). Repurposing Drugs in Oncology (ReDO)-mebendazole as an anti-cancer agent. *Ecancermedicalscience* 8: 443. doi.org/10.3332/ecancer.2014.443.

23 Joe, N.S., Godet, I., Milki, N., Ain, N. U. I., Oza, H. H., Riggins, G. J., & Gilkes, D. M. (2022). Mebendazole prevents distant organ metastases in part by decreasing ITGβ4 expression and cancer stemness. *Breast Cancer Research* 24, no. 98. doi.org/10.1186/s13058-022-01593-7.

24 Pantziarka, P., Bouche, G., Meheus, L., Sukhatme, V., & Sukhatme, V. P. (2014). Repurposing Drugs in Oncology (ReDO)-mebendazole as an anti-cancer agent. *Ecancermedicalscience* 8: 443. doi.org/10.3332/ecancer.2014.443

25 Makis, W., Baghli, I., & Martinez, P. (2025). Fenbendazole as an anticancer agent? A case series of self-administration in three patients. *Case Reports in Oncology* 18, no. 1: 856–863. doi.org/10.1159/000546362.

Chapter 3

1 Mukhopadhyay, T., Sasaki, J., Ramesh, R., & Roth, J. A. (2002). Mebendazole elicits a potent antitumor effect on human cancer cell lines both in vitro and in vivo. *Clinical Cancer Research* 8, no. 9: 2963–69.

2 Bai, R. Y., Staedtke, V., Aprigliano, R., Gallia, G. L., & Riggins, G. J. (2011). Antitumor activity of mebendazole on human glioblastoma cells. *NeuroOncology* 13, no. 9: 974–82. doi.org/10.1093/neuonc/nor077.

3 Bai, R. Y., Staedtke, V., Wanjiku, T., Rudek, M. A., Joshi, A., Gallia, G. L., & Riggins, G. J. (2015). Brain penetration and efficacy of different mebendazole polymorphs in a mouse brain tumor model. *Clinical Cancer Research* 21, no. 15: 3462–70. doi.org/10.1158/1078-0432.CCR-14-2462.

4 Rodrigues, A., Chernikova, S. B., Wang, Y., et al. (2024). Repurposing mebendazole against triple-negative breast cancer leptomeningeal disease. *Research Square* rs.3.rs-3915392. doi.org/10.21203/rs.3.rs-3915392/v1.

5 Choi, H. S., Ko, Y. S., Jin, H., Kang, K. M., Ha, I. B., Jeong, H., Song, H. N., Kim, H. J., & Jeong, B. K. (2021). Anticancer effect of benzimidazole derivatives, especially mebendazole, on triple-negative breast cancer (TNBC) and radiotherapy-resistant TNBC in vivo and in vitro. *Molecules* 26, no. 17: 5118. doi .org/10.3390/molecules26175118.

6 Nguyen, T. Q., Nguyen, D. H., Phan, U. T. T., Tran, G. B., Le, T. H., Doan, C. C., Nguyen, C. T., & Vo, D. V. (2024). Fenbendazole and diisopropylamine dichloroacetate exert synergistic anti-cancer effects by inducing apoptosis and arresting the cell cycle in A549 lung cancer cells. *Anticancer Research* 44, no. 1: 137–48. doi.org/10.21873/anticanres.17704.

7 Lucenda de Silva, E., Mesquita, F., Aragao, D., et al. (2023). Mebendazole targets essential proteins in glucose metabolism leading gastric cancer cells to death. *Toxicology and Applied Pharmacology* 475: 116630. doi.org/10.1016/j .taap.2023.116630.

8 Park, D., Lee, J., & Yoon, S. (2022). Anti-cancer effects of fenbendazole on 5-fluorouracil-resistant colorectal cancer cells. *Korean Journal of Physiology & Pharmacology* 26, no. 5: 377–87. doi.org/10.4196/kjpp.2022.26.5.377.

9 Chang, C. S., Ryu, J. Y., Choi, J. K., et al. (2023). Anti-cancer effect of fenbendazole-incorporated PLGA nanoparticles in ovarian cancer. *Journal of Gynecologic Oncology* 34, no. 5: e58. doi.org/10.3802/jgo.2023.34.e58.

10 Esfahani, M. K. M., Alavi, S. E., Cabot, P. J., Islam, N., & Izake, E. L. (2021). PEGylated mesoporous silica nanoparticles (MCM-41): A promising carrier for the targeted delivery of fenbendazole into prostate cancer cells. *Pharmaceutics* 13, no. 10: 1605. doi.org/10.3390/pharmaceutics13101605.

11 Park, D. (2022). Fenbendazole suppresses growth and induces apoptosis of actively growing H4IIE hepatocellular carcinoma cells via p21-mediated cell-cycle arrest. *Biological & Pharmaceutical Bulletin* 45, no. 2: 184–93. doi.org/10.1248/bpb.b21-00735.

12 Doudican, N. A., Byron, S. A., Pollock, P. M., & Orlow, S. J. (2013). XIAP downregulation accompanies mebendazole growth inhibition in melanoma xenografts. *Anti-Cancer Drugs* 24, no. 2: 181–88. doi.org/10.1097/CAD.0b013e32835a44f2.

13 Simbulan-Rosenthal, C. M., Dakshanamurthy, S., Gaur, A., Chen, Y. S., Fang, H. B., Abdussamad, M. & Rosenthal, D. S. (2017). The repurposed anthelmintic mebendazole in combination with trametinib suppresses refractory NRASQ61K melanoma. *Oncotarget* 8, no. 8: 12576–95. doi.org/10.18632/oncotarget.14031.

14 Li, Y., Thomas, D., Deutzmann, A., Majeti, R., Felsher, D. W., & Dill, D. L. (2019). Mebendazole for differentiation therapy of acute myeloid leukemia identified by a lineage maturation index. *Scientific Reports* 9, no. 1: 16775. doi.org/10.1038/s41598-019-53290-3.

15 He, L., Shi, L., Du, Z., Huang, H., Gong, R., Ma, L. & Gu, H. (2018). Mebendazole exhibits potent anti-leukemia activity on acute myeloid leukemia. *Experimental Cell Research* 369, no. 1: 61–68. doi.org/10.1016/j.yexcr.2018.05.017.

16 Alavi, S. E., & Ebrahimi Shahmabadi, H. (2021). Anthelmintics for drug repurposing: Opportunities and challenges. *Saudi Pharmaceutical Journal* 29, no. 5: 434–445.doi.org/10.1016/j.jsps.2021.04.004.

17 Dogra, N., Kumar, A., & Mukhopadhyay, T. (2018). Fenbendazole acts as a moderate microtubule destabilizing agent and causes cancer cell death by modulating multiple cellular pathways. *Scientific Reports* 8, no. 1: 11926. doi.org/10.1038/s41598-018-30378-6.

18 Jordan, M. A., & Wilson, L. (2004). Microtubules as a target for anticancer drugs. *Nature Reviews Cancer* 4, no. 4: 253–65. doi.org/10.1038/nrc1317.

19 Baghli, I., Makis, W., Marik, P. E., et al. (2024). Targeting the mitochondrial stem cell connection in cancer treatment: a hybrid orthomolecular protocol. *Journal of Orthomolecular Medicine* (published online September 19, 2024). isom.ca/article/targeting-the-mitochondrial-stem-cell-connection-in-cancer-treatment-a-hybrid-orthomolecular-protocol/.

20 Guerini, A. E., Triggiani, L., Maddalo, M., Bonù, M. L., Frassine, F., Baiguini, A., . . . & Buglione, M. (2019). Mebendazole as a candidate for drug repurposing in oncology: An extensive review of current literature. *Cancers* 11, no. 9: 1284. doi.org/10.3390/cancers11091284.

21 Meco, D., Attinà, G., Mastrangelo, S., Navarra, P., & Ruggiero, A. (2023). Emerging Perspectives on the Antiparasitic Mebendazole as a Repurposed Drug for the Treatment of Brain Cancers. *International Journal of Molecular Sciences* 24, no. 2: 1334. doi.org/10.3390/ijms24021334.

22 Liu, C., Yang, M., Zhang, D., Chen, M., & Zhu, D. (2022). Clinical cancer immunotherapy: Current progress and prospects. *Frontiers in Immunotherapy,* 13, 961805. doi.org/10.3389/fimmu.2022.961805.

23 Joe, N. S., Godet, I., Milki, N., Ain, N. U. I., Oza, H. H., Riggins, G. J., & Gilkes, D. M. (2022). Mebendazole prevents distant organ metastases in part by decreasing ITGβ4 expression and cancer stemness. *Breast Cancer Research : BCR,* 24, no. 1: 98. doi.org/10.1186/s13058-022-01591-3.

24 Priyanka, K. B., Ramya, T. S., Swarnalatha, K., Sushmitha, G., Ara, A., Srujana, T. S., Swapna, B. (2023). Cocrystals of fenbendazole with enhanced in vitro dissolution performance. *European Chemical Bulletin* 12, no. 8: 9056–61. doi.org /10.31838/ecb/2023.12.Si8.826.

25 Shrivastava, S., Gidwani, B., & Kaur, C. D. (2020). Development of mebendazole loaded nanostructured lipid carriers for lymphatic targeting: Optimization, characterization, in-vitro and in-vivo evaluation. *Particulate Science and Technology* 39, no. 6: 1–11. doi.org/10.1080/02726351.2020.1751686.

26 Van Cauteren, H., Marsboom, R., Vandenberghe, J., & Will, J. A. (1983). Safety studies evaluating the effect of mebendazole on liver function in dogs. *Journal of the American Veterinary Medical Association* 183, no. 1: 93–98.

27 Ammann, R. W., Fleiner-Hoffmann, A., Grimm, F., & Eckert, J. (1998). Long-term mebendazole therapy may be parasitocidal in alveolar echinococcosis. *Journal of Hepatology* 29, no. 6: 994–98. doi.org/10.1016/s0168-8278(98)80130-9.

28 Meco, D., Attinà, G., Mastrangelo, S., Navarra, P., & Ruggiero, A. (2023). Emerging Perspectives on the Antiparasitic Mebendazole as a Repurposed Drug for the Treatment of Brain Cancers. *International Journal of Molecular Sciences* 24, no. 2: 1334. doi.org/10.3390/ijms24021334.

29 Movahedi, F., Li, L., & Xu, Z. P. (2023). Repurposing anti-parasite benzimidazole drugs as selective anti-cancer chemotherapeutics. *Cancer Insight 2*, no. 1: 17. doi:10.58567/ci02010003.

30 Bai, R. Y., Staedtke, V., Rudin, C. M., Bunz, F., & Riggins, G. J. (2015). Effective treatment of diverse medulloblastoma models with mebendazole and its impact on tumor angiogenesis. *NeuroOncology* 17, no. 4: 545–54. doi.org/10.1093/neuonc /nou234.

31 Williamson, T., de Abreu, M. C., Trembath, D. G., Brayton, C., Kang, B., Mendes, T. B., . . . & Riggins, G. J. (2021). Mebendazole disrupts stromal desmoplasia and tumorigenesis in two models of pancreatic cancer. *Oncotarget* 12, no. 13: 1326–38. doi.org/10.18632/oncotarget.27987.

32 Zhang, L., Bochkur, D. M., Yazal, T., Dong, K., Nguyen, A., Yu, G. & Riggins, G. J. (2019). Mebendazole potentiates radiation therapy in triple-negative breast cancer. *International Journal of Radiation Oncology, Biology, Physics* 103, no. 1: 195–207. doi.org/10.1016/j.ijrobp.2018.08.049.

33 Meco, D., Attinà, G., Mastrangelo, S., Navarra, P., & Ruggiero, A. (2023). Emerging perspectives on the antiparasitic mebendazole as a repurposed drug for

the treatment of brain cancers. *International Journal of Molecular Sciences* 24, no. 2: 1334. doi.org/10.3390/ijms24021334.

34 Navarro, H. J., Saul, J. G., Huckleby, A. E., & Kim, S. K. (2022). Inhibitory effect on hexokinase II by benzimidazoles and the insight into interactions. *Journal of Pharmaceutical Research International* 34, no. 43A: 59–66. journaljpri.com/index.php/JPRI/article/view/8331.

35 Sung, S. J., Kim, H. K., Hong, Y. K., & Joe, Y. A. (2019). Autophagy is a potential target for enhancing the anti-angiogenic effect of mebendazole in endothelial cells. *Biomolecules & Therapeutics* 27, no. 1: 117–25. doi.org/10.4062/biomolther.2018.169.

36 Jo, S. B., Sung, S. J., Choi, H. S., Park, J., Hong, Y., Joe, Y. A. (2022). Modulation of autophagy is a potential strategy for enhancing the anti-tumor effect of mebendazole in glioblastoma cells. *Biomolecules & Therapeutics* 30, no. 6: 616–24. doi.org/10.4062/biomolther.2022.060.

37 Li, Y., Acharya, G., Elahy, M., Xin, H., & Khachigian, L. M. (2019). The anthelmintic flubendazole blocks human melanoma growth and metastasis and suppresses programmed cell death protein-1 and myeloid-derived suppressor cell accumulation. *Cancer Letters*, 459: 268–276. doi.org/10.1016/j.canlet.2019.05.026.

38 Wang, X., Tian, W., Wang, N., Yang, X., Liu, Z., Li, L., & Jia, Y. (2024). Transcriptome analysis reveals the anticancer effects of fenbendazole on ovarian cancer: An in vitro and in vivo study. *BMC Cancer* 24, no. 1: 159. doi.org/10.1186/s12885-024-12593-x.

39 Markowitz, D., Ha, G., Ruggieri, R., & Symons, M. (2017). Microtubule-targeting agents can sensitize cancer cells to ionizing radiation by an interphase-based mechanism. *OncoTargets and Therapy* 10: 5633–42. doi.org/10.2147/OTT.S147103.

40 Sonabend, A. M., Bansal, S., Gu, T., et al. (2022). Fenbendazole synergizes with radiation therapy in a murine model of diffuse intrinsic pontine glioma. *NeuroOncology Advances* 4, no. 1. doi.org/10.1093/noajnl/vdac015.

41 Skibinski, C. G., Williamson, T., & Riggins, G. J. (2018). Mebendazole and radiation in combination increase survival through anticancer mechanisms in an intracranial rodent model of malignant meningioma. *Journal of NeuroOncology* 140, no. 3: 529–38. doi.org/10.1007/s11060-018-03008-z.

42 Pinto, L. C., Moreira-Nunes, C. A., Soares, B. M., Burbano, R. M., Lemos, J. A., & Montenegro, R. C. (2017). Mebendazole, an antiparasitic drug, inhibits drug transporters expression in preclinical model of gastric peritoneal carcinomatosis. *Toxicology in Vitro* 43: 87–91. doi.org/10.1016/j.tiv.2017.06.005.

43 Joe, N. S., Wang, Y., Oza, H. H., Godet, I., Milki, N., Riggins, G. J., & Gilkes, D. M. (2023). Mebendazole treatment disrupts the transcriptional activity of hypoxia-inducible factors 1 and 2 in breast cancer cells. *Cancers* 15, no. 4: 1330. doi.org/10.3390/cancers15041330.

44 Kipper, F. C., Silva, A. O., Marc, A. L., Confortin, G., Junqueira, A. V., Neto, E. P., & Lenz, G. (2018). Vinblastine and antihelmintic mebendazole potentiate temozolomide in resistant gliomas. *Investigational New Drugs* 36, no. 3: 323–31. doi.org/10.1007/s10637-017-0535-9.

45 De Witt, M., Gamble, A., Hanson, D., Markowitz, D., Powell, C., et al., (2017). Repurposing mebendazole as a replacement for vincristine for the treatment of brain tumors. *Molecular Medicine* 23: 50–56. doi.org/10.2119/molmed.2017.00011.

46 Levine, A. J. (1997). p53, the cellular gatekeeper for growth and division. *Cell* 88, no. 3: 323–31. doi:10.1016/s0092-8674(00)81871-1.

47 Muller, P. A., Vousden, K. H. (2014). Mutant p53 in cancer: New functions and therapeutic opportunities. *Cancer Cell* 25, no. 3: 304–17. doi:10.1016/j.ccr.2014.01.021.

48 Doudican, N.,Rodriguez, A., Pavlick, A., et al, (2008). Mebendazole induces apoptosis in distinct melanoma subtypes via Bcl-2 dependent mechanism. *Journal of Clinical Oncology* 26, no. 15_suppl, 20008–20008. doi.org/10.1200/jco.2008.26.15_suppl.20008.

49 Mrkvová, Z., Uldrijan, S., Pombinho, A., Bartůněk, P., & Slaninová, I. (2019). Benzimidazoles Downregulate Mdm2 and MdmX and Activate p53 in MdmX Overexpressing Tumor Cells. *Molecules* (Basel, Switzerland) 24, no.11: 2152. doi.org/10.3390/molecules24112152.

50 Boddu P, et al. (2015). Mebendazole induces differentiation and inhibits proliferation and self-renewal of acute myeloid leukemia cells. *Molecular Cancer Therapeutics* 14, no. 4: 894–904. doi.org/10.1158/1535-7163.MCT-14-0682.

51 Bai, R. Y., Staedtke, V., Aprhys, C. M., Gallia, G. L., and Riggins, G. J. (2011). Antiparasitic mebendazole shows survival benefit in 2 preclinical models of glioblastoma multiforme. *NeuroOncolology* 13, no. 9: 974–82. doi.og/10.1093/neuonc/nor077.

52 Aliabadi, A., Moradi, S. Z., Abdian, S., Fakhri, S., & Echeverría, J. (2025). Critical dysregulated signaling pathways in drug resistance: highlighting the repositioning of mebendazole for cancer therapy. *Frontiers in Pharmacology* 16: 1631419. doi.org/10.3389/fphar.2025.1631419.

53 Elayapillai, S., Ramraj, S., Benbrook, D. M., et al. (2021). Potential and mechanism of mebendazole for treatment and maintenance of ovarian cancer. *Gynecologic Oncology* 160, no. 1: 302–311. doi.org/10.1016/j.ygyno.2020.10.010.

54 Gupta, R., Roy, D., Ghosh, A., Begum, Y., Ghosh, D., & Swarnakar, S. (2025). Mebendazole Exerts Anticancer Activity in Ovarian Cancer Cell Lines via Novel Girdin-Mediated AKT/IKKα/β/NF-κB Signaling Axis. *Cells* 14, no. 2: 113. doi.org/10.3390/cells14020113.

Chapter 4

1 Mukhopadhyay, T., Sasaki, J., Ramesh, R., & Roth, J. A. (2002). Mebendazole elicits a potent antitumor effect on human cancer cell lines both in vitro and in vivo. *Clinical Cancer Research* 8, no. 9: 2963–69. PMID: 12231532.

2 Hoebeke, J., Van Nijen, G., & De Brabander, M. (1976). Interaction of Oncodazole (R17 934), a new antimitotic tumoral drug, with rat brain tubulin. *Biochemical and Biophysical Research Communications* 69, no. 2: 319–24. doi.org/10.1016/0006-291x(76)90615-7.

3 De Brabander, M., Van de Veire, R. M. L., Aerts, F., Borgers, M., & Janssen, P. A. J. (1976). The effects of methyl[5-(2-thienylcarbonyl)-1H-benzimidazole-2-yl] carbamate (R17 934; NSC 238159), a new synthetic antitumoral drug interfering

with microtubules, on mammalian cells cultured in vitro. *Cancer Research* 36, no. 3: 905–16. (PMID: 1253497).

4 Mareel, M., & De Brabander, M. (1978). Effect of microtubule inhibitors on malignant invasion in vitro. *Journal of the National Cancer Institute* 61, no. 3: 787–92. PMID: 690960.

5 De Brabander, M., Geuens, G., Van de Veire, R., Thoné, F., Aerts, F., De Splenter, L., De Cree, J., & Borgers, M. (1977). The effects of R17 934 (NSC 238159), a new antimicrotubular substance, on the ultrastructure of neoplastic cells in vivo. *European Journal of Cancer* 13, no. 4–5: 511–28. doi.org/10.1016/0014-2964 (77)90243-0.

6 Geuens, G. M., Nuydens, R., Willebrords, R. E., Van de Veire, R. M. L., Goossens, F., Dragonetti, C. H., Mareel, M., & De Brabander, M. (1985). Effects of tubulozole on microtubule system of cells in culture and in vivo. *Cancer Research* 45, no. 2: 733–42. (PMID: 3967267).

7 Zimmerman, F. K., Mayer, V. W., & Scheel, I. (1984). Induction of aneuploidy by oncodazole (nocodazole), an anti-tubulin agent, and acetone. *Mutation Research Letters* 141, no. 1: 15–18. doi.org/10.1016/0165-7992(84)90052-0.

8 Hoebeke, J., Van Nijen, G., & De Brabander, M. (1976). Interaction of Oncodazole (R17 934), a new antimitotic tumoral drug, with rat brain tubulin. *Biochemical and Biophysical Research Communications* 69, no. 2: 319–24. doi.org /10.1016/0006-291x(76)90615-7.

9 Mukhopadhyay, T., Sasaki, J., Ramesh, R., & Roth, J. A. (2002). Mebendazole elicits a potent antitumor effect on human cancer cell lines both in vitro and in vivo. *Clinical Cancer Research* 8, no. 9: 2963–69. PMID: 12231532.

10 Manfredi, J. J., & Horwitz, S. B. (1984). Taxol: An antimitotic agent with a new mechanism of action. *Pharmacology & Therapeutics* 25, no. 1: 83–125. doi.org /10.1016/0163-7258(84)90052-8.

11 Delatour, P., & Richard, Y. (1976). Embryotoxic and antimitotic properties of some benzimidazole related compounds. *Therapie* 31, no. 4: 505–15. (PMID: 982082).

12 Bates, D., & Eastman, A. (2017). Microtubule destabilizing agents: Far more than just antimitotic anticancer drugs. *British Journal of Clinical Pharmacology* 83, no. 2: 255–68. doi.org/10.1111/bcp.13071.

13 Zimmerman, F. K., Mayer, V. W., & Scheel, I. (1984). Induction of aneuploidy by oncodazole (nocodazole), an anti-tubulin agent, and acetone. *Mutation Research Letters* 141, no. 1: 15–18. doi.org/10.1016/0165-7992(84)90052-0.

14 Bates, D., & Eastman, A. (2017). Microtubule destabilizing agents: Far more than just antimitotic anticancer drugs. *British Journal of Clinical Pharmacology* 83, no. 2: 255–68. doi.org/10.1111/bcp.13071.

15 Manfredi, J. J., & Horwitz, S. B. (1984). Taxol: An antimitotic agent with a new mechanism of action. *Pharmacology & Therapeutics* 25, no. 1: 83–125. doi.org/10 .1016/0163–7258(84)90052–8.

16 Barok, M., Joensuu, H., & Isola, J. (2014). Trastuzumab emtansine: Mechanisms of action and drug resistance. *Breast Cancer Research* 16, no. 2: 209. doi.org/10 .1186/bcr3621.

17 DeVita, V. T., Jr., & Chu, E. (2008). A history of cancer chemotherapy. *Cancer Research* 68, no. 21: 8643–53. doi.org/10.1158/0008-5472.CAN-07-6611.

18 Yang, R., Zhou, Y., Wang, Y., Du, C., & Wu, Y. (2020). Trends in cancer incidence and mortality rates in the United States from 1975 to 2016. *Annals of Translational Medicine* 8, no. 24: 1671. doi.org/10.21037/atm-20-2378.

Chapter 5

1 Batlle, E., & Clevers, H. (2017). Cancer stem cells revisited. *Nature Medicine* 23, no. 10: 1124–34. doi.org/10.1038/nm.4409.

2 Visvader, J. E., & Lindeman, G. J. (2012). Cancer stem cells: Current status and evolving complexities. *Cell Stem Cell* 10, no. 6: 717–28.

3 Zhou, J., Ji, Q., Li, Q., & Lee, J. Y. (2016). Cancer stem cells and chemoresistance: The smartest survives the raid. *Pharmacology & Therapeutics* 160: 145–58. doi.org/10.1016/j.pharmthera.2016.02.008.

4 Dean, M., Fojo, T., & Bates, S. (2005). Tumour stem cells and drug resistance. *Nature Reviews Cancer* 5, no. 4: 275–84. doi.org/10.1038/nrc1590.

5 Guerini, A. E., Triggiani, L., Maddalo, M., et al. (2019). Mebendazole as a candidate for drug repurposing in oncology: An extensive review of current literature. *Cancers* 11, no. 9: 1284. doi.org/10.3390/cancers11091284.

6 Joe, N. S., Godet, I., Milki, N., Ain, N. U. I., Oza, H. H., Riggins, G. J., & Gilkes, D. M. (2022). Mebendazole prevents distant organ metastases in part by decreasing ITGβ4 expression and cancer stemness. *Breast Cancer Research* 24, no. 1: 98. doi.org/10.1186/s13058-022-01591-3.

7 Dogra, N., Kumar, A., & Mukhopadhyay, T. (2018). Fenbendazole acts as a moderate microtubule destabilizing agent and causes cancer cell death by modulating multiple cellular pathways. *Scientific Reports* 8, no. 1: 11926. doi.org/10.1038/s41598-018-30378.6.

8 Brash, D. E. (2019). Accelerating cancer without mutations. *eLife* 8: e45809. doi.org/10.7554/eLife.45809.

9 Greaves, M., & Maley, C. C. (2012). Clonal evolution in cancer. *Nature* 481 (7381): 306–13. doi.org/10.1038/nature10762.

10 Worsley, C. M., Mayne, E. S., & Veale, R. B. (2016). Clone wars: The evolution of therapeutic resistance in cancer. *Evolution, Medicine, and Public Health* 1: 180–81. doi.org/10.1093/emph/eow015.

11 Nguyen, L. V., Vanner, R., Dirks, P., & Eaves, C. J. (2012). Cancer stem cells: An evolving concept. *Nature Reviews Cancer* 12, no. 2: 133–43. doi.org/10.1038/nrc3184.

12 Govindan, R. (2014). Attack of the clones. *Science* 346, no. 6206: 169–70. doi.org/10.1126/science.1259926.

13 Abdullah, L. N., & Chow, E. K.-H. (2013). Mechanisms of chemoresistance in cancer stem cells. *Clinical and Translational Medicine* 2, no. 1: 3. doi.org/10.1186/2001-1326-2-3.

14 Sung, H., Ferlay, J., Siegel, R. L., Laversanne, M., Soerjomataram, I., Jemal, A., & Bray, F. (2021). Global cancer statistics 2020: GLOBOCAN estimates of incidence and mortality worldwide for 36 cancers in 185 countries. *CA: A Cancer Journal for Clinicians* 71, no. 3: 209–49. doi.org/10.3322/caac.21660.

15 Taherian-Fard, A., Srihari, S., & Ragan, M. A. (2015). Breast cancer classification: Linking molecular mechanisms to disease prognosis. *Briefings in Bioinformatics* 16, no. 3: 461–74. doi.org/10.1093/bib/bbu021.

16 Newton, E. E., Mueller, L. E., Treadwell, S. M., Morris, C. A., & Machado, H. L. (2022). Molecular targets of triple-negative breast cancer: Where do we stand? *Cancers* 14, no. 3: 482. doi.org/10.3390/cancers14030482.

17 Bierie, B., Pierce, S. E., Kroeger, P. T., Stover, D. G., Pattabiraman, D. R., Thiru, P., & Weinberg, R. A. (2017). Integrin-β4 identifies cancer stem cell-enriched populations of partially mesenchymal carcinoma cells. *Proceedings of the National Academy of Sciences* 114, no. 12: E2337–46. doi.org/10.1073/pnas.1618298114.

18 Rodrigues, A. J., Chernikova, S. B., Wang, Y., et al. (2024). Repurposing mebendazole against triple-negative breast cancer CNS metastasis. *Journal of Neurooncology* 168, no. 1: 125–38. doi.org/10.1007/s11060-024-04654-x.

19 De Witt, M., Gamble, A., Hanson, D., Markowitz, D., Markowitz, C., Vogl, W., & Riggins, G. J. (2017). Repurposing mebendazole as a replacement for vincristine for the treatment of brain tumors. *Molecular Medicine* 23: 50–56. doi.org/10.2119/molmed.2017.00011.

20 Bai, R.-Y., Staedtke, V., Aprhys, C. M., Gallia, G. L., & Riggins, G. J. (2011). Antiparasitic mebendazole shows survival benefit in 2 preclinical models of glioblastoma multiforme. *Neuro-Oncology* 13, no. 9: 974–82. doi.org/10.1093/neuonc/nor077.

21 Lei, X., Wang, Y., Chen, Y., Duan, J., Gao, X., & Cong, Z. (2025). Fenbendazole exhibits antitumor activity against cervical cancer through dual targeting of cancer cells and cancer stem cells: Evidence from in vitro and in vivo models. *Molecules 30*, no. 11: 2377. doi.org/10.3390/molecules30112377.

22 Bai, R. Y., Staedtke, V., Wanjiku, T., Rudek, M. A., Joshi, A., Gallia, G. L., & Riggins, G. J. (2015). Brain penetration and efficacy of mebendazole in patients with newly diagnosed high-grade gliomas. *Clinical Cancer Research* 21, no. 15: 3445–53. doi.org/10.1158/1078-0432.CCR-15-0190.

23 Lacey, E. (1988). The role of the cytoskeletal protein, tubulin, in the mode of action and mechanism of drug resistance to benzimidazoles. *International Journal for Parasitology* 18, no. 7: 885–936. doi.org/10.1016/0020-7519(88)90144-8.

24 Makis, M., Baghli, I. & Martinez, P. (2025). Fenbendazole as an anticancer agent? A case series of self-administration in three patients. *Case Reports in Oncology*, 18 (1), 856–863. doi.org/10.1159/000546362.

25 Zhang, L., Bochkur Dratver, M., Yazal, T., Dong, K., Nguyen, A., Yu, G., Dao, A., Bochkur Dratver, M., Duhachek-Muggy, S., Bhat, K., & Sadeghi, S. (2019). Mebendazole potentiates radiation therapy in triple-negative breast cancer. *International Journal of Radiation Oncology, Biology, Physics* 103, no. 1: 195–207. doi.org/10.1016/j.ijrobp.2018.08.049.

26 Zhang, L., Bochkur Dratver, M., Yazal, T., Dong, K., Nguyen, A., Yu, G., Dao, A., Bochkur Dratver, M., Duhachek-Muggy, S., Bhat, K., & Sadeghi, S. (2019). Mebendazole potentiates radiation therapy in triple-negative breast cancer. *International Journal of Radiation Oncology, Biology, Physics* 103, no. 1: 195–207. doi.org/10.1016/j.ijrobp.2018.08.049.

27 Liu, C. S., Zhang, H. B., Jiang, B., Yao, J. M., Tao, Y., Xue, J., & Wen, A. D. (2012). Enhanced bioavailability and cysticidal effect of three mebendazole-oil preparations in mice infected with secondary cysts of *Echinococcus granulosus*. *Parasitology Research* 111, no. 3: 1205–11. doi.org/10.1007/s00436-012-2954-2.

Chapter 6

1 Centers for Disease Control and Prevention. (1981). Pneumocystis pneumonia—Los Angeles. *Morbidity and Mortality Weekly Report* 30, no. 21: 250–52. Retrieved May 1, 2025. cdc.gov/mmwr/preview/mmwrhtml/june_5.htm.
2 McBride, W. G. (1961). Thalidomide and congenital abnormalities. *The Lancet* 278, no. 7216: 1358. doi.org/10.1016/S0140-6736(61)90927-8.
3 Chaffin, J. J., & Davis, S. M. (1994). Stevens-Johnson syndrome associated with lamotrigine. *Journal of the American Academy of Dermatology* 31, no. 5 Pt 1: 777–78. doi.org/10.1016/0190-9622(94)90492-6.
4 Kyle, R. A., Steensma, D. P., & Shampo, M. A. (2016). Barry James Marshall: Discovery of Helicobacter pylori as a cause of peptic ulcer. *Mayo Clinic Proceedings* 91, no. 5: e67–e68. doi.org/10.1016/j.mayocp.2016.01.025.
5 Williams, D. (2019). A Cure for Cancer Hidden in Plain Sight. fenbendazole.s3.amazonaws.com/A-Cure-for-Cancer-Hidden-in-Plain-Sight-July-2019-Dr-David-Williams.pdf. Accessed May 3, 2025.
6 Makis, M., Baghli, I. & Martinez, P. (2025). Fenbendazole as an anticancer agent? A case series of self-administration in three patients. *Case Reports in Oncology* 18, no. 1: 856–63. doi.org/10.1159/000546362.
7 Makis, M., Baghli, I. & Martinez, P. (2025). Fenbendazole as an anticancer agent? A case series of self-administration in three patients. *Case Reports in Oncology* 18, no. 1: 856–63. doi.org/10.1159/000546362.
8 Makis, M., Baghli, I. & Martinez, P. (2025). Fenbendazole as an anticancer agent? A case series of self-administration in three patients. *Case Reports in Oncology* 18, no. 1: 856–63. doi.org/10.1159/000546362.
9 Chiang, R. S., Syed, A. B., Wright, J. L., Montgomery, B., & Srinivas, S. (2021). Fenbendazole enhancing anti-tumor effect: A case series. *Clinical Oncology and Case Reports* 4, no. 2. doi.org/10.17352/2639-8438.000026.
10 Ibid.

Chapter 7

1 Alman, B. (2012). Desmoid tumors: Are they benign or malignant? In: Litchman, C. (eds.) *Desmoid Tumors*. Springer. doi.org/10.1007/978-94-007-1685-8_13.
2 Mayo Clinic. Desmoid Tumors: Symptoms and Causes. mayoclinic.org/diseases-conditions/desmoid-tumors/symptoms-causes/syc-20355083. Retrieved May 13, 2025.
3 Mayo Clinic. Squamous Cell Carcinoma—Symptoms and Causes. mayoclinic.org/diseases-conditions/squamous-cell-carcinoma/symptoms-causes/syc-20352480. Retrieved May 13, 2025.
4 Tang, M., Hu, X., Wang, Y., Yao, X., Zhang, W., Yu, C., Cheng, F., Li, J., & Fang, Q. (2021). Ivermectin, a potential anticancer drug derived from an antiparasitic drug. *Pharmacological Research* 163: 105207. doi.org/10.1016/j.phrs.2020.105207.

Chapter 8

1 Ettinger, S. J., & Feldman, E. C. (eds.). (2017). *Textbook of Veterinary Internal Medicine* (8th ed.). Elsevier.

2 Dobson, J. M. (2013). Breed-predispositions to cancer in pedigree dogs. *ISRN Veterinary Science* 2013: 941275. doi.org/10.1155/2013/941275.

3 Withrow, S. J., Vail, D. M., & Page, R. L. (eds.). (2019). *Withrow & MacEwen's Small Animal Clinical Oncology* (6th ed.). Elsevier.

4 Paoloni, M., & Khanna, C. (2008). Translation of new cancer treatments from pet dogs to humans. *Nature Reviews Cancer* 8, no. 2: 147–56. doi.org/10.1038/nrc2272.

5 Khanna, C., et al. (2014). Genomic approaches to comparative oncology in osteosarcoma. *Veterinary Pathology* 51, no. 1: 181–95. doi.org/10.1177/0300985813517506.

6 Zandvliet M. (2016). Canine lymphoma: a review. *The Veterinary Quarterly* 36, no. 2: 76–104. doi.org/10.1080/01652176.2016.1152633.

7 Marconato, L., Stefanello, D., Valenti, P., et al. (2008). Predictors of long-term survival in dogs with high-grade multicentric lymphoma. *Journal of the American Veterinary Medical Association* 232, no. 6: 886–91. doi.org/10.2460/javma.232.6.886.

8 Efferth, T. (2017). From ancient herb to modern drug: Artemisia annua and artesunate for cancer therapy. *Seminars in Cancer Biology* 46: 65–83. doi.org/10.1016/j.semcancer.2017.02.009.

9 Hohenhaus, A. E., Kelsey, J. L., & Haddad, J. (2016). Canine cutaneous and subcutaneous soft tissue sarcoma: An evidence-based review of case management. *Journal of the American Animal Hospital Association* 52, no. 2: 77–89. doi.org/10.5326/JAAHA-MS-6331.

10 Forrest, L. J., Chun, R., Adams, W. M., et al. (2000). Postoperative radiotherapy for canine soft tissue sarcoma. *Journal of Veterinary Internal Medicine* 14, no. 6: 578–82. doi.org/10.1111/j.1939-1676.2000.tb02271.x.

11 Kuntz, C. A., Dernell, W. S., Powers, B. E., et al. (1997). Prognostic factors for surgical treatment of soft tissue sarcomas in dogs: 75 cases (1986–1996). *Journal of the American Veterinary Medical Association* 211, no. 9: 1147–51. pubmed.ncbi.nlm.nih.gov/9364227.

12 Bergman, P. J. (2013). Canine oral melanoma. In S. J. Withrow & D. M. Vail (eds.), *Withrow & MacEwen's Small Animal Clinical Oncology* (5th ed., pp. 438–43). Elsevier.

13 Spangler, W. L., & Kass, P. H. (2006). The histologic and prognostic significance of tumor depth in canine malignant melanoma of the oral cavity. *Veterinary Pathology* 43, no. 6: 929–35. doi.org/10.1354/vp.43-6-929.

14 Hamzalis, M., Packer, R. M., & Shoemaker, N. J. (2022). Oral malignant melanoma in dogs: Current understanding and future directions. *The Veterinary Journal* 288: 105877. doi.org/10.1016/j.tvjl.2022.105877.

15 Marik, P. E. (2023). The FLCCC Treatment Protocols. Front Line COVID-19 Critical Care Alliance. covid19criticalcare.com/treatment-protocols/.

16 Moore, A. S. (2003). Doxorubicin for the treatment of canine lymphoma: Efficacy and toxicity. *Compendium on Continuing Education for the Practicing Veterinarian,* 25, no. 11, 812–824. doi.org/10.5555/20032995736.

17 Howick, J., Friedemann, C., Tsakek, M., Watson, R., Tsakek, T., et al. (2016). Are treatments more effective than placebos? A systematic review and meta-analysis. *PLOS ONE* 11 no.1: e0147354. doi.org/10.1371/journal.pone.0147354.

18 McMillan F. D. (1999). The placebo effect in animals. *Journal of the American Veterinary Medical Association* 215, no. 7: 992–99.

Chapter 9

1 Cray, C., & Altman, N. H. (2022). An update on the biologic effects of fenbendazole. *Comparative Medicine* 72, no. 4: 215–219. doi.org/10.30802/AALAS-CM-22-000006.

2 Lewis, J. H., Khaldoyanidi, S. K., Britten, C. D., et al. (2022). Clinical significance of transient asymptomatic elevations in aminotransferase (TAEAT) in oncology. *American Journal of Clinical Oncology* 45, no. 8: 352–365. doi.org/10.1097/COC.0000000000000932.

3 Contreras-Zentella, Lucinda M., Hernández-Muñoz, R. (2016). Is liver enzyme release really associated with cell necrosis induced by oxidant stress? *Oxidative Medicine and Cellular Longevity*, 3529149. https://doi.org/10.1155/2016/3529149.

Chapter 10

1 Sung, H., Ferlay, J., Siegel, R. L., Laversanne, M., Soerjomataram, I., Jemal, A., & Bray, F. (2021). Global cancer statistics 2020: GLOBOCAN estimates of incidence and mortality worldwide for 36 cancers in 185 countries. *CA: A Cancer Journal for Clinicians* 71, no. 3: 209–49. doi.org/10.3322/caac.21660.

2 American Cancer Society. (2024). Cancer Statistics, 2024. *CA: A Cancer Journal for Clinicians* 74, no. 1: 12–49. doi.org/10.3322/caac.21820.

3 Greger, M. (2015, September 15). Why are cancer rates so low in India? NutritionFacts.org. Accessed April 21, 2025. nutritionfacts.org/2015/09/15/why-are-cancer-rates-so-low-in-india/.

4 These data were collected and published by the WHO in 2020 without an agenda (we selected 2020 data to exclude any confounding effect of differential covid vaccine uptake on cancer rate). These data are an unbiased record of a global phenomenon accessible by anyone.

5 World Health Organization. (2021). Guideline: Preventive chemotherapy to control soil-transmitted helminth infections in at-risk population groups. World Health Organization. ISBN 978-92-4-004104-4 who.int/publications/i/item/9789240041044.

6 Lacey, E. (1990). Mode of action of benzimidazoles. *Parasitology Today* 6, no. 4: 112–15. doi.org/10.1016/0169-4758(90)90227-U.

7 Florio, R., Carradori, S., Veschi, S., et al. (2021). Screening of Benzimidazole-Based Anthelmintics and Their Enantiomers as Repurposed Drug Candidates in Cancer Therapy. *Pharmaceuticals (Basel, Switzerland)* 14, no. 4: 372. doi.org/10.3390/ph14040372.

8 Ghasemi, F., Black, M., Vizeacoumar, F., Pinto, N., Ruicci, K. M., Fung, K., & Yoo, J. (2017). Repurposing albendazole: New potential as a chemotherapeutic agent with preferential activity against HPV-negative head and neck squamous cell cancer. *Oncotarget* 8, no. 42: 71512. doi.org/10.18632/oncotarget.19569.

9 Pullan, R. L., Smith, J. L., Jasrasaria, R., & Brooker, S. J. (2014). Global numbers of infection and disease burden of soil-transmitted helminth infections in 2010. *Parasites & Vectors* 7, no. 37. doi.org/10.1186/1756-3305-7-37.

10 Ministry of Health and Family Welfare, Government of India. National Deworming Day. Accessed April 10, 2025. nhm.gov.in/index1.php?lang=1&level=2&sublinkid=1319&lid=710.

11 Flisser, A., Valdespino, J. L., García-García, L., Guzman, C., Aguirre, M. T., Manon, M. L., & Gyorkos, T. W. (2008). Using national health weeks to deliver deworming to children: Lessons from Mexico. *Journal of Epidemiology and Community Health* 62, no. 4: 314–17. doi.org/10.1136/jech.2007.068306.

12 Hotez, P. J., & Fenwick, A. (2009). Schistosomiasis in Africa: an emerging tragedy in our new global health decade. *PLoS Neglected Tropical Diseases* 3 no.9, e485. Doi.org/10.137/journal.pntd.0000485.

13 Lo, N. C., Addiss, D. G., Hotez, P. J., King, C. H., Stothard, J. R., Raso, G., & Utzinger, J. (2017). A call to strengthen the global strategy against schistosomiasis and soil-transmitted helminthiasis: The time is now. *The Lancet Infectious Diseases* 17, no. 2: e64–e69. doi.org/10.1016/S1473-3099(16)30235-7.

14 Pan American Health Organization / WHO. Soil-Transmitted Helminthiasis. Accessed April 21, 2025. paho.org/en/topics/soil-transmitted-helminthiasis.

15 World Health Organization, Regional Office for the Western Pacific. Soil-transmitted helminthiasis. Accessed April 21, 2025. who.int/westernpacific/health-topics/soil-transmitted-helminthiasis.

16 Amin, O. M. (2002). Seasonal prevalence of intestinal parasites in the United States during 2000. *The American Journal of Tropical Medicine and Hygiene* 66, no. 6: 799–803. doi.org/10.4269/ajtmh.2002.66.799.

17 McKenna, M. L., McAtee, S., Bryan, P. E., Jeun, R., Ward, T., Kraus, J., & Mejia, R. (2017). Human intestinal parasite burden and poor sanitation in rural Alabama. *The American Journal of Tropical Medicine and Hygiene* 97, no. 5: 1623–28. doi.org/10.4269/ajtmh.17-0396.

18 Parise, M. E., Hotez, P. J., & Slutsker, L. (2014). Neglected parasitic infections in the United States: Needs and opportunities. *The American Journal of Tropical Medicine and Hygiene* 90, no. 5: 783–85. doi.org/10.4269/ajtmh.13-0727.

19 Jones, J. L., Parise, M. E., & Fiore, A. E. (2014). Neglected parasitic infections in the United States: Toxoplasmosis. *The American Journal of Tropical Medicine and Hygiene* 90, no. 5: 794–99. doi.org/10.4269/ajtmh.13-0722.

20 Montgomery, S. P., Starr, M. C., Cantey, P. T., Edwards, M. S., & Meymandi, S. (2014). Neglected parasitic infections in the United States: Chagas disease. *The American Journal of Tropical Medicine and Hygiene* 90, no. 5: 814–18. doi.org/10.4269/ajtmh.13-0729.

21 Cantey, P. T., Coyle, C. M., Sorvillo, F. J., Wilkins, P. P., Starr, M. C., & Nash, T. E. (2014). Neglected parasitic infections in the United States: Cysticercosis. *The American Journal of Tropical Medicine and Hygiene* 90, no. 5: 805–9. doi.org/10.4269/ajtmh.13-0724.

22 Woodhall, D. M., Eberhard, M. L., & Parise, M. E. (2014). Neglected parasitic infections in the United States: Toxocariasis. *The American Journal of Tropical Medicine and Hygiene* 90, no. 5: 810–13. doi.org/10.4269/ajtmh.13-0725.

23 Secor, W. E., Meites, E., Starr, M. C., & Workowski, K. A. (2014). Neglected parasitic infections in the United States: Trichomoniasis. *The American Journal of Tropical Medicine and Hygiene* 90, no. 5: 800–804. doi.org/10.4269/ajtmh.13-0723.

24 Cox, F. E. G. (2002). History of human parasitology. *Clinical Microbiology Reviews* 15, no. 4: 595–612. doi.org/10.1128/CMR.15.4.595-612.2002.

25 Berger, C. N., Sodha, S. V., Shaw, R. K., Griffin, P. M., Pink-Harper, S., Frankel, G., . . . & Tauxe, R. V. (2010). Fresh fruit and vegetables as vehicles for the transmission of human pathogens. *Environmental Microbiology* 12, no. 9: 2385–97. doi.org/10.1111/j.1462-2920.2010.02241.x.

26 Robertson, I. D., Irwin, P. J., Lymbery, A. J., & Thompson, R. C. A. (2000). The role of companion animals in the emergence of parasitic zoonoses. *International Journal for Parasitology* 30, no. 12–13: 1369–77. doi.org/10.1016/S0020-7519(00)00134-X.

27 Over half of pet-owners unaware of infection risks from their pets: Survey. (2024, February 9). *The Korea Herald*. Accessed April 21, 2025. koreaherald.com/view.php?ud=20240209000561.

28 Nwokolo, C. (2021). Health benefits of deworming regularly for adults. Healthguide.ng. Accessed April 21, 2025. healthguide.ng/health-benefits-deworming-regularly-adults/.

29 Sharma, K. (2021). Regular deworming is important for both kids and adults. *The Times of India*. timesofindia.indiatimes.com/life-style/health-fitness/health-news/regular-deworming-is-important-for-both-kids-and-adults/articleshow/80788392.cms. Accessed April 21, 2025.

30 van Tong, H., Brindley, P. J., Meyer, C. G., & Velavan, T. P. (2017). Parasite infection, carcinogenesis and human malignancy. *eBioMedicine* 15: 12–23. doi.org/10.1016/j.ebiom.2016.11.034.

31 Pradas, N. (2020). Deworming among adults: A necessary process. *The New Indian Express*. newindianexpress.com/lifestyle/health/2020/feb/09/deworming-among-adults-a-necessary-process-2100992.html.

32 Medzhitov, R. (2008). Origin and physiological roles of inflammation. *Nature* 454 (7203): 428–35. doi.org/10.1038/nature07201.

33 Maizels, R. M. (2016). Regulation of immunity and allergy by helminth parasites. *Allergy* 71, no. 6: 767–74. doi.org/10.1111/all.12862.

34 Gittleman, A. L. (2001). *Guess What Came to Dinner: Parasites and Your Health*. Penguin Books.

35 Adebajo A. O. (1997). Low frequency of autoimmune disease in tropical Africa. *The Lancet* 349, no. 9048: 361–62. doi.org/10.1016/s0140-6736(05)62867-x.

36 Parise, M. E., Hotez, P. J., & Slutsker, L. (2014). Neglected parasitic infections in the United States: Needs and opportunities. *The American Journal of Tropical Medicine and Hygiene* 90, no. 5: 783–85. doi.org/10.4269/ajtmh.13-0727.

37 Ettling, J. (1981). *The Germ of Laziness: Rockefeller Philanthropy and Public Health in the New South*. Harvard University Press.

38 Centers for Disease Control and Prevention (CDC). Parasites. Accessed April 21, 2025. cdc.gov/parasites/.

39 Meurs, L., Polderman, A. M., Vinkeles, N. et al. (2017). Diagnosing polyparasitism in a high-prevalence setting in Beira, Mozambique: Detection of intestinal parasites in fecal samples by microscopy and real-time PCR. *PLoS Negl Trop Dis* 11, no. 1: e0005310. doi.org/10.1371/journal.pntd.0005310.

40 National Institutes of Health (2023). Financial Burden of Cancer Care. Accessed August 21, 2025. https://progressreport.cancer.gov/after/economic_burden.

41 Afghanistan, Algeria, Angola, Argentina, Armenia, Azerbaijan, Bahrain, Bangladesh, Belize, Benin, Bhutan, Bolivia, Botswana, Burkino Faso, Burundi, Cambodia, Cameroon, Cape Verde, Central Africa Rep., Chad, Chile, Colombia, Comoros, Congo (Dem. Republic), Costa Rica, Cuba, Djibouti, Dominican Republic, Ecuador, Egypt, El Salvador, Eq. Guinea, Eritrea, Eswatini, Ethiopia, Fiji, French Polynesia, Gabon, Gambia, Ghana, Guam, Guatemala, Guinea, Guinea-Bissau, Guyana, Haiti, Honduras, India, Indonesia, Iran, Iraq, Ivory Coast, Jordan, Kazakhstan, Kenya, Kuwait, Kyrgyzstan, Laos, Lebanon, Lesotho, Liberia, Libya, Madagascar, Malawi, Malaysia, Maldives, Mali, Mauritania, Mauritius, Mexico, Moldova, Mongolia, Morocco, Mozambique, Myanmar, Namibia, Nepal, Nicaragua, Niger, Nigeria, North Macedonia, Oman, Pakistan, Panama, Papua New Guinea, Paraguay, Peru, Philippines, Puerto Rico, Qatar, Rep. of Congo, Rwanda, Saint Lucia, Samoa, São Tomé & Principe, Saudi Arabia, Senegal, Sierra Leone, Solomon Isl., Somalia, South Africa, South Sudan, Sri Lanka, Sudan, Suriname, Syria, Tajikistan, Tanzania, Thailand, Timor-Leste, Togo, Trinidad & Tobago, Tunisia, Turkey, Turkmenistan, Uganda, United Arab Emirates, Uzbekistan, Vanuatu, Venezuela, Vietnam, Yemen, Zambia, and Zimbabwe.

42 Albania, Australia, Austria, Bahamas, Barbados, Belarus, Belgium, Bermuda, Bosnia and Herzegovina, Brazil, Brunei, Darussalam, Bulgaria, Canada, China, Croatia, Cyprus, Czechia, Denmark, Estonia, Finland, France, Georgia, Germany, Greece, Greenland, Guadeloupe, Hong Kong, Hungary, Iceland, Ireland, Israel, Italy, Jamaica, Japan, Latvia, Lithuania, Luxembourg, Macao, Malta, Montenegro, Netherlands, New Caledonia, New Zealand, Norway, Poland, Portugal, Romania, Russia, Serbia, Singapore, Slovakia, Slovenia, South Korea, Spain, Sweden, Switzerland, Taiwan, Ukraine, United Kingdom, the United States, and Uruguay.

Chapter 11

1 Plimmer H. G. (1903). The parasitic theory of cancer. *British Medical Journal* 2, no. 2241: 1511–15. doi.org/10.1136/bmj.2.2241.1511.

2 Hanahan, D., & Weinberg, R. A. (2011). Hallmarks of cancer: The next generation. *Cell* 144, no. 5: 646–74. doi.org/10.1016/j.cell.2011.02.013.

3 Hanahan, D. (2022). Hallmarks of cancer: New dimensions. *Cancer Discovery* 12, no. 1: 31–46. doi.org/10.1158/2159-8290.CD-21-1059.

4 Vander Heiden, M. G., Cantley, L. C., & Thompson, C. B. (2009). Understanding the Warburg effect: The metabolic requirements of cell proliferation. *Science* 324, no. 5930: 1029–33. doi.org/10.1126/science.1160809.

5 Cox, F. E. G. (2010). History of human parasitology. *Clinical Microbiology Reviews* 15, no. 4: 595–612. doi.org/10.1128/CMR.15.4.595-612.2002.

6 Bethony, J., Brooker, S., Albonico, M., Geiger, S. M., Loukas, A., Diemert, D., & Hotez, P. J. (2006). Soil-transmitted helminth infections: Ascariasis, trichuriasis, and hookworm. *The Lancet* 367, no. 9521: 1521–32. doi.org/10.1016/S0140-6736(06)68653-4.

7 Liberti, M. V., & Locasale, J. W. (2016). The Warburg effect: How does it benefit cancer cells? *Trends in Biochemical Sciences* 41, no. 3: 211–18. doi.org/10.1016/j.tibs.2015.12.001.

8 DeBerardinis, R. J., Lum, J. J., Hatzivassiliou, G., & Thompson, C. B. (2008). The biology of cancer: Metabolic reprogramming fuels cell growth and proliferation. *Cell Metabolism* 7, no. 1: 11–20. doi.org/10.1016/j.cmet.2007.10.002.

9 Fearon, K., Strasser, F., Anker, S. D., Bosaeus, I., Bruera, E., Fainsinger, R. L., et al. (2011). Definition and classification of cancer cachexia: An international consensus. *The Lancet Oncology* 12, no. 5: 489–95. doi.org/10.1016/S1470-2045(10)70218-7.

10 Ginger, M. L. (2006). Energy metabolism in parasitic protists and helminths. *Acta Tropica* 99 (2–3): 100–11. doi.org/10.1016/j.actatropica.2006.07.001.

11 Gallego-López, G. M., Contreras Guzman, E., Desa, D. E., Knoll, L. J., & Skala, M. C. (2024). Metabolic changes in *Toxoplasma gondii*-infected host cells measured by autofluorescence imaging. *mBio 15* no. 8: e0072724. doi.org/10.1128/mbio.00727-24.

12 Fidler, I. J. (2003). The pathogenesis of cancer metastasis: The "seed and soil" hypothesis revisited. *Nature Reviews Cancer* 3, no. 6: 453–58. doi.org/10.1038/nrc1098.

13 Thiery, J. P., Acloque, H., Huang, R. Y. J., & Nieto, M. A. (2009). Epithelial-mesenchymal transitions in development and disease. *Cell* 139, no. 5: 871–90. doi.org/10.1016/j.cell.2009.11.007.

14 Hotez, P. J., Brooker, S., Bethony, J. M., Bottazzi, M. E., Loukas, A., & Xiao, S. (2004). Hookworm infection. *New England Journal of Medicine* 351, no. 8: 799–807. doi.org/10.1056/NEJMra032492.

15 Gryseels, B., Polman, K., Clerinx, J., & Kestens, L. (2006). Human schistosomiasis. *The Lancet* 368, no. 9541:1106–18. doi.org/10.1016/S0140-6736(06)69440-3.

16 Despommier, D. D. (1998). How does Trichinella spiralis make itself at home? *Parasitology Today* 14, no. 8: 318–23. doi.org/10.1016/s0169-4758(98)01295-7.

17 Schreiber, R. D., Old, L. J., & Smyth, M. J. (2011). Cancer immunoediting: Integrating immunity's roles in cancer suppression and promotion. *Science* 331, no. 6024: 1565–70. doi.org/10.1126/science.1203486.

18 Pardoll, D. M. (2012). The blockade of immune checkpoints in cancer immunotherapy. *Nature Reviews Cancer* 12, no. 4: 252–64. doi.org/10.1038/nrc3239.

19 Topalian, S. L., Hodi, F. S., Brahmer, J. R., Gettinger, S. N., Smith, D. C., McDermott, D. F., . . . & Dong, H. (2012). Safety, activity, and immune correlates of anti-PD-1 antibody in cancer. *New England Journal of Medicine* 366, no. 26: 2443–54. doi.org/10.1056/NEJMoa1200690.

20 Shalapour, S., & Karin, M. (2015). Immunity, inflammation, and cancer: An eternal fight between good and evil. *Journal of Clinical Investigation* 125, no. 9: 3347–55. doi.org/10.1172/JCI80007.

21 Whiteside, T. L. (2008). The tumor microenvironment and its role in promoting tumor growth. *Oncogene* 27, no. 45: 5904–12. doi.org/10.1038/onc.2008.271.

22 Gabrilovich, D. I., & Nagaraj, S. (2009). Myeloid-derived suppressor cells as regulators of the immune system. *Nature Reviews Immunology* 9, no. 3: 162–74. doi.org/10.1038/nri2506.

23 Binnewies, M., Roberts, E. W., Kersten, K., Chan, V., Fearon, D. F., Merad, M., . . . & Coussens, L. M. (2018). Understanding the tumor immune microenvironment (TIME) for effective therapy. *Nature Medicine* 24, no. 5: 541–50. doi.org/10.1038/s41591-018-0014-x.

24 Baruch, D. I., Pasloske, B. L., Singh, H. B., Bi, X., Ma, X. C., Feldman, M., Taraschi, T. F., & Howard, R. J. (1995). Cloning the P. falciparum gene encoding PfEMP1, a malarial variant antigen, and identification of a distinct cross-reactive epitope. *Cell* 82, no. 1: 89–94. doi.org/10.1016/0092-8674(95)90054-x.

25 Horn, D. (2014). Antigenic variation in African trypanosomes. *Molecular and biochemical Parasitology* 195, no. 2: 123–29. doi.org/10.1016/j.molbiopara.2014.05.001.

26 Damian, R. T. (1987). Molecular mimicry: An immunological strategy for parasite evasion. *Immunology Today* 8, no. 6: 184–88. doi.org/10.1016/0167-5699(87)90139-4.

27 van Die, I., & Cummings, R. D. (2010). Glycan gimmickry by parasitic helminths: A strategy for modulating the host immune response? *Glycobiology* 20, no. 1: 2–12. doi.org/10.1093/glycob/cwp140.

28 Maizels, R. M., & Yazdanbakhsh, M. (2003). Immune regulation by helminth parasites: Cellular and molecular mechanisms. *Nature Reviews Immunology* 3, no. 9: 733–44. doi.org/10.1038/nri1183.

29 Aguirre-Ghiso, J. A. (2007). Models, mechanisms and clinical evidence for cancer dormancy. *Nature Reviews Cancer* 7, no. 11: 834–46. doi.org/10.1038/nrc2256.

30 Cox, F. E. G. (2010). History of human parasitology. *Clinical Microbiology Reviews* 15, no. 4: 595–612. doi.org/10.1128/CMR.15.4.595-612.2002.

31 Sacks, D., & Sher, A. (2002). Evasion of innate immunity by parasitic protozoa. *Nature Immunology* 3 , no.11: 1041–1047.

32 Wojtkowiak, J. W., Verduzco, D., Schramm, K. J., & Gillies, R. J. (2011). Drug resistance and cellular adaptation to tumor acidic pH microenvironment. *Molecular Pharmaceutics* 8, no. 6: 2032–38. doi.org/10.1021/mp200291u.

33 Jezweski, A. J., Lin, A., Reisz, J., et al. (2021). Targeting host glycolysis as a strategy for antimalarial development. *Frontiers in Cellular Infectious Microbiology.: Parasite and Host* 11. doi.org/10.3389/fcimb.2021.730413.

34 Miranda-Ozuna, J. F., Hernández-García, M. S., Brieba, L. G. et al. (2016). The glycolytic enzyme triosephosphate isomerase of trichomonas vaginalis is a surface-associated protein induced by glucose That functions as a laminin- and fibronectin-binding protein. *Infection and Immunity* 84 no.10: 2878–2894. doi.org/10.1128/IAI.00538-16.

35 Creek, D. J., Chua, H. H., Cobbold, S. A., Nijagal, B., MacRae, J. I., Dickerman, B. K., . . . & McConville, M. J. (2016). Metabolomics-based screening of the Malaria Box reveals both novel and established mechanisms of action.

Antimicrobial Agents and Chemotherapy 60, no. 11: 6650–63. doi.org/10.1128/AAC.01215-16.

36 Blume, M., Rodriguez, D., & Soldati-Favre, D. (2009). A Toxoplasma gondii protein with a role in histone methylation and DNA replication. *PLoS Pathogens* 5, no. 8: e1000537. doi.org/10.1371/journal.ppat.1000537.

37 Tielens, A. G., & Van Hellemond, J. J. (1998). The electron transport chain in anaerobically functioning eukaryotes. *Biochimica et Biophysica Acta* 1365, no.1–2: 71–78. doi.org/10.1016/s0005-2728(98)00045-0.

38 Anstead, G. M., Chandrasekar, B., Zhao, W., Yang, J., Perez, L. E., & Melby, P. C. (2001). Malnutrition alters the innate immune response and increases early visceralization following Leishmania donovani infection. *Infection and Immunity* 69, no. 8: 4709–18. doi.org/10.1128/IAI.69.8.4709-4718.2001.

39 Abbas, A. K., Lichtman, A. H., & Pillai, S. (2020). *Cellular and Molecular Immunology* (10th ed.). Elsevier.

40 Medzhitov, R. (2008). Origin and physiological roles of inflammation. *Nature* 454, no. 7203: 428–35. doi.org/10.1038/nature07201.

41 White, A. C. Jr., & Robinson, P. (2015). Cestode molecular biology. In *Talaro's Foundations in Microbiology* (10th ed.). McGraw Hill.

42 Hewitson, J. P., Grainger, J. R., & Maizels, R. M. (2009). Helminth immunoregulation: The role of parasite secreted proteins in modulating host immunity. *Molecular and Biochemical Parasitology* 167, no. 1: 1–11. doi.org/10.1016/j.molbiopara.2009.04.008.

43 Maizels, R. M., & Newfeld, S. J. (2023). Convergent evolution in a murine intestinal parasite rapidly created the TGM family of molecular mimics to suppress the host immune response. *Genome Biology and Evolution* 15, no. 9: evad158. doi.org/10.1093/gbe/evad158.

44 Osada, Y., & Kanazawa, T. (2010). Parasitic helminths: New weapons against immunological disorders. *Current Medicinal Chemistry* 17, no. 28: 3116–25. doi.org/10.2174/092986710792231965.

45 Garrido, F., Ruiz-Cabello, F., Cabrera, T., Pérez-Villar, J. J., López-Botet, M., Duggan-Keen, M., & Stern, P. L. (1997). Implications for immunosurveillance of altered HLA class I phenotypes in human tumours. *Immunology Today* 18, no. 2: 89–95. doi.org/10.1016/s0167-5699(97)01004-8.

46 McGranahan, N., & Swanton, C. (2017). Clonal heterogeneity and tumor evolution: Past, present, and the future. *Cell* 168, no. 4: 613–28. doi.org/10.1016/j.cell.2017.01.018.

47 Majeti, R., Chao, M. P., Alizadeh, A. A., Pang, W. W., Jaiswal, S., Gibbs, K. D. Jr., . . . & Weissman, I. L. (2009). CD47 is an adverse prognostic factor and therapeutic antibody target on human acute myeloid leukemia stem cells. *Cell* 138, no. 2: 286–99. doi.org/10.1016/j.cell.2009.05.045.

48 Noy, R., & Pollard, J. W. (2014). Tumor-associated macrophages: From mechanisms to therapy. *Immunity* 41, no. 1: 49–61. doi.org/10.1016/j.immuni.2014.06.010.

49 O'Donnell, J. S., Teng, M. W. L., & Smyth, M. J. (2019). Cancer immunoediting and resistance to T cell-based immunotherapy. *Nature Reviews Clinical Oncology* 16, no. 3: 151–67. doi.org/10.1038/s41571-018-0142-8.

50 Wherry, E. J. (2011). T cell exhaustion. *Nature Immunology* 12, no. 6: 492–99. doi.org/10.1038/ni.2035.

51 Williamson, A. L., Brindley, P. J., Abbenante, G., Prociv, P., & Loukas, A. (2004). Hookworm excretory/secretory products: Potential vaccines and novel chemotherapeutic targets. *Expert Opinion on Biological Therapy* 4, no. 11: 1729–43. doi.org/10.1517/14712598.4.11.1729.

52 Wilson, R. A., & Coulson, P. S. (2009). Immune effector mechanisms against schistosomiasis: looking for a chink in the parasite's armour. *Trends in Parasitology* 25 no. 9: 423–431. doi.org/10.1016/j.pt.2009.05.011.

53 Levin, M., Pezzulo, G., & Finkelstein, J. M. (2017). Endogenous bioelectric signaling networks: Exploiting voltage gradients for control of growth and form. *Annual Review of Biomedical Engineering* 19: 353–387. doi.org/10.1146/annurev-bioeng-071114-040647.

54 Chernet, B. T., & Levin, M. (2013). Transmembrane voltage potential is an essential cellular parameter for the detection and control of tumor development in a Xenopus model. *Disease Models & Mechanisms* 6, no. 3: 595–607. doi.org/10.1242/dmm.010833.

55 Duque-Correa, M. A., Goulding, D., Rodgers, F. H. et al. (2022). Defining the early stages of intestinal colonisation by whipworms. *Nature Communications.* 13: 1725. doi.org/10.1038/s41467-022-29334-0.

56 Evans, S. S., Repasky, E. A., & Fisher, D. T. (2015). Fever and the thermal regulation of immunity: The immune system feels the heat. *Nature Reviews Immunology* 15, no. 6: 335–49. doi.org/10.1038/nri3843.

57 Loeffler, D. A., Lundy, S. K., Singh, K. P., et al. (2002). Soluble egg antigens from Schistosoma mansoni induce angiogenesis-related processes by up-regulating vascular endothelial growth factor in human endothelial cells. *The Journal of Infectious Diseases* 185, no. 11: 1650–1656. doi.org/10.1086/340416.

58 Lu, P., Weaver, V. M., & Werb, Z. (2012). The extracellular matrix: a dynamic niche in cancer progression. *Journal of Cell Biology* 196, no. 4: 395–406. doi.org/10.1083/jcb.201102147.

59 McKerrow, J. H., Caffrey, C., Kelly, B., Loke, P., & Sajid, M. (2006). Proteases in parasitic diseases. *Annual Review of Pathology: Mechanisms of Disease* 1: 497–536. doi.org/10.1146/annurev.pathol.1.110304.100150.

60 Bakhoum, S. F., & Landau, D. A. (2017). Chromosomal instability as a driver of tumor heterogeneity and evolution. *Nature Reviews Cancer* 17, no. 10: 607–19. doi.org/10.1038/nrc.2017.62.

61 Gordon, D. J., Resio, B., & Pellman, D. (2012). Causes and consequences of a neuploidy in cancer. *Nature Reviews Genetics* 13, no. 3: 189–203. doi.org/10.1038/nrg3123.

62 Holland, A. J., & Cleveland, D. W. (2009). Boveri revisited: Chromosomal instability, aneuploidy and tumorigenesis. *Nature Reviews Molecular Cell Biology* 10, no. 7: 478–87. doi.org/10.1038/nrm2718.

63 Sansregret, L., & Swanton, C. (2017). The Role of Aneuploidy in Cancer Evolution. *Cold Spring Harbor Perspectives in Medicine 7* no.1: a028373. doi.org/10.1101/cshperspect.a028373.

64 Sterkers, Y., Lachaud, L., Bourgeois, N., Crobu, L., Bastien, P., & Pagès, M. (2012). Novel insights into genome plasticity in Eukaryotes: Aneuploidy in Leishmania. *MolecularMicrobiology*86,no.1:15–21.doi.org/10.1111/j.1365-2958.2012.08179.x.

65 Negreira, G. H., de Groote, R., Van Giel, D., et al.. (2023). The adaptive roles of aneuploidy and polyclonality in Leishmania in response to environmental stress. *EMBO reports* 24, no. 9: e57413. doi.org/10.15252/embr. 202357413.

66 Rogers, M. B., Hilley, J. D., Dickens, N. J., Wilkes, J., Kube, M., Reinhardt, R., . . . & Mottram, J. C. (2011). Chromosome and gene copy number variation allow Leishmania to adapt to different hosts and environments. *Genome Biology* 12, no. 7: R54. doi.org/10.1186/gb-2011-12-7-r54.

67 Adam, R. D. (2001). Biology of Giardia lamblia. *Clinical Microbiology Reviews* 14, no. 3: 447–75. doi.org/10.1128/CMR.14.3.447-475.2001.

68 Carlton, J. M., et al. (2007). Draft Genome Sequence of the Sexually Transmitted Pathogen Trichomonas vaginalis. *Science* 315, no. 5818: 207–212. doi.org/10.1126/science.1132894.

69 Merrick, C. J. (2015). Aneuploidy in malaria. *Molecular and Biochemical Parasitology* 201, no. 1–2: 43–49. doi.org/10.1016/j.molbiopara.2015.06.002.

70 Mannaert, A., Downing, T., Imamura, H., & Dujardin, J. C. (2012). Adaptive genome evolution in Leishmania. *Molecular and Biochemical Parasitology* 181, no. 2: 75–83. doi.org/10.1016/j.molbiopara.2011.10.010.

71 Ubeda, J. M., Legarda, A., Gualdrón-López, M., Opperdoes, F. R., & Coombs, G. H. (2014). Leishmania's choices during its life cycle. *Clinical Microbiology Reviews* 27, no. 2: 234–51. doi.org/10.1128/CMR.00092-13.

72 Partch, C. L., Green, C. B., & Takahashi, J. S. (2014). Molecular architecture of the mammalian circadian clock. *Trends in Cell Biology* 24, no. 2: 90–99. doi.org/10.1016/j.tcb.2013.07.002.

73 Mohawk, J. A., Green, C. B., & Takahashi, J. S. (2012). Central and peripheral circadian clocks in mammals. *Annual Review of Neuroscience* 35, 445–62. doi.org/10.1146/annurev-neuro-062111-150528.

74 Takahashi, J. S. (2017). Transcriptional architecture of the mammalian circadian clock. *Nature Reviews Genetics* 18, no. 3: 164–79. doi.org/10.1038/nrg.2016.150.

75 Sahar, S., & Sassone-Corsi, P. (2009). Metabolism and cancer: The circadian clock connection. *Nature Reviews Cancer* 9, no. 12: 886–96. doi.org/10.1038/nrc2747.

76 Fu, L., & Kettner, N. M. (2013). The circadian clock in cancer development and therapy. *Progress in Molecular Biology and Translational Science* 119: 221–82. doi.org/10.1016/B978-0-12-396456-4.00009-9.

77 Savvidis, C., & Koutsilieris, M. (2012). Circadian rhythm disruption in cancer biology. *Molecular Medicine* 18, no. 1: 1249–1260. doi.org/10.2119/molmed.2012.00077.

78 Lee, Y., Laothong, U., & Lee, C. (2021). The role of BMAL1 in the regulation of anticancer immunity. *International Journal of Molecular Sciences* 22, no. 21: 11575. doi.org/10.3390/ijms222111575.

79 Ballesta, A., Innominato, P. F., Dallmann, R., Rand, D. A., & Lévi, F. A. (2017). Systems chronotherapeutics. *Pharmacological Reviews* 69, no. 2: 161–97. doi.org/10.1124/pr.116.013441.

80 Sulli, G., Lam, M. T. Y., & Panda, S. (2019). Interplay between circadian clock and cancer: New frontiers for cancer treatment. *Trends in Cancer* 5, no. 8: 475–494. doi.org/10.1016/j.trecan.2019.07.002.

81 Lévi, F., Okyar, A., Dulong, S., Innominato, P. F., & Clairambault, J. (2010). Circadian timing in cancer treatments. *Annual Review of Pharmacology and Toxicology* 50: 377–421. doi.org/10.1146/annurev-pharmtox-010909-105600.

82 Rijo-Ferreira, F., & Takahashi, J. S. (2019). Genomics of circadian rhythms in health and disease. *Genome Medicine* 11, no. 1: 82. doi.org/10.1186/s13073-019-0704-0.

83 Prior, K. F., Rijo-Ferreira, F., Assis, P. A., Hirako, I. C., Weaver, D. R., Gazzinelli, R. T., & Reece, S. E. (2020). Periodic parasites and daily host rhythms. *Cell host & Microbe* 27, no. 2: 176–187. doi.org/10.1016/j.chom.2020.01.005.

84 Ferreria, F. & , Takahashi, J. S. (2020), Sleeping sickness: A tale of two clocks. *Frontiers in Cellular and Infection Microbiology* 10. doi.org/10.3389/fcimb.2020.525097.

85 Hawking, F. (1967). The 24-hour periodicity of microfilariae: Biological mechanisms responsible for its production and control. Proceedings of the Royal Society of London. Series B. *Biological Sciences* 169, no. 1014: 59–76. doi.org/10.1098/rspb.1967.0079.

86 Bhattacharya, R., Stanislav S., Avdieiev, A., et al. (2025). The hallmarks of cancer as eco-evolutionary processes. *Cancer Discovery* 15, no. 4: 685–701. doi.org/10.1158/2159–8290.CD-24-0861.

87 Berriman, M., Haas, B. J., LoVerde, P. T., Wilson, R. A., Dillon, G. P., Cerqueira, G. C., . . . & El-Sayed, N. M. (2009). The genome of the blood fluke Schistosoma mansoni. *Nature* 460, no. 7253: 352–58. doi.org/10.1038/nature08160.

88 Murgia, C., Pritchard, J. K., Kim, S. Y., Fassati, A., & Weiss, R. A. (2006). Clonal origin and evolution of a transmissible cancer. *Cell* 126, no. 3: 477–87. doi.org/10.1016/j.cell.2006.05.051.

89 Pearse, A. M., & Swift, K. (2006). Allograft theory: Transmission of devil facial-tumour disease. *Nature* 439, no. 7076: 549. doi.org/10.1038/439549a.

90 Dujon, A. M., Bramwell, G., Roche, B., Thomas, F., & Ujvari, B. (2021). Transmissible cancers in mammals and bivalves: How many examples are there? *BioEssays* 43, no. 3: e2000222. doi.org/10.1002/bies.202000222.

91 Tissot, S., Gérard, A. L., Boutry, J., Dujon, A. M., Russel, T., Siddle, H., . . . & Thomas, F. (2022). Transmissible cancer evolution: The under-estimated role of environmental factors in the "perfect storm" theory. *Pathogens* 11, no. 2: 241. doi.org/10.3390/pathogens11020241.

92 Laudisi, F., Marônek, M., Di Grazia, A., Monteleone, G., & Stolfi, C. (2020). Repositioning of anthelmintic drugs for the treatment of cancers of the digestive system. *International Journal of Molecular Sciences* 21, no. 14: 4957. doi.org/10.3390/ijms21144957.

93 Lacey, E. (1988). The role of the cytoskeletal protein, tubulin, in the mode of action and mechanism of drug resistance to benzimidazoles. *International Journal for Parasitology* 18, no. 7: 885–936. doi.org/10.1016/0020-7519(88)90111-3.

94 Dogra, N., Kumar, A., & Mukhopadhyay, T. (2018). Fenbendazole acts as a moderate microtubule destabilizing agent and causes cancer cell death by modulating

multiple cellular pathways. *Scientific Reports* 8, no. 1: 11926. doi.org/10.1038/s41598-018-30158-6.

95 Di Santo, N., & Ehrisman, J. (2014). A functional perspective of nitazoxanide as a potential anticancer drug. *Mutation Research* 768: 16–21. doi.org/10.1016/j.mrfmmm.2014.05.005.

96 Juarez, M., Schcolnik-Cabrera, A., & Dueñas-Gonzalez, A. (2018). The multitargeted drug ivermectin: From an antiparasitic agent to a repositioned anticancer drug. *American Journal of Cancer Research* 8, no. 2: 317–31. PMCID: PMC5835698.

97 Mauthe, M., Orhon, I., Rocchi, C., Zhou, X., Luhr, M., Hijlkema, K. J., . . . & Reggiori, F. (2018). Chloroquine inhibits autophagic flux by decreasing autophagosome-lysosome fusion. *Autophagy* 14, no. 9: 1435–55. doi.org/10.1080/15548627.2018.1474314.

98 Tang, M., Hu, X., Wang, Y., et al. (2021). Ivermectin, a potential anticancer drug derived from an antiparasitic drug. *Pharmacological Research* 163: 105207. doi.org/10.1016/j.phrs.2020.105207.

99 Ruffell, B., & Coussens, L. M. (2015). Macrophages and therapeutic resistance in cancer. *Cancer Cell* 27, no. 4: 462–72. doi.org/10.1016/j.ccell.2015.02.015.

100 Ashburn, T. T., & Thor, K. B. (2004). Drug repositioning: Identifying and developing new uses for existing drugs. *Nature Reviews Drug Discovery* 3, no. 8: 673–83. doi.org/10.1038/nrd1468.

101 Guerini, A. E., Triggiani, L., Maddalo, M., Bonù, M. L., Frassine, F., Baiguini, A., . . . & Borghetti, P. (2019). Mebendazole as a candidate for drug repurposing in oncology: An extensive review of current literature. *Cancers* 11, no. 9: 1284. doi.org/10.3390/cancers11091284.

102 Bai, R. Y., Staedtke, V., Aprhys, C. M., Gallia, G. L., & Riggins, G. J. (2011). Antiparasitic mebendazole shows survival benefit in 2 preclinical models of glioblastoma multiforme. *Neuro-oncology* 13, no. 9: 974–82. doi.org/10.1093/neuonc/nor077.

103 Li, Y., Li, P. K., Roberts, M. J., Arend, R. C., Samant, R. S., & Buchsbaum, D. J. (2014). Multi-targeted therapy of cancer by niclosamide: A new application for an old drug. *Cancer Letters* 349, no. 1: 8–14. doi.org/10.1016/j.canlet.2014.04.003.

Chapter 12

1 Holohan, C., Van Schaeybroeck, S., Longley, D. B., & Johnston, P. G. (2013). Cancer drug resistance: An evolving paradigm. *Nature Reviews Cancer* 13, no. 10: 714–26. doi.org/10.1038/nrc3599.

2 Vasan, N., Baselga, J., & Hyman, D. M. (2019). A view on drug resistance in cancer. *Nature* 575 (7782): 299–309. doi.org/10.1038/s41586-019-1730-1.

3 Gottesman, M. M. (2002). Mechanisms of cancer drug resistance. *Annual Review of Medicine* 53 (1): 615–27. doi.org/10.1146/annurev.med.53.082901.103929.

4 Orr, G. A., Verdier-Pinard, P., McDaid, H., & Horwitz, S. B. (2003). Mechanisms of Taxol resistance related to microtubules. *Oncogene* 22, no. 47: 7280–95. doi.org/10.1038/sj.onc.1206931.

5 Siddik, Z. H. (2003). Cisplatin: Mode of cytotoxic action and molecular basis of resistance. *Oncogene* 22, no. 47: 7265–79. doi.org/10.1038/sj.onc.1206933.

6 Gatenby, R. A., & Brown, J. S. (2020). Integrating evolutionary theory into cancer therapy. *Nature Reviews Clinical Oncology* 17, no. 11: 675–86. doi.org/10.1038/s41571-020-0411-1.
7 Boumahdi, S., & de Sauvage, F. J. (2020). The great escape: Tumour cell plasticity in resistance to targeted therapy. *Nature Reviews Drug Discovery* 19, no. 1: 39–56. doi.org/10.1038/s41573–019-0044–1.
8 Marusyk, A., & Polyak, K. (2010). Tumor heterogeneity: Causes and consequences. *Biochimica et Biophysica Acta (BBA)—Reviews on Cancer* 1805, no. 1: 105–17. doi.org/10.1016/j.bbcan.2009.11.002.
9 McGranahan, N., & Swanton, C. (2017). Clonal heterogeneity and tumor evolution: Past, present, and the future. *Cell* 168, no. 4: 613–28. doi.org/10.1016/j.cell.2017.01.018.
10 Easwaran, H., Tsai, H.-C., & Baylin, S. B. (2014). Cancer epigenetics: Tumor heterogeneity, plasticity of stem-like states, and drug resistance. *Molecular Cell* 54, no. 5: 716–27. doi.org/10.1016/j.molcel.2014.05.015.
11 Szakács, G., Paterson, J. K., Ludwig, J. A., Booth-Genthe, C., & Gottesman, M. M. (2006). Targeting multidrug resistance in cancer. *Nature Reviews Drug Discovery* 5, no. 3: 219–34. doi.org/10.1038/nrd1984.
12 Dean, M., Fojo, T., & Bates, S. (2005). Tumour stem cells and drug resistance. *Nature Reviews Cancer* 5, no. 4: 275–84. doi.org/10.1038/nrc1590.
13 Helleday, T., Petermann, E., Lundin, C., Hodgson, B., & Sharma, R. A. (2008). DNA repair pathways as targets for cancer therapy. *Nature Reviews Cancer* 8, no. 3: 193–204. doi.org/10.1038/nrc2342.
14 Marin, J. J. G., Briz, O., Rodriguez-Macias, G., Diez-Martin, J. L., & Macias, R. I. R. (2012). Role of drug transport and metabolism in cancer chemotherapy: Determinants of treatment efficacy and toxicity responses. *Current Cancer Drug Targets* 12, no. 5: 481–501. doi.org/10.2174/156800912800673268.
15 Reya, T., Morrison, S. J., Clarke, M. F., & Weissman, I. L. (2001). Stem cells, cancer, and cancer stem cells. *Nature* 414, no. 6859: 105–11. doi.org/10.1038/35102167.
16 Abdullah, L. N., & Chow, E. K.-H. (2013). Mechanisms of chemoresistance in cancer stem cells. *Clinical and Translational Medicine* 2, no. 1: 3. doi.org/10.1186/2001-1326-2-3.
17 Phi, L. T. H., Sari, I. N., Yang, Y.-G., Lee, S.-H., Jun, N., Kim, K. S., Lee, Y. K., & Kwon, H. Y. (2018). Cancer stem cells in drug resistance and their therapeutic implications in cancer treatment. *Stem Cells International* 2018: 5416923. doi.org/10.1155/2018/5416923.
18 Batlle, E., & Clevers, H. (2017). Cancer stem cells revisited. *Nature Medicine* 23, no. 10: 1124–34. doi.org/10.1038/nm.4409.
19 Mokhtari, R. B., Homayouni, T. S., Baluch, N., Morgatskaya, E., Kumar, S., Das, B., & Yeger, H. (2017). Combination therapy in combating cancer. *Oncotarget* 8, no. 23: 38022–38043. doi.org/10.18632/oncotarget.16723.
20 Ribas, A., & Wolchok, J. D. (2018). Cancer immunotherapy using checkpoint blockade. *Science* 359, no. 6382: 1350–55. doi.org/10.1126/science.aar4060.
21 Visvader, J. E., & Lindeman, G. J. (2012). Cancer stem cells: Current status and evolving complexities. *Cell Stem Cell* 10, no. 6: 717–28. doi.org/10.1016/j.stem.2012.05.007.

22 Zimmermann, G. R., Lehár, J., & Keith, C. T. (2007). Multi-target therapeutics: When the whole is greater than the sum of the parts. *Drug Discovery Today* 12, no. 1–2: 34–42. doi.org/10.1016/j.drudis.2006.11.008.

Chapter 13

1 Gottesman, M. M., Fojo, T., & Bates, S. E. (2002). Multidrug resistance in cancer: Role of ATP-dependent transporters. *Nature Reviews Cancer* 2, no. 1: 48–58. doi.org/10.1038/nrc714.

2 Juliano, R. L., & Ling, V. (1976). A surface glycoprotein modulating drug permeability in Chinese hamster ovary cell mutants. *Biochimica et Biophysica Acta—Biomembranes* 455, no. 1: 152–62. doi.org/10.1016/0005-2736(76)90160-7.

3 Szakács, G., Paterson, J. K., Ludwig, J. A., Booth-Genthe, C., & Gottesman, M. M. (2006). Targeting multidrug resistance in cancer. *Nature Reviews Drug Discovery* 5, no. 3: 219–34. doi.org/10.1038/nrd1984.

4 Ambudkar, S. V., Kimchi-Sarfaty, C., Sauna, Z. E., & Gottesman, M. M. (2003). P-glycoprotein: From genomics to mechanism. *Oncogene* 22, no. 47: 7468–85. doi.org/10.1038/sj.onc.1206948.

5 Trock, B. J., Leonessa, F., & Clarke, R. (1997). Multidrug resistance in breast cancer: A meta-analysis of MDR1/gp170 expression and its relation to clinical outcome. *Journal of the National Cancer Institute* 89, no. 13: 917–31. doi.org/10.1093/jnci/89.13.917.

6 Leith, C. P., Kopecky, K. J., Gottesman, M. M., Pastan, I., et al. (1999). Correlation of multidrug resistance (MDR1) protein expression with functional dye/drug efflux in acute myeloid leukemia by multiparameter flow cytometry: Identification of circumstances where Mdr1 expression is predictive of clinical outcome. *Blood* 94, no. 4: 1432–42. doi.org/10.1182/blood.v94.4.1432.

7 Higgins, C. F. (1992). ABC transporters: From microorganisms to man. *Annual Review of Cell Biology* 8: 67–113. doi.org/10.1146/annurev.cb.08.110192.000435.

8 Thiebaut, F., Tsuruo, T., Hamada, H., Gottesman, M. M., Pastan, I., & Willingham, M. C. (1987). Cellular localization of the multidrug-resistance gene product P-glycoprotein in normal human tissues. *Proceedings of the National Academy of Sciences of the United States of America* 84, no. 21: 7735–38. doi.org/10.1073/pnas.84.21.7735.

9 Aller, S. G., Yu, J., Ward, A., Weng, Y., Chittaboina, S., Zhuo, R., Harrell, P. M., Trinh, Y. T., Zhang, Q., Urbatsch, I. L., & Chang, G. (2009). Structure of P-glycoprotein reveals a molecular basis for poly-specific drug binding. *Science* 323, no. 5922: 1718–22. doi.org/10.1126/science.1168750.

10 Labialle, S., Gayet, L., Marthinet, E., Rigal, D., & Baggetto, L. G. (2002). Transcriptional regulators of the human multidrug resistance 1 gene: recent views. *Biochemical Pharmacology* 64, no. 5: 943–948. doi.org/10.1016/s0006-2952(02)01156-5.

11 Hynes, N. E., & Lane, H. A. (2005). ERBB receptors and cancer: The complexity of targeted inhibitors. *Nature Reviews Cancer* 5, no. 5: 341–54. doi.org/10.1038/nrc1609.

12 Chin, K. V., Ueda, K., Pastan, I., & Gottesman, M. M. (1992). Modulation of activity of the promoter of the human MDR1 gene by Ras and p53. *Science* 255, no. 5043: 460–62. doi.org/10.1126/science.1531507.

13 Mei, W., Mei, B., Chang, J., Liu, Y., Zhou, Y., Zhu, N., & Hu, M. (2024). Role and regulation of FOXO3a: new insights into breast cancer therapy. *Frontiers in Pharmacology* 15: 1346745. doi.org/10.3389/fphar.2024.1346745.

14 Jutten, B., & Rouschop, K. M. (2014). EGFR signaling and autophagy dependence for growth, survival, and therapy resistance. *Cell Cycle* 13, no. 1: 42–51. doi.org/10.4161/cc.27518.

15 Karin, M. (2006). Nuclear factor-kappaB in cancer development and progression. *Nature* 441, no. 7092: 431–36. doi.org/10.1038/nature04870.

16 Bentires-Alj, M., Barbu, V., Fillet, M., et al. (2003). NF-kappaB transcription factor induces drug resistance through MDR1 expression in cancer cells. *Oncogene* 22, no. 1: 90–97. doi.org/10.1038/sj.onc.1206054.

17 Karthika, C., Sureshkumar, R., Zehravi, M., et al. (2022). Multidrug Resistance of Cancer Cells and the Vital Role of P-Glycoprotein. *Life (Basel, Switzerland)* 12, no. 6: 897. doi.org/10.3390/life12060897.

18 Shukla, S., MacLennan, G. T., Fu, P., Patel, M., Marengo, S. R., Resnick, M. I., & Gupta, S. (2004). Nuclear factor-κB/p65 (RelA) is constitutively activated in human prostate adenocarcinoma and correlates with disease progression. *Neoplasia* 6, no. 4: 390–400. doi.org/10.1593/neo.03414.

19 Engelman, J. A., Luo, J., & Cantley, L. C. (2006). The evolution of phosphatidylinositol 3-kinases as regulators of growth and metabolism. *Nature Reviews Genetics* 7, no. 8: 606–19. doi.org/10.1038/nrg1879.

20 Dong, C., Wu, J., Chen, Y., Nie, J., & Chen, C. (2021). Activation of PI3K/AKT/mTOR Pathway Causes Drug Resistance in Breast Cancer. *Frontiers in Pharmacology* 12: 628690. doi.org/10.3389/fphar.2021.628690.

21 Tazzari, P., Cappellini, A., Ricci, F. *et al.* (2007). Multidrug resistance-associated protein 1 expression is under the control of the phosphoinositide 3 kinase/Akt signal transduction network in human acute myelogenous leukemia blasts. *Leukemia* 21: 427–438. doi.org/10.1038/sj.leu.2404523.

22 Ozes, O. N., Mayo, L. D., Gustin, J. A., Pfeffer, S. R., Pfeffer, L. M., & Donner, D. B. (1999). NF-kappaB activation by tumour necrosis factor requires the Akt serine-threonine kinase. *Nature* 401, no. 6748: 82–85. doi.org/10.1038/43476.

23 Comerford, K. M., Wallace, T. J., Karhausen, J., Louis, N. A., Montalto, M. C., & Colgan, S. P. (2002). Hypoxia-inducible factor-1-dependent regulation of the multidrug resistance (MDR1) gene. *Cancer Research* 62, no. 12: 3387–94. PMID: 12067973.

24 Prichard, R. K., & Roulet, A. (2007). ABC transporters and beta-tubulin in macrocyclic lactone resistance: prospects for marker development. *Parasitology* 134, no. 8: 1123–1132. doi.org/10.1017/S0031182007000091.

25 Raza, A., Williams, A. R., & Abeer, M. M. (2023). Importance of ABC Transporters in the Survival of Parasitic Nematodes and the Prospect for the Development of Novel Control Strategies. *Pathogens (Basel, Switzerland)* 12, no. 6: 755. doi.org/10.3390/pathogens12060755.

26 Kaplan, R. M. (2004). Drug resistance in nematodes of veterinary importance: A status report. *Trends in Parasitology* 20, no. 10: 477–81. doi.org/10.1016/j.pt.2004.08.001.

27 Lespine, A., Ménez, C., & Bourguinat, C. (2012). P-glycoproteins and other multidrug resistance transporters in the pharmacology of anthelmintics: Prospects for reversing transport-dependent resistance. *International Journal for Parasitology: Drugs and Drug Resistance* 2: 58–75. doi.org/10.1016/j.ijpddr.2011.10.001.

28 Kaschny, M., Demeler, J., Janssen, I. J. I., et al. (2015). Macrocyclic lactones differ in interaction with recombinant P-glycoprotein 9 of the parasitic nematode Cylicocyclus elongatus and ketoconazole in a yeast growth assay. PLOS Pathogens 11, no. 4: e1004781. https://doi.org/10.1371/journal.ppat.1004781.

29 De Graef, J., Demeler, J., Skuce, P., et al. (2013). Gene expression analysis of ABC transporters in a resistant Cooperia oncophora isolate following in vivo and in vitro exposure to macrocyclic lactones. *Parasitology* 140, no. 4: 499–508. doi.org/10.1017/S0031182012001849.

30 Raza, A., Kopp, S. R., Bagnall, N. H., Jabbar, A., & Kotze, A. C. (2016). Effects of in vitro exposure to ivermectin and levamisole on the expression patterns of ABC transporters in Haemonchus contortus larvae. *International Journal for Parasitology. Drugs and Drug Resistance* 6, no. 2: 103–115. doi.org/10.1016/j.ijpddr.2016.03.001.

31 Peachey, L. E., Pinchbeck, G. L., Matthews, J. B., et al. (2017). P-glycoproteins play a role in ivermectin resistance in cyathostomins. *International Journal for Parasitology. Drugs and Drug Resistance* 7, no. 3: 388–398. doi.org/10.1016/j.ijpddr.2017.10.006.

32 James, C. E., & Davey, M. W. (2009). Increased expression of ABC transport proteins is associated with ivermectin resistance in the model nematode Caenorhabditis elegans. *International Journal for Parasitology* 39, no. 2: 213–220. doi.org/10.1016/j.ijpara.2008.06.009.

33 Kwa, M. S., Veenstra, J. G., & Roos, M. H. (1994). Benzimidazole resistance in Haemonchus contortus is correlated with a conserved mutation at amino acid 200 in beta-tubulin isotype 1. *Molecular and Biochemical Parasitology* 63, no. 2: 299–303. doi.org/10.1016/0166-6851(94)90019-1.

34 Blackhall, W. J., Prichard, R. K., & Beech, R. N. (2008). P-glycoprotein selection in strains of Haemonchus contortus resistant to benzimidazoles. *Veterinary Parasitology* 152, no. 1–2: 101–107. doi.org/10.1016/j.vetpar.2007.12.001.

35 Giglioti, R., Ferreira, J. F. da S., Luciani, G. F., et al. (2022.). Potential of Haemonchus contortus first-stage larvae to characterize anthelmintic resistance through P-glycoprotein gene expression. *Small Ruminant Research* 217: 106864.

36 Cazajous, T., Prevot, F., Kerbiriou, A., Milhes, M., Grisez, C., Tropee, A., Godart, C., Aragon, A., & Jacquiet, P. (2018). Multiple-resistance to ivermectin and benzimidazole of a Haemonchus contortus population in a sheep flock from mainland France, first report. *Veterinary Parasitology, Regional Studies and Reports 14*: 103–105. doi.org/10.1016/j.vprsr.2018.09.005.

37 Kerboeuf, D., & Guégnard, F. (2011). Anthelmintics are substrates and activators of nematode P glycoprotein. *Antimicrobial Agents and Chemotherapy* 55, no. 5: 2224–2232. doi.org/10.1128/AAC.01477-10.

38 Rohrbach, P., Sanchez, C. P., Hayton, K., et al. (2006). Genetic linkage of pfmdr1 with food vacuolar solute import in Plasmodium falciparum. *The EMBO Journal* 25, no. 13: 3000–3011. doi.org/10.1038/sj.emboj.7601193.

39 Sidhu, A. B., Valderramos, S. G., & Fidock, D. A. (2005). Pfmdr1 mutations contribute to quinine resistance and enhance mefloquine and artemisinin sensitivity in Plasmodium falciparum. *Molecular Microbiology* 57, no. 4: 913–26. doi.org/10.1111/j.1365-2958.2005.04721.x.

40 Price, R. N., Uhlemann, A. C., Brockman, A., et al. (2004). Mefloquine resistance in Plasmodium falciparum and increased pfmdr1 gene copy number. *The Lancet* 364, no. 9432: 438–47. doi.org/10.1016/S0140-6736(04)16766-9.

41 Lacey, E. (1990). Mode of action of benzimidazoles. *Parasitology Today* 6, no. 4: 112–15. doi.org/10.1016/0169-4758(90)90227-U.

42 Mukhopadhyay, T., Sasaki, J., Ramesh, R., & Roth, J. A. (2002). Mebendazole elicits a potent antitumor effect on human cancer cell lines both in vitro and in vivo. *Clinical Cancer Research* 8, no. 9: 2963–69. PMID: 12231542.

43 Dogra, N., Kumar, A., & Mukhopadhyay, T. (2018). Fenbendazole acts as a moderate microtubule destabilizing agent and causes cancer cell death by modulating multiple cellular pathways. *Scientific Reports* 8, no. 1: 11926. doi.org/10.1038/s41598-018-30158-6.

44 Monga, J., Ghosh, N. S., Rani, I., Singh, R., Deswal, G., Dhingra, A. K., & Grewal, A. S. (2024). Unlocking the pharmacological potential of benzimidazole derivatives: A pathway to drug development. *Current Topics in Medicinal Chemistry* 24, no. 5: 437–85. doi.org/10.2174/0115680266283641240109080047.

45 Yang, L., Du, Z., Peng, Y., Zhang, W., Feng, W., & Yuan, Y. (2025). Mebendazole effectively overcomes imatinib resistance by dual-targeting BCR/ABL oncoprotein and β-tubulin in chronic myeloid leukemia cells. Korean Journal of Physiology & Pharmacology 29, no. 1: 67–81. doi.org/10.4196/kjpp.24.176.

46 Cray, C., & Altman, N. H. (2022). An Update on the Biologic Effects of Fenbendazole. *Comparative Medicine* 72, no. 4: 215–219. doi.org/10.30802/AALAS-CM-22-000006.

47 Pan, T., Jin, S., Huang, X., Xin, X., Xing, Q., Yang, W., Dong, J., & Li, L. (2025). Fenbendazole induces pyroptosis in breast cancer cells through HK2/caspase-3/GSDME signaling pathway. *Frontiers in Pharmacology* 16: 1596694. doi.org/10.3389/fphar.2025.1596694.

48 Li, Y., Yuan, H., Yang, K., Xu, W., Tang, W., & Li, X. (2010). The structure and functions of P-glycoprotein. *Current Medicinal Chemistry* 17, no. 8: 786–800. doi.org/10.2174/092986710790514507.

49 Melamed, J. R., Morgan, J. T., Ioele, S. A., Gleghorn, J. P., Sims-Mourtada, J., Day, E. S. (2018). Investigating the role of Hedgehog/GLI1 signaling in glioblastoma cell response to temozolomide. *Oncotarget*. 9: 27000–27015.

50 Park, D., Lee, J. H., & Yoon, S. P. (2022). Anti-cancer effects of fenbendazole on 5-fluorouracil-resistant colorectal cancer cells. *The Korean Journal of Physiology & Pharmacology* 26, no. 5: 377–87. doi.org/10.4196/kjpp.2022.26.5.377.

51 Juarez, M., Schcolnik-Cabrera, A., & Dueñas-Gonzalez, A. (2018). The multitargeted drug ivermectin: From an antiparasitic agent to a repositioned anticancer drug. *American Journal of Cancer Research* 8, no. 2: 317–31. PMID: 29511601.

Chapter 14

1 McKellar, Q. A., & Scott, E. W. (1990). The benzimidazole anthelmintic agents—A review. *Journal of Veterinary Pharmacology and Therapeutics* 13, no. 3: 223–47. doi.org/10.1111/j.1365-2885.1990.tb00773.x.

2 Drugs.com. Fenbendazole. (Accessed May 1, 2025) Available from: drugs.com/vet/fenbendazole.html. Drugs.com. Mebendazole. (Accessed May 1, 2025) Available from: drugs.com/mebendazole.html.

3 World Health Organization (WHO). (2023). Soil-transmitted helminth infections. Fact sheet. Available from: who.int/news-room/fact-sheets/detail/soil-transmitted-helminth-infections. Accessed May 1, 2025.

4 Liu, C. S., Zhang, H. B., Jiang, B., Yao, J. M., Tao, Y., Xue, J., & Wen, A. D. (2012). Enhanced bioavailability and cysticidal effect of three mebendazole-oil preparations in mice infected with secondary cysts of Echinococcus granulosus. *Parasitology Research* 111, no. 3: 1205–11. doi.org/10.1007/s00436-012-2954-2.

5 Priyanka, P., Rajarajeshwari, K., Shilpashree, G. R., & Khanum, S. A. (2023). Solubility enhancement of fenbendazole using hydrotropy and mixed hydrotropy techniques. *International Journal of Pharmaceutical Investigation* 13, no. 2: 209–15. doi.org/10.5530/ijpi.2023.2.36.

6 Yamaguchi, T., Shimizu, J., Oya, Y., Horio, Y., & Hida, T. (2021). Drug-induced liver injury in a patient with nonsmall cell lung cancer after the self-administration of fenbendazole based on social media information. *Case Reports in Oncology* 14, no. 2: 886–91. doi.org/10.1159/000516276.

7 Fontana, R. J., Watkins, P. B., Bonkovsky, H. L., et al., (2009). DILIN Study Group. Drug-induced liver injury network (DILIN) prospective study: Rationale, design and conduct. *Drug Safety* 32, no. 1: 55–68. doi.org/10.2165/00002018-200932010-00005.

8 Fogelman I. (2011). The flare phenomenon: still learning after 35 years. *European Journal of Nuclear Medicine and Molecular Imaging* 38, no. 1: 5–6. doi.org/10.1007/s00259-010-1609-8.

9 Smith-Bindman, R., et al. (2019). Radiation dose associated with common computed tomography examinations and the associated lifetime attributable risk of cancer. *JAMA Internal Medicine* 179, no. 12: 1663–71. doi.org/10.1001/jamainternmed.2019.5920.

10 Bosch de Basea, Gomez M., Thierry-Chef, I., Harbron, R., et al. (2023). Risk of hematological malignancies from CT radiation exposure in children, adolescents and young adults. *Nat Medicine* 29, no. 12: 3111–19. doi:10.1038/s41591-023-02620-03.

11 Hauptmann, M., Byrnes, G., Cardis, E., et al. (2023). Brain cancer after radiation exposure from CT examinations of children and young adults:results from the EPI-CT cohort study. *Lancet Oncology* 24, no. 1: 45–53. doi:10.1016/S1470-2045(22)00655-6.

12 Pearce, M. S., Salotti, J. A., Little, M. P., et al. (2012). Radiation exposure from CT scans in childhood and subsequent risk of leukaemia and brain tumours: A retrospective cohort study. *The Lancet* 380, no. 9840: 499–505. doi.org/10.1016/S0140-6736(12)60815-0.

13 Ried, K., Eng, P. and Sali, A. (2017). Screening for circulating tumour cells allows early detection of cancer and monitoring of treatment effectiveness: An observational study. *Asian Pacific Journal of Cancer Prevention* 18, no. 8: 2275–85. doi: 10.22034/APJCP.2017.18.8.2275.

14 Bai, R. Y., Staedtke, V., Aprhys, C. M., Gallia, G. L., & Riggins, G. J. (2011). Antiparasitic mebendazole shows survival benefit in 2 preclinical models of glioblastoma multiforme. *Neuro-oncology* 13, no. 9: 974–82. doi.org/10.1093/neuonc/nor077.

15 Conti, N., Heck, A., Rentsch, K., Zingg, W., Jetter, A., Stieger, B., & Pauli-Magnus, C. (2009). Effect of ritonavir on the pharmacokinetics of the benzimidazoles albendazole and mebendazole: An interaction study in healthy volunteers. *European Journal of Clinical Pharmacology* 65, no. 10: 999–1006. doi.org/10.1007/s00228-009-0683-y.

16 Guerini, A. E., Triggiani, L., Maddalo, M., et al. (2019). Mebendazole as a candidate for drug repurposing in oncology: An extensive review of current literature. *Cancers* 11, no. 9: 1284. doi.org/10.3390/cancers11091284.

17 Drugs.com. Mebendazole. (Accessed May 1, 2025) Available from: drugs.com/mebendazole.html.

18 Milner, C. (2023, September 9). Parasites: An overlooked and underestimated health threat. *Epoch Times*. Accessed May 1, 2025. Available from: theepochtimes.com/health/parasites-how-we-contract-them-and-what-they-do-to-us-5515976.

19 Williams, D. (2019) A cure for cancer hidden in plain sight. fenbendazole.s3.amazonaws.com/A-Cure-for-Cancer-Hidden-in-Plain-Sight-July-2019-Dr-David-Williams.pdf. Accessed April 15, 2025.

20 Mansoori, S., Fryknäs, M., Alvfors, C., Loskog, A., Larsson, R., & Nygren, P. (2021). A phase 2a clinical study on the safety and efficacy of individualized dosed mebendazole in patients with advanced gastrointestinal cancer. *Scientific Reports* 11, no. 1: 8981. doi.org/10.1038/s41598-021-88058-5.

21 Makis, M., Baghli, I. & Martinez, P. (2025). Fenbendazole as an anticancer agent? A case series of self-administration in three patients. *Case Reports in Oncology* 18, no. 1: 856–63. doi.org/10.1159/000546362.

22 Chiang, R. S., Syed, A. B., Wright, J. L., Montgomery, B., & Srinivas, S. (2021). Fenbendazole enhancing anti-tumor effect: A case series. *Clinical Oncology and Case Reports* 4, no. 2. doi.org/10.17352/2639-8438.000026.

Index

M

N

O

P

R

S

T

V

W

X

Read on for an excerpt from William F. Supple Jr.'s upcoming book, *The Sunlight Solution: Reclaiming Vitamin D, Reversing the Chronic Disease Epidemic and Making America Healthy Again*

INTRODUCTION

The Sunshine Hormone: Your Body's Master Key

For millennia, humans have worshipped the sun. We have built monuments to track its journey, oriented our cities toward its light, and instinctively understood its power to give life. In our modern world, however, we have been taught to fear it. We have been told to cover up, seek shade, and slather on sunscreen, casting the sun as a villain responsible for skin cancer and aging. While these risks are real and require sensible precautions, this one-sided story has created a dangerous blind spot. In our flight from the sun, we are starving our bodies of the single most important hormone for overall health: vitamin D. Forget what you have learned about vitamin D being a simple vitamin you can get from a fortified glass of milk. That is a profound understatement of its role.

Vitamin D is not a vitamin at all; it is a potent steroid hormone that your body is designed to produce in abundance when your skin is exposed to sunlight. This book will demonstrate, with undeniable scientific evidence, that sunlight is the primary, intended, and most effective source of this critical hormone. We will explore how maintaining optimal vitamin D levels is fundamental to preventing and managing a vast array of modern diseases that plague our society.

The process of creation of vitamin D is an elegant piece of biological engineering. When ultraviolet B (UVB) light (290-330 nM), from the sun strikes your skin, it converts a cholesterol-like molecule called 7-dehydrocholesterol into pre-vitamin D3. With gentle warmth, this molecule rapidly transforms into vitamin D3. From the skin, it travels to the liver, where it is converted into 25-hydroxyvitamin D, or calcidiol—the form that is measured in the blood. But the process is not finished. For vitamin D to perform its magic, it must make a final stop in the kidneys (and many other cells throughout the body) to be converted into its final, biologically active form: 1,25-dihydroxyvitamin D, or calcitriol. 1,25(OH)D3, as it is known to its friends, is the master key, ready to unlock your body's full potential.

A True Jack of All Trades

The reason vitamin D is so essential for so many different aspects of your health is simple: its influence is coded into the very blueprint of your cells. Throughout your body, on just about every one of your 37 trillion cells, is a receptor for vitamin D. In nearly every tissue and organ, cells are equipped with a special docking station called the Vitamin D Receptor (VDR). Think of the VDR as a lock. The active vitamin D hormone 1,25(OH)D3 is the key. When that key fits into the lock, it sends a powerful signal directly to the cell's nucleus—the command center that holds your DNA. Once inside the nucleus, the vitamin D-VDR complex finds specific locations on your DNA called Vitamin D Responsive Elements (VDREs). By binding to these VDREs, the complex acts as a master switch, turning specific genes on or off. This process, known as gene expression, dictates which proteins your cells will make. These proteins are the workers that carry out every function in your body, from fighting infections to building strong bones and maintaining a healthy brain. Therefore, by controlling which genes are activated, vitamin D directs the fundamental operations of your cells, making it a true jack of all trades for human health. Vitamin D is involved in just every biological process and organ system in our bodies because just about every cell has a receptor for vitamin D.

Sunlight, through its production of vitamin D, is a powerful epigenetic regulator. For our purposes here, epigenetics refers to how the environment, in this case the presence or absence of sunlight and its vitamin D, can affect the expression of various genes in our cells. While you cannot change the DNA sequence you were born with, you can change how it is expressed. Sunlight and vitamin D do not rewrite your genetic code; they act as a conductor, telling your orchestra of genes when to play and how loudly. A body starved of sunlight and vitamin D is like an orchestra without its conductor—the result is cellular chaos and, ultimately, disease.

There is no work-around or life hack to compensate for lack of sunlight and its vitamin D. Our cells are hardwired to "run" on vitamin D. After decades of failing to appreciate and respect this fact of life we have become the sickest, fattest, weakest, and most pathetic of specimens, such that our collective life expectancy is falling dramatically along with our fertility. Our rejection of the sun and its life-sustaining vitamin D has put the human race on the fast track to extinction. Hopefully, after reading this book you will be able to take simple, sensible actions to help reverse this tragedy in your own life and the lives of your loved ones.

CHAPTER 1

The Sun: Humanity's Oldest Ally and Our Modern Blind Spot

For millennia, humanity thrived under the sun's life-giving rays. Our ancestors instinctively understood its power, building civilizations oriented toward its light and incorporating it into their daily lives and spiritual beliefs. Yet, in a profound and dangerous departure from our biological heritage, modern society has been conditioned to fear the sun, viewing it primarily as a threat responsible for skin cancer and premature aging. This distorted view has led us to systematically avoid the sun, inadvertently starving our bodies of a critical, naturally produced steroid hormone: vitamin D. This is not merely a vitamin; it is a master key, fundamentally orchestrating cellular function throughout your entire body. We are not just missing out on a nutrient; we are fundamentally disrupting our biology.

Vitamin D: More Than a Vitamin, a Potent Hormone

To truly grasp the sun's importance, we must first understand vitamin D. Despite its name, vitamin D is not a vitamin at all, but a powerful secosteroid hormone that your body is designed to produce when your skin is exposed to the sun's ultraviolet B (UVB) light. This natural process begins when UVB rays (specifically light rays between 290-330 nM) strike the skin, converting a cholesterol-like molecule, 7-dehydrocholesterol, into pre-vitamin D3. This swiftly transforms into vitamin D3, which then travels to the liver to become 25-hydroxyvitamin D (calcidiol), the form typically measured in blood tests. But the journey isn't complete until it reaches the kidneys (and numerous other cells), where it's converted into its active, hormonal form: 1,25-dihydroxyvitamin D, or calcitriol. This active form, 1,25(OH)D3, is the master key that unlocks your body's inherent potential.

The Master Key and the Blueprint of Life

The pervasive influence of vitamin D stems from its presence in the very genetic blueprint of our cells. Nearly every one of your 37 trillion cells contains a special docking station called the Vitamin D Receptor (VDR). Think of the VDR as a lock, and the active vitamin D hormone, 1,25(OH)D3, as its precisely fitted key. When this key engages its lock, it transmits a potent signal directly to the cell's nucleus, the command center housing your DNA. Once inside the nucleus, the vitamin D-VDR complex locates specific regions on your DNA known as Vitamin D Responsive Elements (VDREs). By binding to these VDREs, the complex acts as a master switch, turning genes on or off. This process, known as gene expression, dictates which proteins your cells manufacture. These proteins are the building blocks of your body and comprise what you are. They are the tireless workers performing every function in your body—from combating infections to building robust bones and maintaining a sharp mind. Therefore, by regulating gene expression, vitamin D directly governs the fundamental operations of your cells, cementing its role as a true jack-of-all-trades for human health.

Beyond individual gene regulation, sunlight, through its production of vitamin D, functions as a powerful epigenetic regulator. Epigenetics describes how environmental factors, like the presence or absence of sunlight and its ensuing vitamin D, influence how your genes are expressed. While your inherent DNA sequence remains unchanged, how it is read and utilized by your cells is dynamic in that can be influenced by many factors including the environment. Sunlight and vitamin D don't rewrite your genetic code; they act as a conductor, guiding your cellular orchestra, dictating which genes play and at what volume. A body deprived of sunlight and vitamin D is akin to an orchestra without its conductor—the inevitable outcome is cellular discord, leading eventually to widespread disease and premature death.

There is no bypass or shortcut for the absence of sunlight and the vitamin D it produces. Our cellular machinery is intrinsically dependent and hardwired to run on vitamin D. Decades of disregard for this fundamental biological reality have rendered Western societies increasingly susceptible to illness, frailty, and a disturbing decline in collective life expectancy and fertility. Our abandonment of the sun and its life-sustaining vitamin D is putting a large segment of the human race on a concerning trajectory toward decline and extinction.

A Preview of the Far-Reaching Power of Vitamin D

The presence of VDRs and VDREs throughout virtually cell and every system in the body explains why a single hormone can exert such a broad and profound impact on health. This ubiquitous presence underscores vitamin D's central role in maintaining optimal physiological function across all organ systems. We will discuss the roles of sunlight and vitamin D in each of the following systems and more, but here is a preview.

Fertility and Reproduction: The very capacity to create new life is intricately linked to vitamin D. VDRs are abundant in the ovaries, uterus, placenta, testes, and even on sperm cells. Vitamin D orchestrates genes involved in crucial hormone production (estrogen and testosterone), fosters a healthy uterine lining for successful pregnancy, and influences sperm motility.

Immune System and Autoimmune Disease: A robust and well-regulated immune system is your primary defense against pathogens and your safeguard against self-attack (autoimmunity). VDRs are densely distributed across all key immune cells, including T-cells, B-cells, macrophages, and dendritic cells. Vitamin D serves as an expert immune modulator, enhancing your ability to fight infections while simultaneously calming the overactive immune responses that drive autoimmune diseases like multiple sclerosis, psoriasis, ulcerative colitis, rheumatoid arthritis, lupus and others.

Cancer: Cancer, characterized by uncontrolled cell proliferation, finds a formidable opponent in vitamin D. VDRs are present in cells of the colon, breast, prostate, skin, and numerous other tissues. When activated by vitamin D, these receptors initiate genes that promote cell differentiation (guiding cells to mature and cease uncontrolled division), inhibit proliferation (curbing cell growth), and induce apoptosis (programmed self-destruction of dangerous cells).

Cardiovascular Disease: A healthy heart and supple blood vessels are paramount for longevity. The entire cardiovascular system is rich in VDRs, found in the endothelial cells lining blood vessels, the smooth muscle cells within vessel walls, and the cardiomyocytes (heart muscle cells). Here, vitamin D plays a vital role in regulating blood pressure, reducing systemic inflammation, and preventing the dangerous stiffening of arteries.

Neurological Disease and Brain Health: Your brain is far from immune to vitamin D's influence. VDRs are distributed throughout the central nervous system in both neurons and glial cells (the brain's essential support cells) (Golan et al., 2013). This explains vitamin D's profound role in protecting against neurological diseases such as multiple sclerosis, where it helps temper the immune system's attack on the nervous system, and Alzheimer's Disease, where it assists in the clearance of neuroinflammatory plaques. Vitamin D also contributes significantly to recovery from traumatic brain injury (TBI) and concussion by mitigating inflammation and fostering neural repair.

Muscle Function: From peak athletic performance to the simple act of rising from a chair in old age, muscle strength is inextricably linked to vitamin D. VDRs are located directly within muscle cells. Vitamin D directly stimulates the synthesis of new muscle proteins, leading to improved muscle strength, enhanced balance, and superior physical performance, thereby significantly reducing the risk of falls, particularly in older adults.

Aging and Inflammaging: The natural process of aging is frequently accompanied by a state of chronic, low-grade inflammation, known as "inflammaging." As discussed, vitamin D is a masterful regulator of inflammation. By maintaining immune system equilibrium and optimizing cellular health across all organ systems, adequate vitamin D levels serve as a cornerstone of healthy aging, helping to defer the onset of age-related chronic diseases. To deprive the body of sunlight and its vital vitamin D is to invite the health scourges that now plague humanity.

Our Skin: An Evolutionary Barometer

The very diversity of human skin color serves as a powerful, living testament to the non-negotiable biological demand for vitamin D. Human skin pigmentation is a brilliant, "on-the-fly" evolutionary adaptation to varying levels of environmental ultraviolet radiation. As human populations migrated away from the equatorial sun, their skin lightened over generations. This wasn't arbitrary; darker pigmentation, while excellent at protecting against UV radiation damage and preserving vital B vitamins like folate, significantly hinders vitamin D synthesis. Lighter skin is a direct evolutionary adaptation designed to maximize vitamin D production in environments with less intense sunlight. Even within an individual, the ability to tan is your body's intelligent mechanism for striking a balance—providing a temporary protective shield only after sufficient vitamin D has been synthesized.

The wide spectrum of human skin color is one of the most visible and compelling proofs of our species' fundamental and non-negotiable biological requirement for sunlight-driven vitamin D. Given that the intricate machinery to utilize vitamin D—the VDR—is present in virtually every cell in the body, it should come as no surprise that depriving the body of sunlight and its essential products, as we have systematically done for the last fifty years or so, has had profound and devastating health consequences.

A History Forged in Light: The Great Forgetting

Our ancestors evolved under the sun's unwavering gaze, their skin naturally producing vitamin D when exposed to specific frequencies of ultraviolet light. Our bodies, with their innate wisdom, seamlessly integrated this readily available natural resource into countless aspects of growth, development, and daily function. As humankind embarked on its great migrations away from the direct and consistent equatorial sun, our skin adapted. This remarkable mutation involved a reduction in melanin content, a strategic evolutionary trade-off designed to maximize essential vitamin D production in environments with less intense sunlight. Over the past half-century, however, a concerted effort has led to the development and widespread adoption of technologies and public health campaigns specifically designed to virtually eliminate all cutaneously-generated vitamin D synthesis.

This systematic vilification of the sun, presented under the guise of health protection, has occurred in stark defiance of our biological heritage. Consequently, the incidence of the chronic diseases that now plague the developed world—cancers, cardiovascular diseases, autoimmune diseases, metabolic disorders, and pervasive frailty—are at the highest levels ever recorded, with no discernible ceiling in sight. This profound disconnect between our biology and our modern lifestyle has had catastrophic health consequences. But fortunately we are at the threshold of finally learning from the hard lessons of denying our biological connections to the sun.

The Sun: Ancient Deity and Primordial Healer

To put into context the extent of the modern perversity of sun phobia, we need to take a step back to see what the ancients knew about the sun and its powers that we have apparently forgotten. Throughout recorded history, and undoubtedly long before, the sun has been a central figure in human consciousness, revered not merely as a celestial object but as a potent deity and a source of life and healing. Ancient civilizations across the globe recognized the sun's indispensable role, from the Egyptians with their sun god Ra, personification of the midday sun and a supreme creator deity, to the Incas who worshipped Inti, the sun god from whom the Sapa Inca emperors were believed to be descended. In ancient Greece, Helios was the Titan god of the sun, often depicted driving a golden chariot across the sky, while Apollo, another Olympian god, became increasingly associated with the sun and, significantly, with healing and medicine. The Roman Sol Invictus, or "Unconquered Sun," became a prominent deity in the later Roman Empire, with his festival on December 25th marking the "rebirth" of the sun.

This deification was not mere superstition; it was an intuitive understanding of the sun's life-sustaining power. Beyond its role in agriculture and warmth, ancient cultures recognized the sun's direct influence on health. The Greek physician Hippocrates, often hailed as the "Father of Medicine" (circa 460–370 B.C.E.), advocated for sunbaths, or "heliosis," for various ailments, recognizing the value of sunlight in promoting health and recovery for conditions ranging from wasting diseases to promoting wound healing (Hippocrates, ca. 400 B.C.E.). Roman physicians, including Celsus and Galen, also prescribed sunbathing for conditions such as epilepsy, paralysis, and jaundice. Pliny the Elder (77–79 C.E.) wrote extensively about the therapeutic benefits of sunlight, terming it "the greatest remedy." These ancient healers observed the sun's power to invigorate, to dispel sickness, and to restore vitality. Their observations, though lacking the biochemical understanding we possess today, were astute. They saw that life flourished under the sun and withered in its absence, a fundamental truth that modern society has perilously chosen to ignore.

Heliotherapy: The Rise and Fall of Sun-Powered Medicine

The empirical observations of these ancient healers provided the foundation for heliotherapy—the therapeutic use of sunlight. While practiced for millennia, heliotherapy experienced a significant revival and systematization in the late nineteenth and early twentieth centuries, driven by physicians who witnessed its profound effects on diseases that defied other treatments of the era. The modern era of heliotherapy is often attributed to figures like Arnold Rikli, a Swiss physician who established a "sun cure" clinic in Austria in the mid-1850s. However, it was Dr. Auguste Rollier, another Swiss physician, who truly popularized and scientifically documented heliotherapy in the early twentieth century. Starting in 1903 in Leysin, Switzerland, Rollier established high-altitude sanatoria where he primarily treated patients suffering from extrapulmonary tuberculosis (TB), such as TB of the bones, joints, and skin (lupus vulgaris).

The justification for heliotherapy was largely empirical: physicians observed remarkable improvements in patients exposed to sunlight, especially in alpine environments with clean air and intense UV radiation. Rollier meticulously documented his methods, emphasizing gradual, whole-body sun exposure while carefully avoiding sunburn. He noted that sunlight appeared to stimulate the body's natural defenses, improve circulation, increase muscle tone, and promote the healing of diseased tissues. Though the exact mechanism (vitamin D synthesis) was not fully understood until later, the clinical outcomes were undeniable. The justification rested on the observed power of the sun to restore health where other methods failed.

The primary application of heliotherapy in the early twentieth century was for tuberculosis, particularly extrapulmonary forms. Dr. Rollier reported astonishing success rates, claiming cure rates as high as 70 to 80 percent for debilitating and often fatal surgical tuberculosis (affecting bones, joints, and lymph nodes. Photographic evidence from his clinics vividly demonstrates patients with severe tuberculous wounds or deformed joints gradually healing under the sun's rays, showcasing profound recoveries involving bone regeneration and tissue repair. Dr. Henry Gauvain in England also achieved significant success using heliotherapy for surgical tuberculosis.

Independently, the connection between sunlight and rickets, a bone-deforming disease in children, was being established. In 1919, Kurt Huldschinsky, a German physician, demonstrated that exposing children with rickets to ultraviolet light from a mercury-vapor quartz lamp could cure the disease. This was followed by the conclusive work of Harriet Chick and her colleagues in Vienna after World War I, who showed that sunlight (or cod liver oil, later identified as rich in vitamin D) could prevent and cure rickets. This discovery provided a crucial biochemical link to the sun's healing power, ultimately leading to the identification of vitamin D.

Heliotherapy was also employed for treating infected wounds, particularly during World War I, where sunlight was used as a disinfectant and to promote healing in soldiers. It also found application in various skin conditions, including psoriasis and eczema.

Decline of Heliotherapy

Despite its documented successes, heliotherapy began to wane in popularity within the medical community by the mid-twentieth century due to several converging factors:

The Rise of Antibiotics: The discovery of streptomycin in 1943, the first effective antibiotic against Mycobacterium tuberculosis, revolutionized TB treatment. Pharmacological interventions offered a seemingly more direct, targeted, and easily administered solution compared to the lengthy and resource-intensive process of heliotherapy.

Focus on Specificity: Medicine was increasingly embracing a reductionist model, seeking specific cures for specific diseases. Heliotherapy, as a broad-spectrum, holistic treatment, did not align neatly with this emerging paradigm.

Logistical Challenges: Operating heliotherapy clinics required specific geographical locations (sunny, high-altitude environments), specialized facilities, and prolonged patient stays, making it less scalable and more expensive in some contexts than drug-based therapies.

Vitamin D Fortification: The discovery of vitamin D and its role in rickets led to widespread food fortification programs (e.g., milk fortified with vitamin D), which largely eradicated rickets in many developed countries. Vitamin D fortification addressed one of the most clear-cut examples of sunlight's benefit, perhaps inadvertently diminishing the perceived need for broader sun exposure.

The undeniable and life-saving success of antibiotics caused the pendulum to swing too far, leading to the neglect of a powerful, natural therapeutic modality that addressed the body's overall physiology in a way that targeted drugs could not. The focus of medicine shifted entirely to fighting the pathogen and its symptoms, overshadowing the importance of strengthening the host—a role the sun had played for millennia.

The Modern View of the Sun: From Healer to Hazard

The latter half of the twentieth century witnessed a dramatic and unprecedented shift in the perception of the sun. Once revered as a life-giver and healer, it was systematically recast as a dangerous carcinogen, something to be feared and meticulously avoided. This modern characterization of the sun as primarily dangerous is profoundly counter to the biological history of all living things on this planet. All life, in its myriad forms, depends directly or indirectly on the sun. Photosynthesis, driven by sunlight, forms the base of most food chains. For humans, beyond the critical synthesis of vitamin D, sunlight plays a role in regulating circadian rhythms, mood, immunity and potentially other physiological processes yet to be fully elucidated. To portray the sun, so fundamental to our evolution and existence, as an outright enemy, is a biological absurdity.

In addition to the shift toward a treatment of-symptom–based model of medicine, the genesis of this man-made attitude of fear toward the sun is multi-faceted, beginning with the dermatology profession. Starting in the mid-twentieth century, dermatology as a specialty increasingly focused on the link between sun exposure, skin aging, and skin cancer, particularly melanoma. While basal cell and squamous cell carcinomas are clearly linked to cumulative sun exposure and are generally treatable and curable, melanoma, though rarer, carries a higher mortality risk. Public health campaigns, often spearheaded by dermatological associations, began to emphasize sun avoidance and the use of sunscreens as primary prevention strategies against all forms of skin cancer. The message became simplified to "sun = bad," neglecting the benefits of sun exposure benefits and the different types of skin cancer.

The broader medical community, influenced by the dermatological perspective and the prevailing risk-averse culture in public health, largely adopted this same anti-sun stance. Advice to avoid sun exposure became standard, often without consideration for an individual's vitamin D status or the broader health benefits of sensible sun exposure. The focus on minimizing one risk (skin cancer) overshadowed the potential for increasing myriad other risks associated with vitamin D deficiency.

Finally, the burgeoning fear of the sun created sun-phobia and a lucrative market for sunscreen products. The sunscreen industry, through extensive marketing, reinforced the message that sun exposure is inherently dangerous and that daily, liberal application of sunscreen is essential for health. Advertising often played on fear, depicting the sun as an aggressor from which one needs constant chemical protection. The industry promoted the idea that sunscreens allowed for "safe" sun exposure, yet the primary effect of broad-spectrum sunscreens is the highly efficient blocking of UVB radiation, the very wavelength necessary for vitamin D synthesis.

This systematic vilification of the sun, driven by a narrow focus on potential skin damage, has had catastrophic and largely unacknowledged adverse consequences on public health. The primary casualty has been population-level vitamin D sufficiency. By convincing populations to shun the sun and diligently apply vitamin D-synthesis-blocking sunscreens, we have effectively engineered widespread vitamin D deficiency and insufficiency across the developed world. Estimates suggest that up to a billion people worldwide may have deficient or insufficient vitamin D levels. Remember that almost all of our 37 trillion cells have receptors for vitamin D and that vitamin D has to come from somewhere. This is not a trivial matter, as vitamin D is not merely a "vitamin" but a potent secosteroid hormone essential for the proper function of virtually every system in the body. Its profound roles in immune system regulation, cardiovascular health, muscle strength and function, brain health, and healthy aging are now well-established.